Immunology of Infection

IMMUNOLOGY AND MEDICINE SERIES

IMMUNOLOGY

SERIES · SERIES · SERIES · SERIES **AND** SERIES · SERIES · SERIES · SERIES

MEDICINE

Volume 25

Immunology of Infection

Edited by

J. G. P. Sissons

Department of Medicine
University of Cambridge
Cambridge, UK

L. K. Borysiewicz

Department of Medicine
University of Wales
College of Medicine
Cardiff, UK

J. Cohen

Department of Infectious Diseases and Bacteriology
Royal Postgraduate Medical School
Hammersmith Hospital
London, UK

Series Editor: K. Whaley

KLUWER ACADEMIC PUBLISHERS
DORDRECHT / BOSTON / LONDON

RB
153
.I46
1994

Distributors

for the United States and Canada: Kluwer Academic Publishers, PO Box 358, Accord Station, Hingham, MA 02018-0358, USA
for all other countries: Kluwer Academic Publishers Group, Distribution Center, PO Box 322, 3300 AH Dordrecht, The Netherlands

A catalogue record for this book is available from the British Library.

ISBN 0-7923-8968-9

Library of Congress Cataloging-in-Publication Data

Immunology of infection / edited by J.G.P. Sissons, L. Borysiewicz, J. Cohen.
    p. cm.—(Immunology and medicine series: v. 25)
   Includes bibliographical references and index.
   ISBN 0-7923-8968-9 (case bound)
   1. Infection—Immunological aspects. I. Sissons, J.G.P. II. Borysiewicz,
L. III. Cohen, J. (Jon), 1949– . IV. Series.
   [DNLM: 1. Infection—immunology. 2. Immunity. W1 IM53BI v. 25
1994 / QW 700 13352 1994]
   RB153.I46   1994
   616'.047—dc20
   DNLM/DLC
   for Library of Congress   94-27318
                                                  CIP

Published in the United Kingdom by Kluwer Academic Publishers, PO Box 55, Lancaster, UK.

Kluwer Academic Publishers BV incorporates the publishing programmes of D. Reidel, Martinus Nijhoff, Dr W. Junk and MTP Press.

Typeset by Lasertext Ltd., Stretford, Manchester, U.K.
Printed and bound in Great Britain by Hartnolls Ltd., Bodmin, Cornwall.

Contents

Series Editor's Note

The interface between clinical immunology and other branches of medical practice is frequently blurred and the general physician is often faced with clinical problems with an immunological basis and is expected to diagnose and manage such patients. The rapid expansion of basic and clinical immunology over the past two decades has resulted in the appearance of increasing numbers of immunology journals and it is impossible for a non-specialist to keep apace with this information overload. The *Immunology and Medicine* series is designed to present individual topics of immunology in a condensed package of information which can be readily assimilated by the busy clinician or pathologist.

K. Whaley, Leicester
May 1994

Preface

The immune system has evolved in large part to enable organisms to resist microbial infection. Given this very fundamental relationship between the immune system and infectious microbial agents it is entirely appropriate that a volume in this series should be devoted to the immunology of infection. Microorganisms have long been used as experimental tools by immunologists, and the study of the immune response to viruses and bacteria has contributed much to our understanding of basic immunological mechanisms (for example of the mechanism by which non-self determinants on cells are recognized). However there are of course important practical and clinical reasons for attempting to understand the immunology of infections – these include the needs for rational design of vaccines and to understand the pathogenesis of human infectious diseases.

The last decade or so has seen a resurgence of interest in infectious diseases and a recognition that they remain of importance and pertinence to all areas of medicine. This is not just because of the advent of AIDS, although that has been a major factor – the rise in drug-resistant mycobacterial infections and the recognition of the infectious aetiology of peptic ulcer disease are other illustrations.

It should be made clear that this volume deals with aspects of the immunolgy of bacteria, viruses and fungi – but it does not deal with parasite immunology which it is planned to cover in a separate volume in the series. The emphasis is in general on human infection with reference to experimental models where appropriate. There is no attempt to deal comprehensively with individual infectious diseases, but rather with the principles involved in the immunolgy of the different classes of infectious agent.

The contributors are all chosen for their active involvement and expertise in the fields on which they write.

List of Contributors

N. ALP
Department of Medicine
University of Cambridge
Cambridge CB2 2QQ
UK

J. D. BAUMGARTNER
Service of Internal Medicine
Hôpital de zone
1110 Morges, Switzerland

K. BAYSTON
Department of Infectious Diseases and
   Bacteriology
Royal Postgraduate Medical School
Hammersmith Hospital
Du Cane Road
London W12 0HS, UK

L. K. BORYSIEWICZ
Department of Medicine
University of Wales College of Medicine
Heath Park
Cardiff, CF4 4XN, UK

J. COHEN
Department of Infectious Diseases and
   Bacteriology
Royal Postgraduate Medical School
Hammersmith Hospital
Du Cane Road
London W12 0HS, UK

M. P. GLAUSER
Division of Infectious Diseases
Department of Internal Medicine
University Medical Center
Lausanne, Switzerland

C. R. HOWARD
Department of Pathology and Infectious
   Diseases
The Royal Veterinary College
Royal College Street
London NW1 0TU, UK

J. R. LAMB
Department of Immunology
St Mary's Hospital Medical School
Praed Street
London W2 1YN, UK

A. MEHLERT
Department of Biochemistry
University of Dundee
Dundee DD1 4HN, UK

A. A. NASH
Division of Immunology
Department of Pathology
University of Cambridge
Cambridge, UK

A. D. M. REES
Department of Genito-Urinary Medicine
   and Communicable Diseases
St Mary's Hospital Medical School
Praed Street
London W2 1YN, UK

G. A. W. ROOK
Department of Medical Microbiology
University College London Medical School
67–73 Riding House Street
London W1P 7PP, UK

S. SHAUNAK
Department of Infectious Diseases and
  Bacteriology
Royal Postgraduate Medical School
Hammersmith Hospital
Du Cane Road
London W12 0HS, UK

J. G. P. SISSONS
Department of Medicine
University of Cambridge
Cambridge, UK

C. TANG
Nuffield Department of Medicine
John Radcliffe Hospital
Headington
Oxford OX3 9DU, UK

A. D. B. WEBSTER
Immunodeficiency Research Group
Clinical Research Centre
Watford Road
Harrow
Middlesex HA1 3UJ, UK

1
Immunity to Bacteria

G. A. W. ROOK

INTRODUCTION

Strategies of pathogenicity

The mechanism required for immunity to any infectious agent depends on the strategy used by that organism to cause disease, and on its structure and vulnerability to the available protective functions. Bacteria are particularly diverse in these respects.

At one extreme there are organisms such as *Corynebacterium diphtheriae* which do not invade the host, but which cause disease by releasing a toxin following attachment to an epithelial surface. The disease is entirely due to the toxin, and antibody able to neutralize that toxin is therefore all that is required for immunity. Theoretically, antibody able to block the establishment of the organism on the epithelium could also be effective.

At the other extreme is *Mycobacterium leprae*, which is invasive, but apparently entirely without toxicity. It causes disease either because a large number of organisms constitute a 'space-occupying lesion' which can be damaging in the constrained space of a nerve sheath, or because the inflammatory response evoked causes tissue damage. In this case much of the disease is classified as immunopathology, attributable to the response of the host which destroys tissues without eliminating the infection.

Most bacterial diseases fall somewhere between these two extremes, with simultaneous elements of toxicity, invasiveness and immunopathology.

Bacterial structure and immunity

The interaction between a given bacterial species and the immune response can be predicted by considering the immunological mechanisms available in relation to the structure of the bacterium (Figure 1)[1]. All bacteria, like any

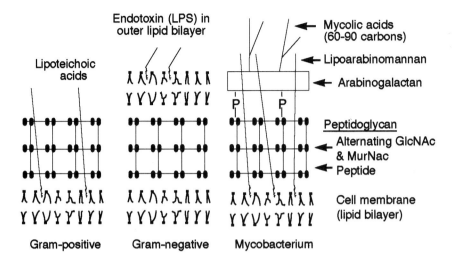

Figure 1 Simplified diagrams of the cell walls of the three major groups of bacteria. Only Gram-negative organisms have an outer lipid bilayer which is a potential target for the lytic pathway of complement. The peptidoglycan layer is common to all three groups, but in the mycobacteria it is covalently bonded to a layer of arabinogalactan, bearing massive waxy mycolic acids. Note the lipoteichoic acids (LTA) and lipoarabinomannan (LAM) inserted in the cell membrane and passing out through the wall of the Gram-positive organisms and mycobacteria respectively. In contrast, Gram-negative organisms have endotoxin (LPS) inserted in the outer bilayer

other type of cell, have an inner lipid bilayer membrane. Outside this is the peptidoglycan. The glycan component of this layer is made up of alternating N-acetylglucosamine and N-acetyl- (or N-glycolyl-) muramic acid. This glycan is cross-linked by short peptides which often contain the characteristic bacterial amino acid, diaminopimelic acid. The glycan structure is susceptible to degradation by lysozyme (muramidase), and some Gram-positive bacteria are rapidly destroyed by this enzyme. In most organisms, however, additional structures protect the peptidoglycan from direct attack. Gram-negative organisms have an outer lipid bilayer into which the lipid moieties of endotoxin (lipopolysaccharide, LPS) are inserted. This lipid bilayer is a potential target for the lytic pathway of complement (C5–C9). It is worth noting that this is the only group of bacteria in which structures sensitive to the lytic C5–C9 complex are potentially accessible to it. Thus many Gram-negative bacteria are rapidly killed by fresh serum, though pathogenic organisms avoid this fate (see below).

The mycobacterial peptidoglycan is covalently linked to a layer of arabinogalactan, outside which are covalently linked mycolic acids – large waxy molecules up to 90 carbon atoms long. Further high molecular weight lipids and glycolipids are also present in this outer layer[2]. It is evident therefore that the mycobacterial wall will be remarkably resistant to complement or other mammalian enzyme systems attacking from outside.

Most bacteria also have capsules which can further impede the access of complement to vulnerable sites, the adhesion to phagocytes, and the functions of phagocytes.

In spite of these complex structures, bacteria cannot isolate themselves completely from their environment. There are inevitably 'holes' in all cell walls, including those of mycobacteria, since some substances, such as toxins, enzymes and transport molecules must be secreted and nutrients must be taken in. Moreover some structures (the lipoteichoic acids of Gram-positive bacteria, and the lipoarabinomannan (LAM) of mycobacteria) appear to be inserted in the inner membrane while the polysaccharide component extends out through the peptidoglycan layer.

NON-SPECIFIC DEFENCES

Barriers to the establishment of bacterial infection

Before actually confronting the immune mechanisms, an organism must pass a number of obvious but important non-specific barriers. The skin excludes most bacteria, and its barrier function is aided by the presence of toxic fatty acids and of commensal organisms which may occupy an ecological niche and so deny it to a pathogen. Commensals play a similar role in the gut and vagina, where disease due to overgrowth of pathogens can result from depletion of commensals by antibiotic therapy. The acidity of the stomach and vagina also limit the growth of many species. The respiratory system is protected by the entrapment of particulate matter on the turbinates and in the mucus of the upper respiratory tract, and its removal by the action of cilia, although smoking damages this mechanism.

Lysozyme (muramidase) in tears and other secretions may damage some bacterial species and secretory antibody, particularly IgA, may help to inhibit the establishment of infection on epithelial surfaces[3].

Another general mechanism of defence is deprivation of iron. In the presence of oxygen this is present only as the immensely insoluble ferric form. Concentrations of free iron in biological fluids, where it is bound to transferrin, are too low for bacterial growth. All organisms release iron-chelating compounds in an attempt to obtain and solubilize iron from their environments.

The protective role of non-specific recognition of common microbial components

If an organism manages to penetrate the defences outlined above and gains entry to the tissues, it is confronted by a series of mechanisms which detect the presence of conserved bacterial structures. These early recognition events have several important functions: first, they immediately activate protective mechanisms that can operate before specific T cell or antibody-mediated responses are initiated; second, they help to determine the nature of the immune response that is subsequently activated. This immunoregulatory

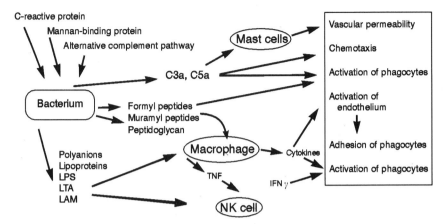

Figure 2 Recognition of common microbial components by acute phase reactants, complement and phagocytes. These non-specific recognition systems promote rapid attraction and activation of phagocytes before the specific immune response develops. Note the triggering of cytokine release by LPS, LTA and LAM which are shown also on Figure 1

'decision' can determine the outcome of the infection, and is discussed in detail later.

Protective mechanisms following non-specific recognition of common bacterial structures

Some of the non-specific protective mechanisms are phylogenetically very ancient, and much of the defence against bacteria depends on pathways which have nothing to do with the specific antigen receptors of either B cells or T cells, and which probably antedate these in evolution. Examples of such bacterial structures, and the responses which they evoke, are shown in Figure 2. Thus the organisms may be recognized by complement[4], and by two acute phase proteins, C-reactive protein[5] and mannose-binding protein[6] which also fix complement. Similarly, phagocytes have receptors for the formyl peptides released by bacteria: these are chemoattractants and activators of these cells. Other components, considered in greater detail below, trigger cytokine release, and directly or indirectly activate endothelial cells, phagocytes and lymphocytes.

It is interesting to note that the Limulus assay used to detect contaminating LPS in preparations for use in man is based on one such recognition pathway. In *Limulus polyphemus* (the horse-shoe crab) tiny quantities of LPS trigger formation of fibrin which walls off the LPS-bearing infectious agent.

The triggering of cytokine release by microbial products

One of the most important types of recognition system for common microbial components, particularly during the very early stages of infection, results in

4

the triggering of release of cytokines, particularly interleukin-1 (IL-1) and tumour necrosis factor alpha (TNFα) (Figure 2). These cytokines have rapid protective effects, but if their release is excessive or prolonged they can cause severe immunopathology and even death. Direct evidence for the protective role of TNFα *in vivo* has been obtained by the injection of recombinant TNFα. This cytokine protects mice from *Mycobacterium avium* infection[7], and accelerates clearance of *Legionella pneumophila*[8]. It will also protect mice from infection by *Streptococcus pneumoniae* and *Klebsiella*[9]. C3H/HeJ mice, which produce little cytokine in response to the LPS of Gram-negative bacteria, are 1000-fold more susceptible to lethal infection with *Escherichia coli* than are the congenic, LPS-sensitive C3H/HeN mice. The C3H/HeJ mice could be protected from infection with a dose of *E. coli* equivalent to >20 LD_{50} by pretreatment with a combination of IL-1 and TNFα[10]. In this model of Gram-negative infection, TNFα itself seems to be protective. The mechanisms mediating cytokine release, and the subsequent protective effects are discussed below.

The bacterial components responsible for cytokine release

The lipopolysaccharides of Gram-negative organisms are the most studied triggers of cytokine release, but the somewhat analogous (but structurally quite different) lipoteichoic acids (LTA) of Gram-positive cocci[11] and the phosphatidyl inositol mannosides (LAM) of the mycobacteria[12] are equally potent. Muramyl dipeptide (MDP), a synthetic analogue of part of the ubiquitous bacterial cell wall peptidoglycan appears to prime for enhanced release of TNFα by other bacterial components[13]. It is possible that all micro-organisms trigger release of TNFα: in addition to the organisms already discussed above, *Legionella*[8], *Listeria*[14] and a streptococcal cell wall preparation[15] all have this property, though the active components have not been identified.

Another important class of bacterial (and viral) components that trigger cytokine release are known as superantigens, though in this case cytokine release appears to be of benefit to the bacterium rather than to the host. They are discussed later in relation to immunopathology.

Rapid enhancement of the arrival of phagocytes at the site of infection

Cytokines rapidly induce increased adhesion of neutrophils to endothelial cells (Figure 3)[16]. This effect is apparent within 5 min of exposure to TNFα, and is partly due to increased expression of the complement receptor CR3. Some bacterial components such as LPS also increase neutrophil adhesion directly. Cytokines also increase the expression of adhesion molecules on the endothelium[17]. Adhesion of myeloid cells to the endothelium is a prerequisite for their passage from the circulation into the tissues. In mice a monoclonal antibody directed against CR3 which is able to block such adhesion, exacerbates infection with *Listeria monocytogenes*[18] and reduces endotoxin-

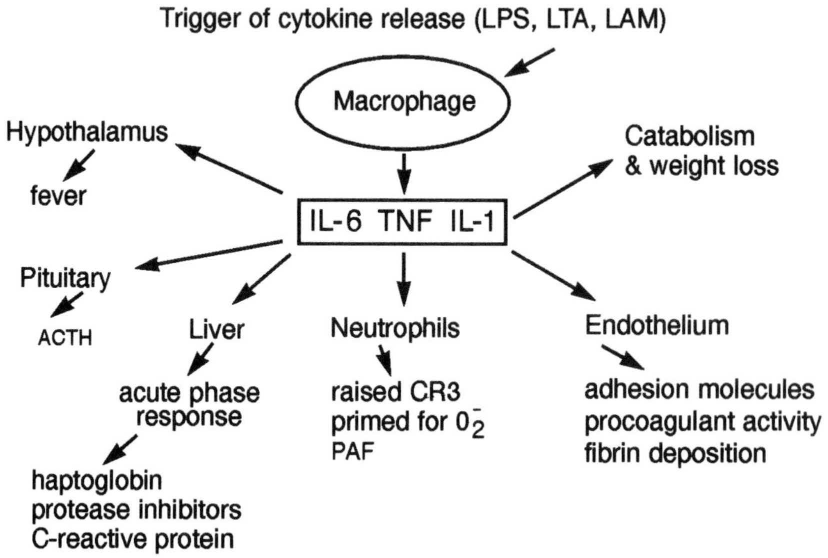

Figure 3 Some of the effects of cytokines released from macrophages triggered by bacterial components. Note that in the short term these are protective responses, but if excessive or prolonged the changes in endothelial cells and in neutrophil adhesiveness and activation can result in local or systemic tissue damage

induced entry of neutrophils into the lung (H. Rosen, personal communication). These adhesion events are in fact crucial and involve the integrins, selectins and members of the immunoglobulin superfamily such as intercellular adhesion molecule (ICAM)-1 and VCAM-1[19,20].

Rapid activation of microbicidal mechanisms in neutrophils by cytokines

TNFα can prime neutrophils so that they subsequently give an exaggerated burst of superoxide or H_2O_2 when exposed to stimuli such as zymosan (Figure 3)[21], phorbol myristate acetate (PMA) or f-met-leu-phe[22]. The increased oxidative response to zymosan[21] and to opsonized organisms[23] has been attributed to increased expression of CR3[21]. Priming for enhanced superoxide production is apparent within 20 min. These effects could explain the enhanced clearance of *Legionella* induced by TNFα *in vivo*[8].

Activation of macrophages by cytokines

TNFα-exposed macrophages have increased activity against various organisms *in vitro*. There is, therefore, a direct activating effect of TNFα on macrophages. There is also, however, an important indirect effect which operates via natural killer (NK) cells which, in the presence of bacterial components, are induced by TNFα to release interferon (IFN)-γ[24]. This pathway is discussed in greater detail in a later section.

The effect of TNFα on growth of organisms in tumour cells and fibroblasts

Exposure of HEp-2 cells (derived from a human carinoma of the larynx) to TNFα renders them resistant to invasion by *Salmonella typhimurium*[25] and inhibits intracellular growth of *Chlamydia trachomatis*[26]. The latter effect is partly reversed by addition of tryptophan, suggesting that TNFα augments tryptophan-depleting enzyme activity.

We have found recently that cells infected with *M. tuberculosis* become very sensitive to the toxic effects of TNFα[27]. Since TNFα was already known to kill some transformed or virus-infected cells, it now seems possible that a general function of TNFα is the elimination of cells which have become abnormal for whatever reason.

Cytokines and the endocrine system

The cytokines are also responsible for enhanced production of glucocorticoid hormones from the adrenal gland, secondary to increased output of adreno-corticotrophin (ACTH) from the pituitary. At first sight it seems odd that cytokines released early in an infection should promptly suppress the immune response. This dilemma is nearing resolution since it is now clear that a major product of the adrenal gland, dehydroepiandrosterone, is a genuine anti-glucocorticoid[28], the receptors for which are found in T cells[29]. The regulation and impact of this hormone is providing an exciting new area of research.

Cytokines and the acute phase response

Cytokines (particularly IL-6) also drive the acute phase response, in synergy with glucocorticoids. When exposed to these stimuli the liver increases production of a range of glycoproteins, the function of some of which remains unknown. C-reactive protein[5] and mannose-binding protein[6] may be involved in recognition of organisms, while haptoglobin, caeruloplasmin and the protease inhibitors probably help to limit tissue damage.

Interactions between bacteria and complement

The second major group of stimuli for the arrival of phagocytes is provided by the complement system. Numerous bacterial components can activate the alternative pathway. This results in three categories of protective function[4]:

(i) Release of the complement components C3a and C5a. These cause smooth muscle contraction, mast cell degranulation, and neutrophil chemotaxis and activation. Histamine and leukotriene release induced by this component contribute to further increases in vascular permeability.

(ii) Attachment to the organism of derivatives of C3 which play an important role in the subsequent interaction with phagocytes described below.

(iii) Some Gram-negative organisms may be killed if the lytic complex C5–C9 gains access to the outer lipid bilayer.

Many organisms have devised strategies to resist these detrimental effects of complement[30]. Some capsules are very poor activators of the alternative pathway. Alternatively, long side-chains (O antigens) on LPS may fix C3b at a distance from the vulnerable lipid bilayer. Similarly, smooth Gram-negative organisms such as *E. coli*, *Salmonella* and *Pseudomonas* may fix and then rapidly shed the C5b–C9 membrane complex. Other organisms exploit the physiological mechanisms which block destruction of host cells by complement. When C3b has attached to a surface it can either interact with factor B, leading to further amplification and eventually to generation of the lytic complex, or it can become inactivated by factors H and I. Capsules rich in sialic acid (such as host cell membranes) seem to promote the interaction with factors H and I: *Neisseria meningitidis*, *Escherichia coli* K1, and Group B *Streptococcus* resist complement attachment in this way. The M protein of Group A *Streptococcus* acts as an acceptor for factor H, and there is a gene for a C5a protease close to the M protein gene.

The role of non-specific recognition of common bacterial components in adjuvanticity, and in the selection of response mechanisms

Non-specific bacterial recognition pathways are conceptually important, and help to explain not only the phenomenon of 'adjuvanticity', but also the ability of the immune system to select the appropriate mechanism of response.

If a purified antigen of the type often used by immunologists is injected into an animal by itself there may be little response. However, if it is injected into a site previously infected with, for instance, a mycobacterium such as the Bacillus Calmette Guèrin (BCG), or if it is injected with cell wall peptidoglycan, muramyl dipeptide, trehalose dimycolate, LPS or various capsular polysaccharides, a much greater immune response may be evoked. This effect, which is routinely exploited in the 'adjuvants' used by immunologists to boost immune responses, makes sense from an evolutionary point of view. The specific T cell and B cell receptors did not evolve in isolation to recognize purified antigens: they evolved as an adjunct to pre-existing systems for recognizing common microbial components, and seem to operate best when these systems are active. However the non-specific recognition mechanisms do not merely boost the response, they also help to direct it. It has been established in the mouse, and more recently in man[31], that the pattern of cytokines secreted by T helper (T_H) cells is variable, and determines

8

the nature of the immune response that occurs. The T_{H1} 'subset' (this may not be the correct word to use, since these phenotypes seem to be at least partly susceptible to modulation) secretes IL-2 and IFNγ and promotes cell-mediated immunity to a wide range of intracellular parasites. The second 'subset' (T_{H2}) secretes IL-4, IL-5 and IL-10 and preferentially drives antibody responses, including that of the IgE and IgA isotypes. In general there is a tendency for the cytokines secreted by each subset to inhibit the other. It has become clear from numerous studies that immunity to infectious agents depends on the activation of helper T cells secreting the appropriate pattern of cytokines. Immunization that leads to activation of the wrong T_H subset can lead to enhanced susceptibility rather than to immunity[32]. The subset of T_H cells that is activated depends on endocrine[33] and cytokine[34] factors present before and during the activation process. These in turn are determined largely by the non-specific recognition pathways.

THE SPECIFIC IMMUNE RESPONSE

The role of antibody

Antibody clearly plays a crucial role during infection with toxigenic organisms. It neutralizes diphtheria toxin by blocking the attachment of the binding portion of the molecule to its target cells. Similarly it may block locally acting toxins, extracellular matrix-degrading enzymes which act as spreading factors, and motility due to flagellae. An important function on external surfaces, often performed by secretory IgA, is inhibition of bacterial binding to epithelial cells. It is also likely that some antibodies to the bacterial surface can block functional requirements of the organism such as the binding of iron-chelating compounds or the intake of nutrients. However the most important role of antibody in immunity to non-toxigenic bacteria is the more efficient targeting of complement so that even organisms which resist the alternative pathway by the mechanisms described above[30] are damaged by complement, or become coated with C3 products. The most efficient complement-fixing antibodies in man are IgG1, IgG3 and IgM. IgG1 and IgG3 are also the subclasses with the highest affinity for Fc receptors.

Interactions between bacteria and phagocytic cells

The important consequences of the inflammatory and chemotactic events triggered by bacteria in the tissues is the enhanced exposure of the bacteria to phagocytic cells.

Binding to the phagocyte surface

The first stage in intracellular killing is the attachment of the organism to the surface of the phagocyte. This important and complex interaction determines whether uptake occurs and whether killing mechanisms are triggered. The acute phase reactant, C-reactive protein, can bind to some organisms, and then to receptors on monocytes[5]. Many micro-organisms express carbohydrate-binding molecules (lectins) which are important for their attachment to target cells. The same lectin sometimes mediates attachment to phagocytes. For instance the mannose-binding lectin on Type 1 fimbriae of *E. coli* stimulates uptake and subsequent killing, possibly by cross-linking the CR3 receptor for C3bi[35]. The reverse type of interaction occurs when a lectin on the macrophage membrane binds to carbohydrate on the organism[35]. Particularly relevant in this context is the family of adhesion-promoting receptors CR3, LFA-1 and p150,95. These receptors have multiple binding sites with different specificities[36] and can bind to β-glucans, *Histoplasma capsulatum*[37] and to the LPS endotoxin of Gram-negative bacteria[38]. In addition to normal phagocytosis, congenital defects of these receptors lead to failure of phagocytes to arrive at the site of the lesion, and are associated with increased susceptibility to infection.

Organisms coated with complement components, including C3bi, bind to CR3 and other complement receptors. The interaction with complement can be direct or secondary to the binding of antibody, or to the binding of a mannose-binding lectin which is an acute phase reactant in human sera[6]. This lectin can fix complement by the classical pathway. It is becoming clear that many interactions between organisms and phagocytes use CR3; this may thus be one of the major pathways of macrophage activation[39].

Triggering of uptake

The binding of a micro-organism to a macrophage receptor does not always lead to its uptake: zymosan particles and red cells coated with C3bi both bind to CR3, but only the zymosan particles are ingested[36]. However exposure of a monocyte to C5a or fibronectin activates the receptor and causes phagocytosis of coated erythrocytes. These studies show that the cellular response triggered by a receptor can depend on the ligand which has bound to that receptor, and also that a receptor can become 'uncoupled' from its function.

Triggering of microbicidal activity

Phagocytosis of an organism does not always activate killing mechanisms. Some killing mechanisms are only triggered by binding of the micro-organism to a receptor such as CR3, when the monocyte has been previously activated by exposure to agents such as LPS. Other killing mechanisms may require two distinct signals: antibody is required for optimal intake of *Candida albicans* by human neutrophils, but killing requires the presence of complement[40].

Activation of antimicrobial functions

Monocytes and polymorphonuclear cells possess a number of oxygen-dependent and -independent antimicrobial mechanisms. Most monocyte antimicrobial mechanisms decline when the cells are cultured *in vitro* and allowed to mature into macrophages. This decline can be prevented, and the killing mechanisms of fresh neutrophils and monocytes can be enhanced by certain bacterial products (Figure 2), by cytokines, the release of which from macrophages is induced by bacterial products (Figure 2), and by lymphokines such as IFNγ. Some of the ways in which this may enhance killing mechanisms are discussed below.

Antimicrobial mechanisms of phagocytic cells

Oxygen-dependent pathways

1. Superoxide anion

Activation of this microbicidal pathway requires a triggering event, usually the binding of various ligands to membrane receptors. Following triggering, oxygen is reduced by a membrane-associated cytochrome system which transfers an electron onto molecular oxygen to form the superoxide anion (O_2^-). Subsequent interactions give rise to hydrogen peroxide (H_2O_2), hydroxyl radicals (OH'), and perhaps singlet oxygen ($\Delta^1 gO_2$), which is oxygen with one electron in a high energy state. These toxic intermediates are generated in the absence of myeloperoxidase (MPO), and therefore may not require fusion of the MPO-containing lysosomes with the phagosome. If fusion does occur MPO catalyses the formation of hypohalous acids from H_2O_2 and halides: in effect, this is intraphagosomal bleach. Since triggering via membrane receptors is required, oxygen-dependent killing usually occurs at the time of phagocytosis.

Monocytes are very active in generating these reactive oxygen intermediates. This capacity increases during the first 3 days *in vitro*, but then decreases rapidly and is virtually absent by 6 days. Levels of MPO are high in monocytes and fall within 24 h, becoming absent by 6 days of culture[41,42]. Production of OH' also seems to decline early, possibly because of a decline in the availability of iron, which is a catalyst for its formation. It is unlikely that oxygen reduction products are involved when the *in vitro* maturation of monocytes has no effect on killing of the organism in question. The complexity of these interactions is illustrated by the fact that closely related variants of *Chlamydia trachomatis* differ in their susceptibility to killing by mature macrophages[43].

2. Nitric oxide (NO)

Recently a second oxygen-dependent pathway has been recognized. It has been known for some years that nitric oxide (NO) can be released by various cell types, and it is an important regulator of blood vessel dilatation. It is now clear that murine macrophages produce nitric oxide synthase which, in the presence of co-factors including tetrahydrobiopterin, can oxidize the guanidino nitrogen of L-arginine to yield citrulline and NO[44]. This seems to be relevant to some antimicrobial effects of mouse macrophages[45-47]. However the importance of this mechanism in man is less clear, because human macrophages contain low levels of tetrahydrobiopterin, and without this co-factor very little NO is formed.

Evidence for oxygen-independent pathways

Cells from patients with chronic granulomatous disease (CGD) are incapable of generating reactive oxygen intermediates but can kill a wide range of organisms. Moreover, the cells of these patients develop additional non-oxidative antimicrobial activity after incubation with lymphokines[48]. Similarly, cells cultured under strictly anaerobic conditions can kill many Gram-negative and Gram-positive organisms, including obligate anaerobes, and human alveolar and peritoneal macrophages take up and kill *Toxoplasma gondii* without any oxidative burst. This killing is not affected by scavengers of superoxide, peroxide, singlet oxygen or hydroxyl radicals[49].

Further evidence for the existence of different antimicrobial mechanisms comes from the clinically important effects of glucocorticoid hormones. Exposure of monocytes to 10^{-8} M dexamethasone, or 10^{-7} M cortisol inhibits killing of *Aspergillus* spores, *Listeria*, *Nocardia* or *Salmonella*. IFNγ restores activity against *Listeria* and *Salmonella*: this is probably due to its enhancement of the oxygen-dependent pathway which is not glucocorticoid sensitive. However, IFNγ does not restore activity against *Aspergillus* or *Nocardia*[50] which are sensitive to unidentified oxygen-independent mechanisms. Glucocorticoids also eliminate the ability of fresh human monocytes to slow down the rate of replication of *M. tuberculosis*[51].

Oxygen-independent mechanisms

Some oxygen-independent killing may be due to sequential exposure to neutral proteases at pH 7.0–8.0, followed by acid hydrolases after the acidification step. Acidification itself may also be more important than previously realized. Other specific mechanisms are discussed below.

Nutritional deprivation

Additional bacteriostasis may be due to deprivation of essential nutrients. One important unknown is the availability of iron within macrophages, which do not normally contain lactoferrin, though this may be acquired from polymorphonuclear cells. Normal monocytes contain tryptophan: this is available to ingested organisms, and tryptophan-requiring auxotrophic mutants of *Legionella pneumophila* grow well in these cells[52]. However exposure to IFNγ causes degradation of tryptophan in monocytes[53,54] and fibroblasts, and depletion of this amino acid has been implicated in the subsequent inhibition of replication of *Toxoplasma gondii*[55].

Cationic proteins

Odeberg and Olssen[56] reported that human granulocytes contain cationic proteins with microbicidal activity. Six have been sequenced: they are cysteine- and arginine-rich peptides of 32–34 amino acids with a molecular weight of about 4 kD, and are represenative of a conserved family of related mammalian 'antibiotics' which have been named defensins. Similar proteins have been found in the granules of rabbit alveolar macrophages but not in human macrophages, though these contain other cationic antibacterial substances. Defensins will kill organisms as diverse as *Staphylococcus aureus*, *Pseudomonas aeruginosa*, *Escherichia coli*, *Crytococcus neoformans* and even the enveloped *herpes simplex* virus[57]. There are also chymotrypsin-like proteins which kill Gram-positive and Gram-negative bacteria and fungi by mechanisms quite independent of their enzymatic activity and a cationic protein named BPI because it increases bacterial permeability in some Gram-negative bacteria. It has recently become apparent that this molecule can neutralize some of the effects of LPS[58]. Similarly, lysozyme has a limited spectrum of antibacterial activity, due partly to its ability to cleave the $\beta1$–4 linkage between the N-acetylglucosamine and N-acetylmuramic acid residues which form the carbohydrate component of cell wall peptidoglycan, and partly to its cationic nature (discussed in ref. 57). The bactericidal activity of cationic proteins is greatest at pH 7.0–8.0: the pH in phagosomes rises transiently to this level. At this pH, the cationic proteins displace the divalent cations (such as Ca^{2+}) which cross-link the endotoxin molecules in the outer membrane of Gram-negative organisms[59]. At a lower pH, the major effect seems to be permeabilization of the outer membrane, perhaps allowing entry of other microbicidal molecules. The mechanisms by which they damage Gram-positive organisms and fungi are not so obvious.

Uptake of microbicidal material from other cells

Monocytes can take in the products of neutrophils, presumably including defensins and lactoferrin, and this can enhance their antimicrobial activity[60]. Addition of eosinophil peroxidase, which is cationic and binds to organisms, enhances the killing of *Toxoplasma* and *Leishmania* by macrophages[42]. It is likely that the uptake of enzymes and cations from other cells also plays a significant role in the antibacterial function of macrophages *in vivo*.

Cell-mediated immunity (CMI)

This term is usually reserved for immunity which involves direct intervention of T lymphocytes. These recognize antigen peptides displayed on the membranes of antigen-presenting cells in association with products of the major histocompatibility complex (discussed in detail in Chapter 2). One of their functions is then to release lymphokines, which have several effects.

First, they provide yet another mechanism which attracts monocytes and polymorphonuclear cells to the site of infection. Enhanced localization of phagocytes in the lesion seems to be the most significant role of CMI in immunity to *Listeria monocytogenes* infection in mice. This organism is readily killed by oxygen-dependent mechanisms in both monocytes and neutrophils without a requirement for activation[61], but it will overwhelm the host if arrival of phagocytes is not accelerated by CMI.

Second, lymphokine release activates the antimicrobial functions of phagocytic cells. As discussed above, these cells express numerous antimicrobial activities in the absence of lymphokine-mediated activation, but lymphokines make a critical difference to the stasis or killing of certain bacteria. Organisms which are not killed by freshly isolated monocytes but which are killed, or at least inhibited, by activated cells include *Legionella pneumophila*[62], *Leishmania donovani* amastigotes[48] and *Mycobacterium tuberculosis* in murine macrophages[63]. Recombinant IFNγ, or CD4[+], MHC Class II-restricted T cell lines recognizing mycobacterial antigen will induce total stasis of *M. tuberculosis* in murine macrophages[63]. IFNγ, however, has a variable effect on growth of *M. tuberculosis* in human monocytes and sometimes significantly increases the growth of this organism[64,65].

The role of IFNγ in enhancement of the microbicidal pathways has been briefly discussed above. There may well be many other undefined antibacterial mechanisms which are activated by lymphokines. Similarly, although IFNγ is probably the major phagocyte-activating lymphokine, the role of other lymphokines is gradually being revealed. For instance, granulocyte-macrophage colony stimulating factor (GM-CSF) causes monocytes to differentiate into macrophages and activates them for killing *Leishmania donovai*[66], and murine bone-marrow macrophages show enhanced inhibition of mycobacterial growth when exposed to IL-4 or IL-6[67]. In our hands inhibition of *M. tuberculosis* growth by murine peritoneal macrophages is not enhanced when cultured with IL-4, so it is possible that the results with bone-marrow cells are attributable to maturation rather than activation, though this is an obscure distinction. The situation is further complicated by the fact that recent work with murine macrophages has shown that some antimicrobial functions may require the synergistic action of two or more lymphokines, each of which may be completely inactive alone[68]. Therefore many published studies with defined or recombinant lymphokines may reveal only part of the truth.

Third, it is likely that the mechanisms described above, including accumulation and activation of lymphocytes and macrophages at a site where antigen is present, constitute the basis for the delayed hypersensitivity reaction to skin-test challenge with soluble antigen, typified by the Mantoux test.

Fourth, when release of lymphokines and accumulation of mononuclear cells is persistent, characteristic T cell-dependent tuberculoid granulomata are formed. These granulomata can be isolated and the release of cytokines monitored *in vitro*[69]. It is likely that they serve to isolate organisms within a focus of activated macrophages. However, when there is a vigorous cell-mediated response to bacterial components which are difficult to metabolize, such as the cell wall debris of *M. leprae*, the granuloma can persist in spite of an almost total lack of live organisms. The distribution of T cell subsets within such granulomata has been studied in detail in leprosy[70]. In tuberculosis the T cell-dependent granulomata tend to be necrotic. Possible explanations of this phenomenon are discussed below.

Lastly, IFNγ also evokes antimicrobial mechanisms in other cells, such as endothelial cells which are incapable of the oxidative burst, as shown with *Rickettsia* and *Chlamydia psittaci*[71,72].

Interaction between lymphokines and vitamin D3 metabolites in the regulation of macrophages and T cells in man

IFNγ causes human macrophages to express a 1-α hydroxylase which converts the circulating inactive form of vitamin D3 (25(OH)-vitamin D3) into the active 1,25-dihydroxy metabolite (calcitriol). Leakage of calcitriol from sites of macrophage activation into the systemic circulation accounts for the hypercalcaemia sometimes seen in sarcoidosis, tuberculosis or histoplasmosis. What is its function in chronic granulomatous inflammation? At physiological concentrations *in vitro* (10^{-9}–10^{-7} M) calcitriol activates antimycobacterial mechanisms in monocytes rather more efficiently than does IFNγ[73]. This may account for the fact that in the 1940s vitamin D was shown to cure chronic skin tuberculosis[74]. Alternatively, the physiological target may be the lymphocyte rather than the macrophage, as suggested below.

Avoidance of macrophage antimicrobial mechanisms

The T_{H1} to T_{H2} switch; avoidance of macrophage activation

Every stage of the interaction between organisms and macrophages is potentially opposed. One mechanism is the down-regulation of macrophage activation. In chronic inflammatory states there tends to be a switch from T_{H1} to T_{H2}, and the possible importance of this in relation to progression from positivity for human immunodeficiency virus (HIV)[75] to AIDS has been highlighted recently[75]. The same thing happens in other infections[76] including syphilis[77]: the T cells in the lesions of lepromatous leprosy are predominantly of the T_{H2} type[78] and may allow unopposed proliferation of *M. leprae*. Since calcitriol tends to down-regulate T_{H1} lymphocyte function[79] the IFNγ released by T_{H1} cells may exert an indirect negative feedback on T_{H1} activity via the formation of calcitriol, as described above.

Avoidance of macrophage functions

Some organisms secrete toxins which repel or kill the phagocytes. Capsules of carbohydrate (*Streptococcus pneumoniae*) or polypeptide (*Bacillus anthracis*) may impede complement deposition and phagocytosis[30]. The M proteins of Group A streptococci limit uptake of the organism by phagocytes, while permitting its specific attachment to the epithelium of the oropharynx. Other organisms are taken up, but fail to trigger the oxidative burst[49]. In general the avoidance mechanism is unknown, but *Chlamydia psittaci* seems to avoid the usual type of endocytosis by a mechanism resembling the internalization of polypeptide hormones via receptors in clathrin-coated pits[80]. Secretion of polyanions or ammonia have been reported to block phagolysosome fusion, though the methods used to demonstrate these phenomena have recently been re-evaluated[81]. It now seems that polyanions may cause differential inhibition of transfer of lysosomal components into phagosomes rather than complete blockage of fusion, and presumably they may help to block the action of cationic proteins. Similarly, superoxide dismutase and catalase can degrade oxygen intermediates, and the phenolic glycolipid secreted by *M. leprae* may act as a scavenger of oxygen radicals[82]. Another obvious strategy would be inhibition of lymphokine-mediated macrophage activation, and it has recently been suggested that the LAM released from mycobacteria can do this. Murine macrophages heavily infected with *M. leprae* cannot be activated to kill protozoa[83]. Other organisms avoid antimicrobial mechanisms by escaping from the phagosome. *M. leprae* and *Shigella flexneri* can multiply free in the cytoplasm, while *Brucella abortus* and *Legionella pneumophila* are found in the rough endoplasmic reticulum[84]. Finally, some organisms, such as *M. tuberculosis* tend to kill the macrophage. We have observed recently that cells infected with *M. tuberculosis* become exquisitely sensitive to the toxic effects of TNFα[27]. It is therefore possible that infected macrophages are killed by the TNFα which they themselves are induced to release by the mycobacterial LAM.

Other cell-mediated antibacterial pathways

NK cells

NK cells can directly damage some bacteria[85]. However, a more striking role for NK cells in bacterial infection was mentioned briefly above. In synergy with microbial components, TNFα causes murine NK cells to release IFNγ[24]. This may be an important pathway, providing the source of IFNγ in severe combined immunodeficiency (SCID) mice which are unexpectedly resistant to many infections[24]. It also provides a simple explanation for the observation that if given very early (before day 3 of infection) a neutralizing antibody to TNFα exacerbates infection with *Listeria*[14,86] and BCG[87] *in vivo*. It also provides a possible explanation for the protective effect of TNFα against *M. avium*[7] and *Toxoplasma*[88] in mice. This pathway is interesting from an evolutionary point of view because it means that IFNγ is available early after infection, before the T cell response has developed. It should be noted that if this is how TNFα protects mice against *M. avium*, it is of doubtful relevance to human infections with mycobacteria, since all authors agree that IFNγ has no effect on the growth of these organisms in human macrophages[64,65].

Cytotoxic T cells

Cytotoxic T cells are generated during the cell-mediated response to intracellular pathogens[89,90] and can kill infected or antigen-pulsed macrophages. It is becoming apparent that this phenomenon may be of greater importance than was previously realized. In view of the absence of any convincing evidence that human macrophages can be induced to kill *M. tuberculosis*, or even the less pathogenic *M. avium*, it seems possible that mycobacteria which survive the killing mechanisms operating at the moment of phagocytosis (and most do survive or fail to trigger them) are then safe within the macrophage. If so, immunity may require the destruction of the infected cell so that the bacteria can be exposed to repeated cycles of phagocytosis. It is therefore interesting that recent studies have confirmed an earlier claim that *M. tuberculosis* can escape from the phagolysosome (B.R. Bloom, personal communication) since that would facilitate presentation of antigen by Class I MHC, and therefore the activation of CD8$^+$ cytotoxic T cells. This train of thought is made still more exciting by the recent observation that β_2-microglobulin knockout mice, which cannot express Class I MHC, are very susceptible to tuberculosis (B.R. Bloom, personal communication; I. Orme, personal communication).

γ/δ T cells

In the mouse at least, mycobacterial infection leads to a disproportionate increase in the γ/δ T cell population[91,92]. γ/δ T cells which respond to mycobacterial antigens can be isolated from the lesions of some types of leprosy[93], but their role in human bacterial disease is unclear. Nevertheless, a strikingly high proportion of the circulating γ/δ T cells from normal donors respond to *M. tuberculosis*[94]. This interaction is not MHC-restricted. It seems likely that these cells play a role early in infection, and they appear to recognize components that are present in many bacterial species.

MECHANISMS OF IMMUNOPATHOLOGY

Superantigens

Although early cytokine release by bacterial components is clearly part of a rapid protective pathway, as described earlier, excessive release is an important cause of pathology. An important class of bacterial (and viral) components that cause such excessive release is the superantigens. Superantigens are particularly common in the staphylococci and streptococci. They include the enterotoxins, exfoliative toxin and toxic shock syndrome toxin of staphylococci (TSST-1)[95], and the scarlet fever toxins, pyrogenic toxins and M proteins of streptococci[96]. Superantigens interact with the Class II major histocompatibility complex on antigen-presenting cells, and cross-link this onto the T cell receptor complex by binding to the products of particular T cell receptor Vβ gene families. This interaction bypasses the conventional mechanism of antigen presentation, because the superantigen is not engaged in the peptide-binding groove of the Class II MHC antigen, and does not interact with the parts of the T cell receptor α or β chains that are involved in recognition of such peptides. The toxicity of these compounds results from their ability to activate essentially all T cells bearing products of the relevant Vβ gene family, whatever their specificity. This leads to massive cytokine

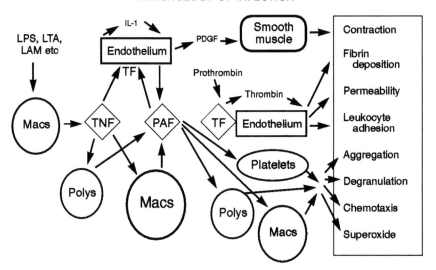

Figure 4 Pathways of cytokine-mediated tissue damage in endotoxin shock, the Shwartzman reaction and probably, the Koch phenomenon. The crucial mediators, tumour necrosis factor (TNF), platelet activating factor (PAF), and tissue thromboplastin (TF) are written inside diamonds. IL-1, interleukin-1; PDGF, platelet-derived growth factor; numerous other relevant mediators are omitted. TF is expressed on endothelial cells in response to TNF and PAF. It then promotes thrombin formation and fibrin deposition. Proof that these are critical events has been obtained with neutralizing antibodies to TNF and TF, and with inhibitors of PAF

release, and since the genes for superantigens are strongly conserved, it must also subvert the immune response in a way that is helpful for bacterial survival[97].

Septicaemic shock and the adult respiratory distress syndrome

The previous sections have discussed the protective roles of cytokine release triggered by bacterial infection. These cytokines are also essential components of the lethal events which accompany gram-negative septicaemia. This is shown by the fact that a neutralizing antibody to TNFα is protective in a model of septicaemic shock in the baboon[98]. Similarly, administration of TNFα can induce cachexia, anaemia, inflammation and haemorrhagic necrosis[99]. The systemic toxicity of TNFα is greatly increased in the presence of IL-1 or LPS[100], both of which are likely to be present during bacterial infections. Thus when present in excessive concentrations, and especially if accompanied by IL-1 or LPS, the effects of TNFα on phagocytes and endothelial cells can lead to the cascade of events shown in simplified form in Figure 4. The critical events, which can be determined with appropriate blockers and neutralizing antibodies, are the release of platelet activating factor (PAF), the switch of endothelial cell surfaces from anticoagulant to procoagulant and the increased adhesiveness of phagocytes. The end results are endothelial damage, fluid loss and diffuse intravascular coagulation.

Since TNFα can also be protective, the timing and level of TNFα must be critical. High serum levels of TNFα correlate with a poor clinical outcome in septicaemia[101], and in the adult respiratory distress syndrome[102].

The Shwartzman reaction

Cytokine release can also cause local rather than systemic pathology. Microbial products, and certain types of inflammatory response 'prepare' tissue sites so that they become exquisitely sensitive to cytokines, particularly TNFα, and are liable to undergo haemorrhagic necrosis in their presence[103,104]. This 'preparation' of an inflamed site involves changes in the properties of endothelial cells (reviewed in ref. 17), and the accumulation of phagocytic cells. It can be brought about both by T cell-independent (LPS)[103] and T cell-dependent (low doses of soluble mycobacterial antigen)[105] responses to microbial products. This phenomenon probably explains the Shwartzman reaction[104,106] in which a skin site prepared by an injection of bacteria (LPS alone can be used) undergoes necrosis when a further dose of LPS-rich bacteria is given intravenously 24 h later. It may also explain the rash often seen during *Meningococcus* septicaemia. If bacteria released during a previous subclinical septicaemic episode have lodged in skin capillaries, these will become prepared sites, and a later septicaemic episode severe enough to trigger massive cytokine release will cause these sites to undergo necrosis. The final pathway of tissue damage is probably similar to that shown in Figure 4.

The Koch phenomenon and necrotizing T cell-dependent granulomata

Some of the immunopathology seen during T cell-dependent granulomatous inflammation is due to the space-occupying nature of the lesions or to chronic non-specific inflammatory effects. However in other situations frank necrosis occurs, and the mechanism is important.

Robert Koch observed that tuberculous guinea-pigs skin-tested with tuberculosis bacilli or culture supernatant showed necrotic reaction at the skin-test site within 24–48 h[107]. This phenomenon is also seen in individuals with previous or current tuberculosis, but it is not an inevitable component of a cell-mediated reaction to mycobacterial antigen because it does not occur in tuberculoid leprosy patients or BCG-vaccinated individuals, even when there is vigorous positive induration. It has been suggested elsewhere that this phenomenon, and some of the necrosis seen in the tuberculous lesions themselves, may be related to the Shwartzman reaction[106,108]. Thus the mycobacterial antigens may first 'prepare' the site as described above. Local T cell-mediated macrophage activation, reinforced by the calcitriol positive feed-back loop described earlier, may then provide a source of TNFα[73,108]. Finally, the mycobacterial LAM and peptidoglycan fragments may trigger local release of TNFα, resulting in necrosis[12,108].

Interestingly, the alveolar lavage macrophages of tuberculosis patients release TNFα spontaneously *in vitro*[108] and although TNFα is not usually detectable in the serum elevated levels of an inhibitor of the toxicity of TNFα are present[109].

TNF release and activation of HIV

One important consequence of the release of cytokines, particularly TNFα, may be the activation of HIV. If T cell lines latently infected with HIV are exposed to TNFα, virus production is enhanced[110]. It seems likely that this is one reason for the rapid progression of AIDS in patients infected with *M. tuberculosis*, since the activated macrophages, triggered by LAM will provide a source of TNFα.

THE INDUCTION OF AUTOIMMUNITY BY BACTERIAL INFECTIONS

Autoantibodies

Autoimmunity is another form of immunopathology that may be important in some infections. Chronic bacterial infections are accompanied by the production of a spectrum of autoantibodies similar to that seen in diseases usually assumed to be autoimmune[111]. This may be due to cross-reactivity, to polyclonal activation, or simply to 'adjuvant' effects or 'second signals' provided by bacterial components. Several other possible mechanisms have also been suggested.

Heat-shock proteins (hsp)

It was discovered recently that several dominant antigens of infectious agents are homologues of heat-shock or stress proteins (hsp)[112]. These molecules are encoded by several gene families and they play essential roles in the transport, assembly and folding of other proteins, particularly in stressed cells. The functions of these proteins are similar, in all pro- and eukaryotes and are essential to survival, and there is remarkable conservation of their amino acid sequences. Responses to some of these hsp may mediate protective immunity. Because hsp are so strongly conserved, generating an immune response to them has the advantage for the host that any micro-organism will be recognizable. However in view of the strong homology between bacterial and human proteins, there are other possible consequences of such responses. For example, induction of strong responses to hsp during mycobacterial (and other) infections could result in autoimmune responses to autologous hsp. These may play a pathogenetic role during infections, and perhaps in rheumatoid arthritis[113]. Also, infected (and therefore stressed) cells, or cells stressed by exposure to cytokines or free radicals might process their own hsps and present peptides derived from them in association with MHC molecules, becoming targets of cross-reactive T cell responses[86]. Alternatively some γ/δ T cells may recognize a form of the hsp65 associated with the cell membrane, though the evidence for this is weak.

It is possible that the latter two mechanisms form the basis of a physiological mechanism for the removal of stressed cells.

Membrane-associated forms of some hsp exist, and members of the 70 kD hsp gene family are found in the MHC. Since the function of hsp includes the binding of unfolded or abnormally folded proteins, these molecules could be involved in novel types of antigen presentation to T cells[113,114].

Superantigens

Superantigens could theoretically lead to autoimmunity by polyclonally activating all the T cells bearing products of a particular $V\beta$ gene. Some of the T cells activated could be specific for self components.

CONCLUSIONS

In recent years there has been a tendency to consider the specific immune response to bacteria mediated by antibodies and T cell receptors, in complete isolation from the overall physiology of the host–parasite interaction. In fact antibody and specific T cells form only one, rather recently evolved part of this interaction. In order to provide immunological understanding that is relevant to the clinician and to the patient, this review has deliberately tipped the balance away from the areas of antigenic peptides and antigen presentation by the MHC, towards cytokines, endocrinology, and the mechanisms involved in the recognition of common bacterial components. These are the factors which determine much of bacterial immunity and pathology. However in order to complete the picture, this chapter should be read in conjunction with other chapters in this volume dealing with new approaches to vaccine design, and the recognition of mycobacterial antigens by T lymphocytes.

References

1. Esser RE, Schwab JH, Eisenberg RA. Immunology of peptidoglycan–polysaccharide polymers from cell walls of Group A streptococci. In: Stewart-Tull DES, Davies M, eds. Immunology of the bacterial cell envelope. New York: Wiley; 1985: 91–118.
2. Brennan PJ. Structure of mycobacteria: recent developments in defining cell wall carbohydrates and proteins. Rev Infect Dis. 1989; 11: S420–S430.
3. Mestecky J, McGhee JR. Immunoglobulin A: molecular and cellular interactions involved in biosynthesis and immune response. Adv Immunol. 1987; 40: 153–245.
4. Walport M. Complement. In: Roitt I, Brostoff J, Male D, eds. Immunology. London: Gower Medical Publishing; 1989: 13.1–13.16.
5. Tebo JM, Mortensen RF. Characterisation and isolation of a C-reactive protein receptor from the human monocyte cell line U937. J Immunol. 1990; 144: 231–238.
6. Ezekowitz RAB, Day LE, Herman GA. A human mannose-binding protein is an acute-phase reactant that shares sequence homology with other vertebrate lectins. J Exp Med. 1988; 167: 1034–1046.
7. Bermudez LEM, Stevens P, Kolonoski P, Wu M, Young LS. Treatment of experimental disseminated *Mycobacterium avium* complex infection in mice with recombinant IL-2 and tumour necrosis factor. J Immunol. 1989; 143: 2996–3000.

8. Blanchard DK, Djeu JY, Klein TW, Friedman H, Stewart WE. Protective effects of tumor necrosis factor in experimental *Legionella pneumophila* infections in mice via activation of PMN function. J Leukoc Biol. 1988; 43: 429–435.

9. Parent M. Effects of TNF in bacterial infections. Ann Inst Pasteur Immunol. 1988; 139: 301–304.

10. Cross AS, Sadoff JC, Kelly N, Bernton E, Gemski P. Pretreatment with recombinant murine tumor necrosis factor alpha/cachectin and murine interleukin 1 alpha protects mice from lethal bacterial infection. J Exp Med. 1989; 169: 2021–2027.

11. Usami H, Yamamoto A, Yamashita W, Sugawara Y, Hamada S, Yamamoto T, Kato K, Kokeguchi S, Ohokuni H, Kotani S. Antitumour effects of streptococcal lipoteichoic acids on Meth A fibrosarcoma. Br J Cancer. 1988; 57: 70–73.

12. Moreno C, Taverne J, Mehlert A, Bate CA, Brealey RJ, Meager A, Rook GAW, Playfair JHL. Lipoarabinomannan from *Mycobacterium tuberculosis* induces the production of tumour necrosis factor from human and murine macrophages. Clin Exp Immunol. 1989; 76: 240–245.

13. Noso Y, Parent M, Parent F, Chedid L. Production of tumour necrosis factor in nude mice by muramyl peptides associated with bacterial vaccines. Cancer Res. 1988; 48: 5766–5769.

14. Havell EA. Production of tumor necrosis factor during murine listeriosis. J Immunol. 1987; 139: 4225–4231.

15. Yamamoto A, Nagamuta M, Usami H, Sugawara Y, Watanabe N, Niitsu Y, Urushizaki I. Release of tumour necrosis factor (TNF) into mouse peritoneal fluids by OK432, a streptococcal preparation. Immunopharmacology. 1986; 11: 79–86.

16. Gamble JR, Harlan JM, Klebanoff SJ, Vadas MA. Stimulation of the adherence of neutrophils to umbilical vein endothelium by human recombinant tumour necrosis factor. Proc Natl Acad Sci USA. 1985; 82: 8667–8671.

17. Pober JS. TNF as an activator of vascular endothelium. Ann Inst Pasteur Immunol. 1988; 139: 317–323.

18. Rosen H, Gordon S, North RJ. Exacerbation of murine listeriosis by a monoclonal antibody specific for the type 3 complement receptor of myelomonocytic cells. Absence of monocytes at infective foci allows *Listeria* to multiply in nonphagocytic cells. J Exp Med. 1989; 170: 27–37.

19. Springer TA. Adhesion receptors of the immune system. Nature. 1990; 346: 425–434.

20. Bevilacqua MP. Endothelial-leukocyte adhesion molecules. Annu Rev Immunol. 1993; 11: 767–804.

21. Klebanoff SJ, Vadas MA, Harlan JM, Sparks LH, Gamble JR, Agosti JM, Waltersdorf AM. Stimulation of neutrophils by tumour necrosis factor. J Immunol. 1986; 136: 4220–4225.

22. Berkow RL, Dodson MR. Biochemical mechanisms in the priming of neutrophils by tumour necrosis factor. J Leukocyte Biol. 1988; 44: 345–352.

23. Ferrante A. Tumor necrosis factor alpha potentiates neutrophil antimicrobial and *Candida albicans* and associated increases in oxygen and radical production and lysosomal enzyme release. Infect Immun. 1989; 57: 2115–2122.

24. Bancroft GJ, Sheehan KC, Schreiber RD, Unanue ER. Tumor necrosis factor is involved in the T cell-independent pathway of macrophage activation in scid mice. J Immunol. 1989; 143: 127–130.

25. Deare M, Bukholm G, Czariecki CW. In vitro treatment of HEp-2 cells with human tumour necrosis factor alpha and human interferons reduces invasiveness of *Salmonella typhimurium*. J Biol Regul Homeost Agents. 1989; 3: 1–7.

26. Shemer-Avni Y, Wallach D, Sarov I. Reversion of the antichlamydial effect of tumour necrosis factor by tryptophan and antibodies to beta interferon. Infect Immun. 1989; 57: 3484–3490.

27. Filley EA, Rook GAW. Effect of mycobacteria on sensitivity to the cytotoxic effects of tumor necrosis factor. Infect Immun. 1991; 59: 2567–2572.

28. Blauer KL, Poth M, Rogers WM, Bernton W. Dehydroepiandrosterone antagonises the suppressive effects of dexamethasone on lymphocyte proliferation. Endocrinology. 1991; 129: 3174–3179.

29. Meikle AW, Dorchuck RW, Araneo BA, et al. The presence of a dehydroepiandrosterone-specific receptor-binding complex in murine T cells. J Steroid Biochem Mol Biol. 1992; 42:

293–304.
30. Frank MM. Evasion strategies of microorganisms. Prog Immunol. 1989; VII: 194–201.
31. Romagnani S. Human TH1 and TH2 subsets: doubt no more. Immunol Today. 1991; 12: 256–257.
32. Sher A, Gazzinelli RT, Oswald IP, et al. Role of T-cell derived cytokines in the downregulation of immune responses in parasitic and retroviral infection. Immunol Rev. 1992; 127: 183–204.
33. Daynes RA, Araneo BA, Dowell TA, Huang K, Dudley D. Regulation of murine lymphokine production in vivo. III. The lymphoid tissue microenvironment exerts regulatory influences over T helper cell function. J Exp Med. 1990; 171: 979–996.
34. Maggi E, Parronchi P, Manetti R, et al. Reciprocal regulatory effects of IFN-gamma and IL-4 on the in vitro development of human Th1 and Th2 clones. J Immunol. 1992; 148: 2142–2147.
35. Ofek I, Sharon N. Lectinophagocytosis: a molecular mechanism of recognition between cell surface sugars and lectins in the phagocytosis of bacteria. Infect Immun. 1988; 56: 539–547.
36. Ross GD, Cain JA, Myones BL, Newman SL, Lachmann PJ. Specificity of membrane complement receptor type 3 (CR3) for beta-glucans. Complement. 1987; 4: 61–74.
37. Bullock WE, Wright SD. Role of the adherence-promoting receptors CR3, LFA-1 and p150,95 in binding of Histoplasma capsulatum by human macrophages. J Exp Med. 1987; 165: 195–210.
38. Wright SD, Jong MTC. Adhesion-promoting receptors on human macrophages recognises E. coli by binding to lipopolysaccharide. J Exp Med. 1986; 164: 1876–1888.
39. Ding A, Wright S, Nathan C. Activation of mouse peritoneal macrophages by monoclonal antibodies to MAC-1 (complement receptor type 3). J Exp Med. 1987; 165: 733–749.
40. Bridges CG, Dasilva GL, Yamamura M, Valdimarsson H. A radiometric assay for the combined measurement of phagocytosis and intracellular killing of Candida albicans. Clin Exp Immunol. 1980; 42: 226–233.
41. Nakagawara A, Nathan CF, Cohn Z. Hydrogen peroxide metabolism in human monocytes during differentiation in vitro. J Clin Invest. 1981; 68: 1243–1252.
42. Locksley RM, Nelson CS, Fankhauser JE, Klebanoff SJ. Loss of granule myeloperoxidase during in vitro culture of human monocytes correlates with decay in antiprotozoa activity. Am J Trop Med Hyg. 1987; 36: 541–548.
43. Yong EC, Chi EY, Kuo CC. Differential antimicrobial activity of human mononuclear phagocytes against human biovars of Chlamydia trachomatis. J Immunol. 1987; 139: 1287–1302.
44. Nathan CF, Hibbs JB. Role of nitric oxide synthesis in macrophage antimicrobial activity. Curr Opin Immunol. 1991; 3: 65–70.
45. Hibbs JB Jr, Taintor RR, Vavrin Z. Macrophage cytotoxicity: role for L-arginine deiminase and imino nitrogen oxidation to nitrate. Science. 1987; 235: 473–476.
46. Green SJ, Meltzer MS, Hibbs JB, Nacy CA. Activated macrophages destroy intracellular Leishmania major amastigotes by an L-arginine-dependent killing mechanism. J Immunol. 1990; 144: 278–283.
47. Chan J, Xing Y, Magliozzo RS, Bloom BR. Killing of virulent Mycobacterium tuberculosis by reactive nitrogen intermediates produced by activated murine macrophages. J Exp Med. 1992; 175: 1111–1122.
48. Murray HW, Cartelli DM. Killing of intracellular Leishmania donovani by human mononuclear phagocytes. Evidence for oxygen-dependent and -independent leishmanicidal activity. J Clin Invest. 1984; 72: 32–44.
49. Catterall JR, Black CM, Leventhal JP, Rizk NW, Wachtel JS, Remington JS. Nonoxidative microbial activity in normal human alveolar and peritoneal macrophages. Infect Immun. 1987; 55: 1635–1640.
50. Schaffner A. Therapeutic concentrations of glucocorticoids suppress the antimicrobial activity of human macrophages without impairing their responsiveness to gamma interferon. J Clin Invest. 1985; 76: 1755–1764.
51. Rook GAW, Steele J, Ainsworth M, Leveton C. A direct effect of glucocorticoid hormones on the ability of human and murine macrophages to control the growth of M. tuberculosis. Eur J Resp Dis. 1987; 71: 286–291.
52. Mintz CS, Chen JX, Shuman HA. Isolation and characterisation of auxotrophic mutants

of *Legionella pneumophila* that fail to multiply in human monocytes. Infect Immun. 1988; 56: 1449–1455.

53. Ozaki Y, Edelstein MP, Duch DS. The actions of interferon and antiinflammatory agents of induction of indoleamine 2,3-dioxygenase in human peripheral blood monocytes. Biochem Biophys Res Commun. 1987; 144: 1147–1153.

54. Bitterlich G, Szabo G., Werner ER, Larcher C, Fuchs D, Hausen A, Reibnegger G, Schulz TF, Troppmair J, Wachter H. Selective induction of mononuclear phagocytes to produce neopterin by interferons. Immunobiology. 1988; 176: 228–235.

55. Pfefferkorn ER. Interferon gamma blocks the growth of *Toxoplasma gondii* in human fibroblasts by inducing the host cells to degrade tryptophan. Proc Natl Acad Sci USA. 1984; 81: 908–912.

56. Odeberg H, Olsson I. Mechanisms for the microbicidal activity of cationic proteins of human granulocytes. Infect Immun. 1976; 14: 1269–1275.

57. Ganz T, Selsted ME, Szklarek D, Harwig SS, Daher K, Bainton DF, Lehrer RI. Defensins. Natural peptide antibiotics of human neutrophils. J Clin Invest. 1985; 76: 1427–1435.

58. Marra MN, Wilde CG, Griffith JE, Snable JL, Scott RW. Bactericidal/permeability-increasing protein has endotoxin-neutralising activity. J Immunol. 1990; 144: 662–666.

59. Sawyer JG, Martin NL, Hancock RE. Interaction of macrophages cationic proteins with the outer membrane of *Pseudomonas aeruginosa*. Infect Immun. 1988; 56: 693–698.

60. Pruzanski W, Ranadive NS, Saito S. Modulation of phagocytosis and intracellular bactericidal activity of polymorphonuclear and mononuclear cells by cationic proteins from human granulocytes: alternative pathway of phagocytic enhancement. Inflammation. 1984; 8: 445–457.

61. Czupyrnski CJ, Campbell PA, Henson PM. Killing of Listeria monocytogenes by human neutrophils and monocytes but not by monocyte-derived macrophages. J Reticuloendothel Soc. 1984; 34: 29–44.

62. Horwitz M. Cell-mediated immunity in Legionnaire's disease. J Clin Invest. 1983; 71: 1686–1697.

63. Rook GA, Champion BR, Steele J, Varey AM, Stanford JL. I-A restricted activation by T cell lines of anti-tuberculosis activity in murine macrophages. Clin Exp Immunol. 1985; 59: 414–420.

64. Douvas GS, Looker DL, Vatter AE, Crowle AJ. Gamma interferon activates human macrophages to become tumoricidal and leishmanicidal but enhances replication of macrophage-associated mycobacteria. Infect Immun. 1985; 50: 1–8.

65. Rook GAW, Steele J, Ainsworth M, Champion BR. Activation of macrophages to inhibit proliferation of *Mycobacterium tuberculosis*: comparison of the effects of recombinant gamma interferon on human monocytes and murine peritoneal macrophages. Immunology. 1986; 59: 333–338.

66. Weiser WY, van-Niel A, Clark SC, David JR, Remold HG. Recombinant human granulocyte/macrophage colony-stimulating factor activates intracellular killing of *Leishmania donovani* by human monocyte-derived macrophages. J Exp Med. 1987; 166: 1436–1446.

67. Kaufmann SHE, Munk ME, Koga T, Steinhoff U, Wand-Wurttenberger A, Gatrill AJ, Flesch I, Schoel B. Effector T cells in bacterial infections. Prog Immunol. 1989; VII: 963–970.

68. Belosevic M, Davis CE, Meltzer MS, Nacy CA. Regulation of activated macrophage antimicrobial activities. Identification of lymphokines that cooperate with IFN-gamma for induction of resistance to infection. J Immunol. 1988; 141: 890–896.

69. Elliott DE, Righthand VF, Boros DL. Characterization of regulatory (interferon-alpha/beta) and accessory (LAF/IL-1) monokine activities from liver granuloma macrophages of *Schistosoma mansoni*-infected mice. J Immunol. 1987; 138: 2653–2662.

70. Rea TH, Modlin RL. Immunopathology of leprosy skin lesions. Semin Dermatol. 1991; 10: 188–193.

71. Wisseman CL Jr, Wadell A. Interferon-like factors from antigen and mitogen-stimulated human leukocytes with anti-rickettsial and cytolytic on *Rickettsia prowazekii* infected human endothelial cells, fibroblasts and macrophages. J Exp Med. 1983; 157: 1780.

72. Rothermel CD, Rubin BY, Jaffe EA, Murray HW. Oxygen-independent inhibition of intracellular *Chlamydia psittaci* growth by human monocytes and interferon-activated macrophages. J Immunol. 1986; 137: 689–692.

73. Rook GA, Steele J, Fraher L, Barker S, Karmali R, O'Riordan J, Stanford JL. Vitamin D3, gamma interferon and control of proliferation of *Mycobacterium tuberculosis* by human monocytes. Immunology. 1986; 57: 159–163.
74. Rook GAW. The role of vitamin D in tuberculosis. Am Rev Resp Dis. 1988; 138: 768–770.
75. Clerici M, Shearer GM. A TH1 to TH2 switch is a critical step in the etiology of HIV infection. Immunol Today. 1993; 14: 107–111.
76. Grzych JM, Pearce JE, Cheever A, et al. Egg deposition is the stimulus for the production of Th2 cytokines in murine schistosomiasis mansoni. J Immunol. 1991; 146: 1332–1340.
77. Fitzgerald TJ. The Th1/Th2 switch in syphilitic infection: is it detrimental? Infect Immun. 1992; 60: 3475–3479.
78. Sieling PA, Modlin RL. T cell and cytokine patterns in leprosy skin lesions. Semin Immunopathol. 1992; 13: 413–426.
79. Daynes RA, Meikle AW, Araneo BA. Locally active steroid hormones may facilitate compartmentalization of immunity by regulating the types of lymphokines produced by helper T cells. Res Immunol. 1991; 142: 40–45.
80. Hodinka RL, Davis CH, Choong J, Wyrick PB. Ultrastructural study of endocytosis of *Chlamydia trachomatis* by McCoy cells. Infect Immun. 1988; 56: 1456–1463.
81. Goren MB, Vatter AE, Fiscus J. Polyanionic agents do not inhibit phagosome-lysosome fusion in culture macrophages. J Leukoc Biol. 1987; 41: 122–129.
82. Neill MA, Klebanoff SJ. The effect of phenolic glycolipid-1 from *Mycobacterium leprae* on the antimicrobial activity of human macrophages. J Exp Med. 1988; 167: 30–42.
83. Sibley LD, Krahenbuhl JL. Mycobacterium leprae-burdened macrophages are refractory to activation by gamma interferon. Infect Immun. 1987; 55: 446–450.
84. Oldham LJ, Rodgers FG. Adhesion, penetration and intracellular replication of *Legionella pneumophila*: an *in vitro* model of pathogenesis. J Gen Microbiol. 1985; 131: 697–706.
85. Garcia-Penarrubia P, Koster FT, Kelley RO, McDowell TD, Bankhurst AD. Antibacterial activity of human natural killer cells. J Exp Med. 1989; 169: 99–113.
86. Nakane A, Minagawa T, Kato K. Endogenous tumour necrosis factor (cachectin) is essential to host resistance against *Listeria monocytogenes* infection. Infect Immun. 1988; 56: 2563–2569.
87. Kindler V, Sappino AP, Grau GE, Piguet PF, Vassallia P. The inducing role of tumor necrosis factor in the development of bactericidal granulomas during BCG infection. Cell. 1989; 56: 731–740.
88. Black CM, Israelski DM, Suzuki Y, Remington JS. Effect of recombinant tumour necrosis factor on acute infection in mice with *Toxoplasma gondii* or *Trypanosoma cruzi*. Immunology. 1989; 68: 570–574.
89. Koga T, Wand-Wurttenberger A, DeBruyn J, Munk ME, Schoel B, Kaufmann SH. T cells against a bacterial heat shock protein recognize stressed macrophages. Science. 1989; 245: 1112–1115.
90. Ottenhoff TH, Ab BK, van-Embden JD, Thole JE, Kiessling R. The recombinant 65kDa heat shock protein of *Mycobacterium bovis*/Bacillus Calmette Guèrin/*M. tuberculosis* is a target molecule for CD4+ cytotoxic T lymphocytes that lyse human monocytes. J Exp Med. 1988; 168: 1947–1952.
91. Augustin A, Kubo RT, Sim GK. Resident pulmonary lymphocytes expressing the gamma/delta T-cell receptor. Nature. 1989; 340: 239–241.
92. Janis EM, Kaufmann SH, Schwartz RH, Pardoll DM. Activation of gamma delta T cells in the primary immune response to *Mycobacterium tuberculosis*. Science. 1989; 244: 713–716.
93. Modlin RL, Pirmez C, Hofman FM, Torigian V, Uyemura K, Rea TH, Bloom BR, Brenner MB. Lymphocytes bearing antigen-specific gamma delta T-cell receptors accumulate in human infectious disease lesions. Nature. 1989; 339: 544–548.
94. Kabelitz D, Bender A, Schondelmaier S, Schoel B, Kaufmann SHE. A large fraction of human peripheral blood gamma/delta T cells is activated by *Mycobacterium tuberculosis* but not by its 65kDa heat shock protein. J Exp Med. 1990; 1000: 667–679.
95. Jupin C, Anderson S, Damais C, Alouf JE, Parant M. Toxic shock syndrome toxin 1 as an inducer of human tumor necrosis factors and gamma interferon. J Exp Med. 1988; 167: 752–761.
96. Schlievert PM. Role of superantigens in human disease. J Infect Dis. 1993; 167: 997–1002.

97. Cantor H, Crump AL, Raman VK, et al. Immunoregulatory effects of superantigens: interactions of staphylococcal enterotoxins with host MHC and non-MHC products. Immunol Rev. 1993; 131: 27–42.

98. Tracey KJ, Fong Y, Hesse DG, Manogue KR, Lee AT, Kuo GC, Lowry SF, Cerami A. Anti-cachectin/TNF monoclonal antibodies prevent septic shock during lethal bacteraemia. Nature. 1987; 330: 662–664.

99. Tracey KJ, Wei H, Manogue KR, Fong Y, Hesse DG, Nguyen HT, Kuo GC, Beutler B, Cotran RS, Cerami A. et al. Cachetin/tumor necrosis factor induces cachexia anemia, and inflammation. J Exp Med. 1988; 167: 1211–1227.

100. Waage A, Espevik T. Interleukin 1 potentiates the lethal effect of tumor necrosis factor alpha/cachectin in mice. J Exp Med. 1988; 167: 1987–1992.

101. Waage A, Halstensen A, Espevik T. Association between tumour necrosis factor in serum and fatal outcome in patients with meningococcal disease. Lancet. 1987; 1: 355–357.

102. Millar AB, Foley NM, Singer M, Johnson NMcI, Meager A, Rook GAW. TNF in bronchopulmonary secretions of patients with adult respiratory distress syndrome. Lancet. 1989; ii: 712–714.

103. Rothstein J, Schreiber H. Synergy between tumour necrosis factor and bacterial products causes haemorrhagic necrosis and lethal shock in normal mice. Proc Natl Acad Sci. 1988; 85: 607–611.

104. Shwartzman G. Phenomenon of local tissue reactivity and its immunological, pathological, and clinical significance. New York: Paul B. Hoeber; 1937.

105. Al Attiyah R, Moreno C, Rook GAW. TNF-alpha-mediated tissue damage in mouse foot-pads primed with mycobacterial preparations. Res Immunol. 1992; 143: 601–610.

106. Rook GAW. Mechanisms of immunologically mediated tissue damage during infection. In: Champion R, Pye R, eds. Recent advances in dermatology. Edinburgh: Churchill Livingstone; 1990: 193–210.

107. KKoch R. Forsetzung der Mittheilungen uber ein Heilmittel gegen Tuberculose. Deutsche Med Wschr. 1991; 17: 101–102.

108. Rook GAW, Al Attiyah R. Cytokines and the Koch phenomenon. Tubercle. 1991; 72: 13–20.

109. Foley N, Lambert C, McNicol M, Johnson NMcI, Rook GAW. An inhibitor of the toxicity of tumour necrosis factor in the serum patients with sarcoidosis, tuberculosis and Crohn's disease. Clin Exp Immunol. 1990; 80: 395–399.

110. Folks TM, Clouse KA, Justement J, Rabson A, Duh E, Kehrl JH, Fauci AS. Tumor necrosis factor alpha induces expression of human immunodeficiency virus in a chronically infected T-cell clone. Proc Natl Acad Sci USA. 1989; 86: 2365–2368.

111. Schoenfeld Y, Isenberg DA. Mycobacteria and autoimmunity. Immunol Today. 1988; 9: 178–182.

112. Young DB, Lathigra R, Hendrix R, Sweetser D, Young RA. Stress proteins are immune targets in leprosy and tuberculosis. Proc Natl Acad Sci USA. 1988; 85: 4267–4270.

113. Winfield JB. Stress proteins, arthritis, and autoimmunity. Arthritis Rheum. 1989; 32: 1497–1504.

114. Vanbuskirk A, Crump BL, Margoliash E, Pierce SK. A peptide binding protein having a role in antigen presentation is a member of the hsp70 heat shock family. J Exp Med. 1989; 170: 1799–1809.

2
Molecular Structure and Immune Recognition of Mycobacteria

A. D. M. REES, A. MEHLERT and J. R. LAMB

INTRODUCTION

Mycobacteria are the causative organisms of diseases such as leprosy and tuberculosis which have always been and continue to be a major world health problem. Immunologically, perhaps their most important characteristic is the fact that they are intracellular parasites. The degree to which this habit is facultative (*Mycobacterium tuberculosis*) or obligate (*Mycobacterium leprae*) varies within the species. As a consequence, these organisms are not susceptible to antibody-mediated mechanisms of immunity. In the 1960s the pioneering work of George Mackaness[1,2] demonstrated that immunity to *Listeria monocytogenes*, which is also a facultative intracellular parasite, was primarily dependent on two cell types, the T cell and the phagocytic macrophage. Cell transfer experiments showed that while macrophage-mediated mechanisms were non-specific, T cell responses were specific to the inducing organism. The fine specificity of these cells and the relationship between this and effector mechanisms have implications for the design of vaccines, diagnosis and treatment. Technologies such as T cell cloning, together with improvements in the methodology available to assess T cell antigenic specificity, have generated more information on the nature of T cell epitopes, and have improved our understanding of the biological importance of particular specificities. This chapter will address three aspects of mycobacterial immunity. First, the antigens of *M. tuberculosis* will be described in some detail. Mycobacteria are antigenically highly complex mixtures, not just in terms of the numbers of different proteins they contain, but also in the presence of significant levels of immunomodulatory lipids and carbohydrates. Nevertheless, it has recently become clear that, at least as far as protein antigens are concerned, mycobacteria have a lot in common with other infectious and parasitic organisms. This observation may prove to be of fundamental importance to our understanding of the immune response to such organisms. Second, the various methods available to determine the fine specificity of T cells and some of their applications are described in some detail. These methods are the basic tools for determining T cell specificity both in mono- and polyclonal T cell populations. Finally, some aspects of the immune mechanisms involved are discussed.

ANTIGENS

History

Although tubercle bacilli were one of the first micro-organisms to be recognized as causative agents of human disease, characterization of their components has always been hampered by the slow growth of the organisms in vitro. Indeed *M. leprae* has yet to be successfully grown under laboratory conditions. Until recently, researchers in the mycobacteria field were still relying on very crude mixtures of mycobacterial extracts on which to base their immunological studies.

The first of these extracts was made by Koch in the last century, and it is still known as 'old tuberculin'. This was enthusiastically advocated by Koch as an enhancer of the immune response in tuberculosis patients. It could, however, cause necrotic lesions in some circumstances thus showing, very early on in mycobacterial research, that despite prolonged degradation, components of *M. tuberculosis* can cause severe pathological effects. In 1932 Seibert introduced purified protein derivative (PPD), an extract of *M. tuberculosis* which was meant to be more reproducible than the old tuberculin extracts. Unfortunately, the name PPD is now known to be incorrect except for the last word; however this heterogenous mixture is still used to test delayed-type hypersensitivity (DTH) responses in human populations.

An attempt to standardize mycobacterial components was made in 1980 (US–Japan reference system) using culture filtrates of *M. tuberculosis* and goat anti-filtrate antisera. With this reference system 11 major antigens were detected by immunoelectrophoresis; however most of these were shared between *M. tuberculosis* and the non-pathogenic *M. bovis*. Indeed, antigens 1 and 2 were later found to be arabinomannan and arabinogalactan which are common components of cell walls in many bacterial genera. The crossed immunoelectrophoresis (CIE) reference system covers a broad range of antigens, but problems with reproducing results in different laboratories were often encountered. However, some *M. bovis* BCG antigens identified by this reference system have been purified, and some sequence data obtained. The complete sequence of the 18 kD protein, and the partial sequence of the 28 kD and the 23 kD proteins were published in 1986[3]. The two main types of mycobacterial antigens are carbohydrate and protein in nature.

Carbohydrate antigens

There has been a great deal of research on various aspects of mycobacterial polysaccharides, glycolipids and glycopeptidolipids. The capsule (which is responsible for acid-fast staining) and cell walls are very complex structures, and much interest has been shown in their components because of the adjuvant activity associated with mycobacterial cell walls. It has been known for many years that mycobacterial cells are very potent enhancers of the immune system[4]. In the 1950s Freund developed the adjuvant which bears his name (complete Freund's adjuvant; CFA), composed of killed tubercle bacilli in mineral oil, in an oil and water emulsion. The carbohydrate antigens were classified by Brennan[5] into three groups: glycopeptidolipids, lipo-oligosaccharides and phenolic glycolipids. The glycopeptidolipids are primarily important surface antigens in the *M. avium*, *M. intracellulare* and *M. scrofulaceum* (MAIS) group of organisms.

A great deal of interest has been shown in the third group of carbohydrate antigens, the phenolic glycolipids. These antigens comprise a phenol–thioglycerol core with one to four saccharide units forming the species determinant. The antigenic determinant of the phenolic glycolipid of *M. leprae* has been identified as the terminal sugar residue 3,6-dio-methyl glucose[6]: this is a key determinant involved in antibody recognition and suppression in leprosy patients[7].

Lipoarabinomannan (LAM) has recently been recognized as a major antigen of *M. leprae* and *M. tuberculosis*, and it is now understood to be the same as antigen 1 in the US–Japan reference system. Many monoclonal antibodies directed against LAM have been raised, and the molecule has some promise as a diagnostic reagent in sputum-negative tuberculosis patients[8].

Proteins

The problems associated with purifying individual proteins from mycobacterial extracts are legion[9]. Biochemical separations have been attempted using many methods but the effort involved in these experiments is tremendous. Goren[4] quotes the example of a final yield of 0.4 mg of tuberculin active 'peptide A' recovered from 752 g of defatted dry *M. tuberculosis* cells! Purification of this 12 kD protein subsequently gave an improved yield of 1.5 g from 676 g cells, but this product was still no more active than PPD in skin tests.

During the last decade dramatic developments in molecular biology and hybridoma technology have increased our understanding of the mycobacterial protein antigens. Sera from infected patients or immune individuals have been used in immunoprecipitation and immunoblotting experiments, to investigate which antigens are important in the humoral response to mycobacteria. However the advent of monoclonal antibody technology has permitted a more thorough analysis of immunogenic mycobacterial components. Several laboratories have successfully produced monoclonal antibodies using spleen cells from mice immunized with soluble preparations of *M. leprae* and/or *M. tuberculosis*. In 1984 and 1985, WHO held workshops to exchange information concerning the monoclonal antibodies produced in eight different laboratories[10,11]. The antigen specificities and cross-reactivities of 55 monoclonal antibodies were examined. Surprisingly, although the complicated mixture of proteins contained in the preparations used to immunize the mice varied, the monoclonal antibodies generated in different laboratories often had overlapping specificities. For example, antibodies which recognized the 65 kD protein were found in every laboratory, and four separate groups reported antibodies directed towards the 19 kD protein of *M. tuberculosis*. These findings suggested that these proteins may be immunodominant, at least for the mouse B cell repertoire. Monoclonal antibodies have also been used in the purification of small quantities of mycobacterial proteins by affinity chromatography[12,13].

Recombinant DNA technology has also advanced our understanding of the immune recognition of mycobacterial antigens. The mycobacterial proteins recognized by monoclonal antibodies have been expressed from the *M. leprae* and the *M. tuberculosis* genomic libraries, using the λgt11 system[14,15]. The DNA clones expressing the 65 kD protein, or parts of it, were found at a high frequency, and the promoter for this protein has been shown to function in *E. coli*[16]. The sequence of the 65 kD proteins has been determined for *M. bovis* BCG, *M. leprae* and *M. tuberculosis*[17,18].

A great deal of interest has been shown in the 65 kD antigen. This was thought to be a common bacterial antigen, since monoclonal antibodies directed against it recognize epitopes on many other bacterial proteins from such diverse genera as *Nocardia* and *Actinomyces*[12]. Eventually, the 65 kD protein was shown by antibody cross-reactivity, and later by sequence analysis, to be a homologue of the *E. coli* GroEL gene product[19]. GroEL is a stress protein, the expression of which is constitutive under normal conditions but greatly up-regulated by heat shock, oxidative radicals and heavy metals. It is a highly conserved protein: every bacterial species examined contains a GroEL homologue (see ref. 20 for review). Like GroEL, the 65 kD mycobacterial protein of the rapidly growing species *M. smegmatis* is also inducible by heat[17]. GroEL is required for the assembly of bacteriophage particles in *E. coli*[21] and appears to be transiently associated with newly synthesized unfolded polypeptides[22], suggesting that the mycobacterial 65 kD protein may also be involved in protein folding or oligomeric assembly. More evidence for the function of this family of proteins was provided by Hemmingsen et al.[23], who reported that Rubisco binding protein shared 50% sequence identity with *E. coli* GroEL. GroEL and Rubisco binding protein have been termed 'molecular chaperones': they take no part in the final oligomeric structure, but are necessary for its assembly. The mycobacterial 65 kD protein fits into the same pattern of quaternary structure in that the recombinant protein is a dimer, and the native protein, purified from zinc-deficient cultures of *M. bovis* BCG[24] is a tetramer (Rees et al., unpublished observations). Several groups are currently working on various aspects of the structure of GroEL and its role in responses to stress and infection.

Recently obtained sequence data have revealed that the 12 kD protein of *M. tuberculosis* is homologous to *E. coli* GroES, the gene for which is on the same operon as GroEL[25]. GroEL and GroES are known to interact with each other and with ATP in the assembly of bateriophage particles, and they are co-transcribed.

Further evidence for a link between stress proteins and antigenicity was provided by the mycobacterial 70 kD protein, which is homologous to DnaK, the *E. coli* member of the hsp70 family[19,26]. Several monoclonal antibodies to this protein have been produced[10,11] (Rees et al., unpublished work), and it is induced by heat shock in *M. bovis* BCG[27]. The protein was shown to be a major extracellular component of short-term *M. tuberculosis* cultures[28]. It has been proposed that antigens which accumulate in the culture supernatant could be particularly accessible for immune recognition, and could therefore play a role in protective immunity to intracellular mycobacteria. Interestingly, the 64 kD protein of *M. bovis* BCG was shown to accumulate in zinc-deficient cultures[24]. However it is not possible to assess how similar the pattern of protein secretion into synthetic laboratory media is to the proteins produced by mycobacteria growing in a phagocytic cell.

Members of the hsp70 group of stress proteins are known to play a role in the translocation of proteins through membranes in eukaryotic cells[29,30]. The ubiquity of these proteins suggests that they are essential for normal growth. Fibroblasts injected with monoclonal anti-hsp70 are unable to withstand heating to 43°C, a temperature normally tolerated by the same cells, suggesting that they may have an essential role during stress[31]. The mammalian group of hsp70 proteins is well characterized[20]. It comprises several very similar proteins which are expressed constitutively (the hsc group) and others which are induced by stress conditions such as increased temperature, viral infection, the presence of active oxygen intermediates, heavy metals or alcohol (the hsp group). The molecular weights of these proteins are in the 71–73 kD range, and they all have a high affinity for nucleotides, especially ATP: the mammalian homologue was originally described as a clathrin-uncoating ATPase[32]. They are easily cleaved into stable fragments, with loss of the amino terminal. The N-terminal fragment, which is protease sensitive, contains the clathrin binding site while the core 44 kD protein contains the ATP binding site. The structure of this molecule is being investigated, and crystals of this protein have recently been grown[33].

Many proteins which are important in the immune response to a variety of bacterial and parasitic infections are members of stress protein families (reviewed in ref. 34). Mycobacteria are so far the only organisms shown to contain immunogenic proteins from three different groups, (hsp70, GroEL, and the low molecular weight heat shock proteins). However, other homologues of GroEL which are important in the immune response include the homologue of *Coxiella burnettii*, the causative agent of Q fever, *Treponema pallidum* which causes syphilis, and *Borrelia burgdorferi*, which causes Lyme disease. Among the helminthic parasites *Brugia malayi*, the organisms which causes filariasis, and two species of schistosomes have been shown to induce antibodies to their hsp70 homologues. The hsp70 homologues of the protozoa *Plasmodium*, *Trypanosoma* and *Leishmania* all feature in the immune response to those organisms. It seems, therefore, that immunodominant antigens in many infectious or parasitic organisms belong to the stress protein families. The high degree of homology between molecules derived from many sources, taken together with their immunodominance, is consistent with an important role for these antigens in immune responsiveness.

The protein antigens of mycobacteria differ in their subcellular location depending upon their function in the organism (reviewed in ref. 35). Thus the heat shock proteins which act as molecular chaperones are cytoplasmic. Lipoproteins form another class of protein that has recently become of interest[36]. These are associated with the cell wall of mycobacteria and have biochemical and sequence characteristics suggesting involvement in the transport of nutrients through the mycobacterial cell wall. They possess a potential signal peptide preceding the N-terminus of the mature protein, which would permit post-translational modification and secretion of the protein. Two lipoproteins have so far been identified in mycobacteria, the 19 and 38 kD antigens. The latter has a high degree of sequence homology with the Phos protein of *E. coli*[37] which transports nutrients across the cell wall into the micro-organism. As the lipoproteins are secreted early in the growth of mycobacteria they may be accessible for immune recognition at an earlier stage than other antigens which are released by the breakdown of the organism.

ANALYSIS OF T CELL ANTIGEN RECOGNITION

The application of different strains of mycobacteria

Prior to the generation of monoclonal antibodies[10,11] and the cloning of the major protein antigens in the λgt11 expression system[14,15], the specificity of T cell responses to mycobacteria was primarily investigated using distant or related strains of mycobacteria to induce proliferation or DTH. T cells that discriminated between *M. tuberculosis* and *M. leprae* were readily observed. T cells with unique specificity for *M. tuberculosis* as opposed to *M. bovis* have, however, proved more difficult to identify[38,39]. It appears from animal models that, with the exception of *M. leprae*, protection is only elicited by immunization with viable organisms[2]. Comparison of the antigen specificity of the T cell repertoire induced by viable and nonviable mycobacteria would therefore require the use of intact organisms rather than subcellular components. Although, this approach allows the relative proportions of the T cell repertoire that are species-specific and cross-reactive to be examined, its limitation is that it provides no information on the actual determinant being recognized.

Nitrocellulose immunoblasts

The identification of the components of mycobacteria that are potentially antigenic for T cells presents a major problem because these cells only recognize antigen complexed with MHC proteins on the surface of antigen-presenting cells[40,41]. Generally, the primary means of identifying these determinants has been to add biochemically purified antigens to cell cultures. The limitation of this approach is the difficulty encountered in purifying each of the mycobacterial proteins. In addition, the antigens selected for screening of T cell responses were those identified by murine monoclonal antibodies. This may bias the analysis, since the specificity of T and B cell repertoires need not necessarily overlap[42]. A procedure for probing the T cell repertoire with unfractionated antigens would avoid this problem. This was achieved by modifying the Western blotting technique[43] established for antibody/antigen analysis for application in T cell proliferation cultures[38]. Complex antigenic mixtures fractionated by polyacrylamide gel electrophoresis and transferred to nitrocellulose, when added as individual segments or an emulsion, could induce T cell proliferation in the presence of accessory cells. In this way, it was possible to determine the specificity of the overall T cell responses to mycobacteria without extensive purification or serological preselection[38].

Using this method, the antigenic specificity of polyclonal T cells from the ascitic effusion of a patient with reactive tuberculosis was analysed. Both *M. tuberculosis* and *M. leprae* fractionated and immunoblotted on nitrocellulose were used, in order to identify antigenic components potentially unique to one of these two closely related species of mycobacteria[38]. Both qualitative and quantitative differences in the profiles or reactivity to the two antigenic preparations were observed. These may, however, be due in part to technical factors such as modification of the antigen content of the organisms by variable growth conditions or unequal transfer of proteins. Some fractions of the immunoblots failed to activate T cells, generating a trough in the profile of the proliferative responses. These fractions may contain either non-specific inhibitory elements or specific suppressor determinants. One such trough occurred at fractions co-migrating with a molecular weight of approximately 35 kD: these failed to induce proliferation in all individuals tested. The high frequency with which this occurred in an outbred population suggested that the inhibition or suppression was not under immune response gene control[44]. Furthermore, this effect was antigen non-specific, as the addition of these fractions to the antigen-dependent response of cloned influenza virus-reactive T cells inhibited proliferation[38].

It has been proposed that the presence of suppresor determinants in *M. leprae* may account for the specific anergy found in lepromatous leprosy[45]. If this is the case it is possible that physical separation of potential suppressor and helper determinants on immunoblots would uncover CD4$^+$ T cell responses. This does seem to occur in some, but not all, leprosy patients[38]. Another potential application of this method is the possibility of identifying 'protective' or 'pathogenic' determinants by comparing the immunoblot profiles in different populations, e.g. vaccinated, healthy contacts and individuals with disease. When this was undertaken in seven patients with leprosy and 22 family contacts, using either immunoblotted *M. tuberculosis* or *M. leprae* as a stimulus, response profiles were very similar in each group. Three main peaks were found, with molecular weights corresponding to 12–22, 35–40 and 65 kD[46]. In some instances, however, species-specific responses were evident. These results suggested that MHC haplotype, and not exposure to the infectious agent, had the greatest effect on immune responses. Other investigators[47] have also found that responses in healthy leprosy contacts are associated with protons with similar molecular weights.

Immunoblots have also been successful in identifying the determinants recognized by T cell clones initially induced with an antigenic mixture. Although the antigenic specificities of the majority of the T cell clones examined corresponded to components that could be serologically defined, one T cell clone was found to recognize a 52–55 kD determinant that appeared not to contain a dominant B cell epitope[38]. The preselection of antigens for serological study may, therefore, exclude some T cell epitopes. In this study not all the T cell clones responded to solid phase antigens. The reason for this is unknown but it could be due to a number of factors, including differential processing of solid-phase antigens, the nature of the responding subset, or receptor affinity.

In conclusion this approach has been a very useful tool for providing much new information on T cell specificity in mycobacterial responses. We have indicated some of the possible uses but there is no doubt that it has many other applications.

Affinity purified and recombinant DNA antigens

The isolation and purification of components of mycobacteria using monoclonal antibodies has provided a number of antigens[35,48] that have been tested for their ability to stimulate T cell responses. All of these antigens (70, 65, 38, 23, 19, 18, 14 and 12 kD) stimulate polyclonal T cell responses in both leprosy and tuberculosis patients, as well as in control subjects[13,49–54]. Some are also recognized by T cell clones isolated from healthy BCG-vaccinated subjects as well as from tuberculosis patients[50,55–61]. While responses to most antigens have been demonstrated some, such as the 65 kD antigen appear to be more immunodominant for CD4$^+$ T cells[62]. Interestingly, another of the M. leprae antigens, with a molecular weight of 36 kD stimulates both CD4$^+$ and CD8$^+$ T cells[57,63]. CD8$^+$ T cell clones[64] and CD4$^+$ T cell lines[19,20] specific to the 70 kD antigen have also been described. There are not, however, enough of these reports to enable any conclusion to be reached as to the relative importance of antigens in stimulating the different T cell subsets.

Although population studies suggest the existence of an association between HLA-DR3 and HLA-DQw1 and leprosy[65] the nature of the antigens which stimulate cells isolated from leprosy patients with different MHC haplotypes is not well understood. Some studies with T cell clones have suggested some interesting associations, however. Preliminary studies on the restriction specificities of CD4$^+$ T cell clones from a patient with the HLA-DR2,3 haplotype suggested that the M. leprae-specific determinants were more often recognized in association with HLA-DR3 than with HLA-DR2[66]. In these experiments the individual antigens recognized by the T cell clones were not defined. Similarly, while population studies of serum antibodies reactive with the 38 kD protein of M. tuberculosis suggest that the HLA-DR2 allele may be linked with increased susceptibility to tuberculosis[67], there is as yet no evidence of an association at the level of T cell recognition. To date the clearest evidence for linkage between the response to particular antigens and MHC haplotype comes from studies of the HLA class 1 restricted responses to influenza virus proteins. It was found, for example, that the nucleoprotein is preferentially recognized in the context of HLA-B37 whereas the response to the matrix protein is associated with HLA-A2[68]. It is obviously of some importance that similar studies are performed for the responses to mycobacterial antigens.

The use of affinity purified antigens in the analysis of the cellular immune response has been hindered by the practical limitations of in vitro culture of mycobacteria, particularly *M. leprae*. The molecular cloning of genomic fragments of DNA for the major proteins of both *M. leprae* and *M. tuberculosis* using the λgt11 expression system[14,15] has, however, considerably improved the situation.

A large number of laboratories have now successfully used recombinant DNA antigens, expressed as free antigen or β-galactosidase fusion proteins, in the investigation of the specificity of anti-mycobacterial T cell responses at both the clonal and the polyclonal level. This followed the initial report that cloned human T cells induced with *M. leprae* proliferated specifically in response to *E. coli* lysates containing the 18 kD protein[69]. The use of recombinant sub-libraries and truncated genes has also been of great value in the mapping of T cell epitopes with a protein[70].

T cell recognition of synthetic peptides derived from mycobacterial antigens

It is well documented that the T cells recognize short linear sequences of amino acids. Consequently, in those diseases where T cells are implicated in pathology or protection, interest has been generated in the potential of synthetic peptides as components of subunit vaccines and as tools for diagnosis.

As a major part of the CD4[+] T cell response in both man[56,60,71,72] and mouse[62] appears to be directed against the 65 kD (mycobacterial GroEL) and 19 kD proteins, these two molecules have been the primary targets of investigation. Additional interest in the mycobacterial GroEL has arisen from the observation that cloned T cells capable of inducing adjuvant arthritis in the rat are reactive with mycobacterial GroEL[73]. T cells from the synovial infiltrate of chronic arthritis patients also respond to this antigen[26,74-76]. In addition, human T cell clones specific for the 65 kD antigen have also been generated from the synovial fluid of patients with arthritis[77-79]. The specificity of both polyclonal and clonal human T cells isolated from an ascitic effusion was analysed using peptides selected for synthesis because they contained a distinctive amino acid pattern (motif) consisting of a glycine or charged residue followed by two or three hydrophobic residues and terminating with a polar amino acid[80]. Although a total of 31 potential T cell epitopes bearing this motif were identified in the mycobacterial GroEL only six, which were similar to sequences known to stimulate T cells, were actually synthesized. From these, two epitopes were identified mapping to residues 65–85 and 390–412, the location of which was confirmed with the DNA sub-library[70]. These peptides were also used to investigate the species specificity of responding T cells at both the clonal and polyclonal level[26]. T cells reactive with residues 65–85 to 116–137 failed to recognize the corresponding sequence in either *E. coli* or human GroEL, whereas the response to residues 153–171 was cross-reactive with *E. coli* GroEL. In contrast, residues 195–219 and 390–412 of mycobacterial *E. coli* and human GroEL were cross-reactive at the T cell level and must, therefore, contain sufficient sequence identity to allow binding to both MHC Class II proteins and the T cell receptor. This was confirmed by demonstrating that cloned human T cells reactive with mycobacterial GroEL (residues 195–208) were stimulated by a synthetic peptide corresponding to the human sequence[81]. The presence of non-cross-reactive T cell epitopes, even at sites of inflammation, has also been demonstrated for synovial fluid-derived 65 kD-specific human T cell clones[77].

The allele-specific motif[80] was also used to predict DR1-restricted epitopes in the 19 kD protein. A peptide based on one such motif in the N-terminus of the protein was synthesized[59]. Peripheral blood lymphocytes from tuberculosis patients and BCG-vaccinated subjects expressing either the HLA-DR1 or -DR4 class 2 haplotype proliferated in response to this peptide[59]. Recognition of the peptide in association with DR1 and DR4 was confirmed using T cell clones and transfected murine fibroblasts expressing appropriate MHC Class II molecules.

A similar, but not identical, epitope was also identified by the use of overlapping sets of peptides spanning the sequence of this antigen[54]. This study also identified 16 other epitopes, only a proportion of which bore either the Rothbard–Taylor motif, or the amphipathic algorithm[82]. More recently, the ability to elute peptides from Class II antigens has enabled motifs evident in naturally processed peptides to be defined[83]. Many epitopes bearing the DR1 motif can be identified by spanning the 19 kD sequence[83]. Not all are recognized, so other factors probably play a role in selecting epitopes. The capacity to bind to human Class II molecules is unlikely to be the limiting factor as peptide binding appears to be highly degenerate[84]. Polyclonal responses to the 19 kD antigen[84] show that the N-terminal is strongly and dominantly recognized by the majority of donors, irrespective of HLA type. This kind of degenerate recognition has also been observed in the T cell responses to other extrinsic antigens[85,86] and is consistent with the presence of multiple epitopes, each recognized in the context of related families of HLA molecules, within a T cell epitope 'hot spot' in a protein. Other areas may be recognized in a more restricted fashion[54,87]. Why some areas of a protein are the focus for T cell recognition in this way is as yet unclear. Various mechanisms could introduce such a bias. Susceptibility to key proteases, such as cathepsins[88,89] could for example, focus immune recognition on certain regions of proteins. It has proved difficult to predict the precise cleavage sites for the thiol proteases, and analysis of the 19 kD N-terminal sequence does not reveal any clear correlation with the motifs available[90]. Nevertheless, whatever the mechanism, the degeneracy of the restriction observed in these and other responses suggests that peptide vaccines may not be as limited as was initially thought.

T cell recognition of mycobacterial carbohydrates

Although there have been occasional reports of T cell recognition of mycobacterial carbohydrates[7,91], it is not at all clear that this was solely due to the carbohydrate moiety and that contaminating peptides were not involved[56]. Furthermore, pure carbohydrates do not appear to interact with MHC in a detectable manner[92]. Nevertheless, glycopeptides can interact with MHC at concentrations which, although higher than those of the unmodified peptide, are still stimulatory. Under these circumstances T cell responses were specific to the glycopeptide suggesting the carbohydrate moiety was playing a role in recognition[92].

Carbohydrate components of mycobacteria are also able to modulate T cell responses through mechanisms independent of the T cell receptor. For example, Kaplan and colleagues[93] demonstrated that lipoarabinomannan (LAM) can induce CD8$^+$ T cells capable of suppressing the T cell responses of lepromatous and tuberculoid leprosy patients to PPD. Lipopolysaccharides such as LAM are also capable of inhibiting antigen dependent T cell proliferation in vitro at the level of the antigen-presenting cell[94].

T$\gamma\delta$ and mycobacterial antigens

A small proportion of T cells recognize antigen using a receptor composed of $\gamma\delta$ rather than $\alpha\beta$ chains[95]. These T cells are found in all tissues, generally within epithelial spaces, and also in the thymus, where they may be a distinct subpopulation[96]. They have also been found in the skin lesions of leprosy patients, where they are at their most numerous during reversion[97]. T$\gamma\delta$ cells generated from leprosy and other patients (reviewed in ref. 98) have shown specificity for mycobacterial antigens. In at least two of these studies the stimulating antigen was the 65 kD heat shock protein, which has led to the hypothesis that, rather than representing a specialized anti-mycobacterial mechaism, T$\gamma\delta$ cells respond to self-hsp molecules displayed on damaged or infected cells at sites of local invasion[99].

Increases in T$\gamma\delta$ recognition have been observed following heat stress[100]. However, as stress also enhances autoreactive T cell recognition through increased expression of MHC Class II antigens[101] this may be due to a similar effect on the non-classical MHC molecule, and not to altered levels of the peptide ligand. Whatever, the mechanism T$\gamma\delta$ cells appear to accumulate at inflammatory sites and may be implicated in pathogenesis[102]. Consistent with this, reactivity to mycobacteria appears to be largely restricted to certain T$\gamma\delta$ cell receptors[103,104]. On the other hand other mycobacterial components apart from hsp, which are not yet fully defined[105], are also involved. In this context it is of interest that T$\gamma\delta$ are restricted by non-polymorphic MHC molecules such as CD1, which are known to be expressed only on certain cells, such as dendritic Langerhans cells in man (reviewed in refs. 106, 107). Human CD4$^-$ CD8$^-$ TCR$^+$ T$^-$ cells specific for M. tuberculosis have also been shown to be restricted by CD1b and to have similar processing requirements to the MHC Class II-restricted pathway[108]. Recent evidence showing that only a few of the T$\gamma\delta$ cells stimulated in culture are specific for the hsp65[109], taken together with reports showing that these cells can respond to other antigens such as tetanus toxoid[110], suggests that their function is not exclusively related to stress proteins. Although the actual antigen has not yet been identified, $CD4^- CD8^- \alpha\beta TCR^+ T^-$ cells are also not specific to heat shock protein peptides. The possibility that superantigens may be involved in the recognition of $T\gamma\delta$ cells has not been excluded, although the finding that at least one $T\gamma\delta$ cell clone can be stimulated by a synthetic peptide corresponding to a part of the hsp65 sequence[111] would seem to make this less likely. $T\gamma\delta$ cell receptors in tissues do, however, have limited heterogeneity, which might support the notion of a role for superantigens and would be in keeping with their putative role as a primitive defence mechanism.

IMMUNE MECHANISMS

Mycobacteria and autoimmunity

The observation that T cells induced by mycobacterial GroEL can also recognize self stress peptides is consistent with the hypothesis that auto-immunity results from inappropriate activation of these cells[112]. In contrast, those T cells with specificity for the variable epitopes in mycobacterial GroEL may be able to induce potentially protective immune responses[113]. Several factors may influence the development of autoimmunity. First, as T cells recognize peptide fragments of antigen complexed with MHC molecules[114] the binding avidity of peptide with a sequence specific to self or shared with extrinsic antigens[115] will be influential. Second, while studies in the mouse suggest that low responsiveness to *M. leprae* may result from tolerance to self MHC proteins that are cross-reactive with *M. leprae*[116] a failure to develop tolerance to self hsp may lead to a T cell repertoire able to recognize the self peptide–MHC complex. Studies with synthetic peptides based on human hsp65 have suggested that such T cells may be very common[53]. This has led to the suggestion[117] that a complex immunoregulatory network exists that 'normally' regulates the activity of these cells. Other more quantitative assessments, however, failed to show the expected frequency differences between the blood and synovial fluid[118]. Third, some infectious agents may break tolerance in potentially autoreactive $CD4^+$ T cells by activation of alternative pathways[119]. Lastly, activation of these T cells will also depend on the presence of the self peptide ligand, which may only occur in disease sites under certain circumstances.

The conditions leading to the expression of self hsp peptide ligands are likely to occur when cells are exposed to stress such as viral infection, oxygen radical production and inflammation (heat)[120]. All of these conditions result in the enhanced synthesis of one or other member of the hsp family[20]. It is worth bearing in mind, however, that the biochemical stress response is heterogeneous, and varies both with the stress, and the cell lineage involved[121]. Thus the 65 kD protein is strongly produced following virus infection of murine macrophages[122] but not in human B cell lines subjected to heat or oxygen radical stress[101]. Interestingly, stressed murine macrophages were recognized by Class I-restricted CD8[+] T cells, suggesting that the self hsp peptide ligand can interact with the endogenous processing pathway[122]. There is also evidence for 65 kD-specific CD4[+] T cell-specific recognition of heat-stressed antigen-presenting cells[79]. These cells can also be cytotoxic suggesting a mechanism for autopathogenesis[63]. Stress does not, however, always enhance recognition[101] and some stressed antigen-presenting cells are tolerogenic[124]. The factors predisposing to the development of autoimmunity are, therefore, highly complex and a cause and effect relationship is difficult to establish.

Cytotoxic mechanisms

It was first demonstrated by George Mackaness in the 1960s that resistance to intracellular pathogens is mediated by T cells and expressed in activated macrophages[1,2]. Since then the paradigm that CD4[+] T cells, either directly or through the release of lymphokines, were the main effector subset has prevailed[125]. In this scheme the role of CD8[+] T cells is viewed as primarily regulatory, controlling CD4[+] T cell mechanisms that otherwise result in irreparable fibrotic tissue damage. Support for this view comes from histological studies of the location of these cells within the architecture of the tuberculoid leprosy granulomas. CD4[+] T cells are to be found in the centre in close contact with the phagocytic cells whilst CD8[+] T cells surround them[126]. In lepromatous leprosy, in contrast, these subsets were admixed.

More recent evidence, however, suggests that CD8[+] T cells may also play a more active role in anti-mycobacterial immunity. For example, Naher and colleagues[127] showed that while macrophage activation was MHC Class II restricted and dependent on CD4[+] T cells, granuloma formation in listerial infection was MHC Class I restricted and CD8[+] T cell dependent. Both cell types were required for the full expression of protective immunity. Similar observations have been made for *M. leprae*[128]. The mechanism by which CD8[+] T cells stimulate granuloma formation is unknown, but they may facilitate CD4[+] T cell recruitment, possibly by releasing organisms from sequestered sites[129].

MHC Class I responses are most readily generated by viral infection[123] while soluble exogenous antigens generated by the processing of phagocytosed organisms such as mycobacteria, are generally presented in the context of Class II antigens. A number of scattered reports[64,130] have suggested that exogenous mycobacterial antigens can interact with the Class I-restricted pathway. Recently, it has been shown that while CD4[+] cells are stimulated by both heat-killed and live bacteria[131], only live *Listeria monocytogenes* replicating in the cytosolic compartment can activate CD8[+] T cells, suggesting that in certain intracellular locations mycobacterial antigens could also intersect the Class I-restricted pathway. 'Regurgitated' peptides could also bind to post-Golgi Class I MHC molecules[132]. The first pathway would provide an explanation for Mackaness'[1] original observation that live organisms were required for protective immunity. Endogenous stress proteins could, of course, be processed in both pathways. It has also been shown that phagocytosed bacterial antigens which do not penetrate the cytosol can also be presented in the context of Class I molecules[132]. The antigens of mycobacteria contained within phagosomes could also gain access to Class I molecules via this pathway. There are, therefore, a number of different ways in which mycobacterial antigens could prime CD8[+] T cells. The paucity of evidence for the production of these cells following mycobacterial infection is probably a consequence of the difficulty encountered in reproducing the appropriate priming conditions in vivo and in vitro. It was, therefore, both interesting and important for future vaccine prospects that the BCG recombinant vaccine[133] induced both subsets.

Cytokines

The most informative tool for the dissection of mechanisms for antimycobacterial immunity is likely to be the genetically engineered mouse. Recently, two groups have described mice lacking either expression of the interferon-γ gene[134], or its receptor[135]. Interferon-γ is a pleiotrophic cytokine long implicated in antimicrobial immunity[136]. It induces macrophages to produce nitric oxide[137] and reactive oxygen intermediates that enhance intracellular killing of mycobacteria[138]. While other cytokines can also increase the production of reactive oxygen intermediates[139], studies in interferon-γ-deficient mice[134] indicate that nitric oxide production is uniquely enhanced by this cytokine. Thus while the respiratory burst is still present, albeit diminished, nitric oxide production is absent. As a consequence these mice are also highly susceptible to normally sublethal infection with *M. bovis*. Expression of MHC Class II antigens is also reduced, thus compromising CD4[+] T cell activation. These experiments definitively illustrate the central role of interferon-γ and suggest that this cytokine is an obvious target for therapeutic intervention.

Tumour necrosis factor alpha (TNFα) has also been shown to play a role in anti-mycobacterial immunity[140]. Antibodies to this cytokine inhibit granuloma formation: as this response is essential to the containment of the organisms, this results in a marked increase in the numbers of mycobacteria in the tissues. TNFα has toxic effects, however, which may limit its therapeutic potential. The use of modified cytokines or specific inhibitors in the future may lessen these effects[141]. TNFα is also involved in the formation of granuloma in response to schistosome eggs[142]. In this murine model, cytokines secreted by the T_{H2} subset of lymphocytes were important in recruiting cells to the granuloma. T_{H2} cytokines also played a role, although this may have been indirectly due to their recruitment by T_{H1} cytokines. Differential recognition of mycobacterial antigens by CD4[+] T cell subsets has been demonstrated[143] and could be important, particularly in a disease such as leprosy where a polar spectrum of disease exists.

CONCLUSIONS

An overall scheme of antimycobacterial immunity is complicated by the multiplicity and the complexity of mechanisms involved. In terms of the main effector mechanisms it is clear that the view revolving around macrophage activation by T cells or their products was too simple and we now have to consider the active role of CD8$^+$ T cells as well as the regulatory interactions between CD8$^+$ and CD4$^+$ cells. In addition to this kind of T–T cell interaction the different types of phagocytic cells and the nature of the lesion in which the immune response is occurring must be of some importance to the nature and type of response. We need to know considerably more about the cellular milieux in these lesions and studies of this kind are being carried out[144]. The influence of the local environment is likely to be considerable and to affect the response at many different levels: factors involved include the types of antigen presenting cells present, whether they are MHC Class I and II positive, if they can phagocytose mycobacteria and present mycobacterial antigens correctly and deliver an appropriate second signal required for activation or alternatively, whether they are tolerogenic. Our ideas on T cells have also changed as it becomes clear that, at least for T cell clones, functional divisions such as cytotoxicity and macrophage activating factor production are not absolute but may rather depend upon the way in which the cells are activated. The immune response, then, is likely to be complex and regulated by interactions that we do not understand very well as yet. An understanding of these elements would help us to address important problems, such as why AIDS patients develop mycobacteriosis, why some heavily exposed individuals are protected while others are susceptible to infection, and the difference between a pathogenic and a protective response.

References

1. Mackaness GB. Cellular resistance to infection. J Exp Med. 1962; 116: 381.
2. Mackaness GB. The influence of immunologically committed lymphoid cells on macrophage activity in vitro. J Exp Med. 1969; 129: 973.
3. Harboe M, Nagai S, Patarro ME, Torres ML, Ramirez C, Cruz N. Properties of proteins MPB64, MPB70 and MP80 of *M. bovis* BCG. Infect Immun. 1986; 52: 293–302.
4. Goren MB. Immunoreactive substances of mycobacteria. Am Rev Resp Dis. 1982; 125: 50.
5. Brennan PT. Mycobacterial glycolipids. In: Lieve L, Schlessinger D, eds. Microbiology. Washington, ASM Press; 1984: 366–375.
6. Fujiwara T, Hunter SW, Chos N, Aspinall GO, Brennan PJ. Chemical synthesis and serology of disaccharides and trisaccharides of phenolic glycolipid antigens from the leprosy bacillus and preparation of a disaccharide protein conjugate for serodiagnosis of leprosy. Infect Immun. 1984; 43: 245.
7. Mehra V, Brennan PJ, Rada E, Convit J, Bloom BR. Lymphocyte suppression in leprosy induced by a unique M. leprae glycolipid. Nature. 1984; 308: 194.
8. Bothamley G, Udani P, Rudd R, Festenstein F, Ivanyi J. Humoral response to defined epitopes of tubercle bacilli in adult pulmonary and child tuberculosis. Eur J Clin Infect Dis. 1988; 7: 639–645.
9. Daniel TM, Janicki BW. Mycobacterial antigens: D. a review of their isolation chemistry and immunological properties. Microbiol Rev. 1978; 42: 84.
10. Engers HD. Results of WHO sponsored workshop on monoclonal antibodies to *M. leprae*.

Infect Immun. 1985; 48: 603–605.

11. Engers HD. Results of a WHO sponsored workshop to characterize antigens recognized by mycobacteria specific monoclonal antibodies. Infect Immun. 1986; 51: 718.

12. Young DB, Ivanyi J, Cox JH, Lamb JR. The 65 kDa antigen of mycobacteria – a common bacterial protein? Immunol Today. 1987; 8: 1215–1219.

13. Britton WJ, Hellqvist L, Basten A, Inglis AS. Immunoreactivity of a 70 kD protein purified from *Mycobacterium bovis* Bacillus Calmette-Guerin by monoclonal antibody affinity chromatography. J Exp Med. 1986; 164: 695.

14. Young RA, Mehra V, Sweetses D, Buchanen T, Clarke-Davis J, Davis RW, Bloom BR. Genes for the major protein antigens of the leprosy parasite. Nature. 1985; 316: 450.

15. Young RA, Bloom BR, Grosskinsky CM, Ivanyi J, Thomas D, Davis RW. Dissection of *Mycobacterium tuberculosis* antigens using recombinant DNA. Proc Natl Acad Sci USA. 1985; 82: 2583.

16. Shinnick T. The 65 kDa antigen of *M. tuberculosis*. J. Bacteriol. 1987; 169: 188.

17. Shinnick TM, Vodkin MH, Williams JL. The *M. tuberculosis* 65 kDa antigen in a heat shock protein which corresponds to common antigen and to the E. coli GroEL protein. Infect Immun. 1988; 56: 446–451.

18. Mehra V, Sweetser D, Young RA. Efficient mapping protein antigenic determinants. Proc Natl Acad Sci USA. 1986; 83: 7013.

19. Young DB, Lathigra R, Hendrix R, Sweetser D, Young RA. Stress proteins are immune targets in leprosy and tuberculosis. Proc Natl Acad Sci USA. 1988; 85: 4267–4270.

20. Lindquist S. The heat shock response. Annu Rev Biochem. 1986; 55: 1151.

21. Hendrix R. Purification and properties of GroE a host protein involved in bacteriophage assembly. J Mol Biol. 1979; 129: 375–392.

22. Bochkareva ES, Lissin NM, Girshovich AS. Transient association of newly synthesized unfolded protein with the heat-shock GroEL protein. Nature. 1988; 332: 254.

23. Hemmingsen S, Woolford C, Van der Vies SM, Tilly K, Dennis DT, Georgopolilos CP, Hendrix RW, Ellis RJ. Homologous plant and bacterial proteins chaperon oligomeric protein assembly. Nature. 1988; 333: 330.

24. de Bruyn J, Bosmans R, Turner M, Weckx M, Nyabenda J, Van Voorlen J-P, Falmagne P, Wiker HG, Harboe M. Purification and partial characterization of a skin-reactive protein antigen from *M. bovis* BCG. Infect Immun. 1987; 55: 245–252.

25. Baird PN, Hall LMC, Coates ARM. A major antigen from *M. tuberculosis* which is homologous to the heat shock protein GroES from *E. coli* and the LtpA gene product of Coxiella burnetti. Nucleic Acids Res. 1988; 16: 9047.

26. Young DB, Mehlert A, Bal V, Mendez-Samperio P, Ivanyi J, Lamb JR. Stress proteins and the immune response to mycobacteria antigens as virulence factors. J Microbiol. 1988; 54: 431.

27. Mehlert A, Young D. Biochemical and antigenic characterization of the *M. tuberculosis* 71 kDa antigen a member of the 70 kDa hsp family. Mol Microbiol. 1989; 3: 125.

28. Abou-Zeid C, Smith I, Grange JM, Ratcliffe TL, Steele J, Rook GAW. The secreted antigens of *M. tuberculosis* and the relationship to those recognized by the available antibodies. J Gen Microbiol. 1988; 134: 531.

29. DeShaies RJ, Rock BD, Werner-Washburn M, Craig EA, Schekman R. A subfamily of stress proteins facilitates translocation of secretory and mitochondrial precursor polypeptides. Nature. 1988; 332: 800.

30. Chirico WJ, Waters MG, Blobel G. 70 kD heat shock related proteins stimulate protein translocation into microsomes. Nature. 1988; 332: 805.

31. Riabowol KT, Mizzen LA, Welch WJ. Heat shock is lethal to fibroblasts microinjected with antibodies against hsp70. Science. 1988; 242: 433.

32. Schlossman DM, Schmid SC, Braell WA, Rothman JE. An enzyme that removes clathrin coats; purification of an uncoating ATPase. J Cell Biol. 1984; 99: 723.

33. DeLuca Flaherty C, Flaherty KM, McIntosh LJ, Bahrami B, McKay DB. Crystals of an ATPase fragment of bovine clathrin uncoating ATPase. J Mol Biol. 1988; 200: 749.

34. Young DB, Mehlert A, Smith DF. Stress proteins and infectious diseases. In: Stress proteins in biology and medicine. Cold Spring Harbour Laboratory press; 1989.

35. Young DB, Garbe TR, Lathigra R, Abou-Zeid C. Protein antigens: structure, function and regulation. In: McFadden J, ed. Biology of the Mycobacteria. Surrey Univ. Seminars;

1991: 1.
36. Young DB, Garbe T. Lipoprotein antigens of *Mycobacterium tuberculosis*. Res Microbiol. 1991; 142: 5.
37. Anderson AB, Hansen EB. Structure and mapping of antigenic domains of protein antigen b, a 38 kDa protein of *M. tuberculosis*. Infect Immun. 1989; 57: 2481.
38. Lamb JR, O'Hehir RE, Young DB. The use of nitrocellulose immunoblots for the analysis of antigen recognition by T lymphocytes. J Immunol Methods. 1988; 110; 1.
39. Mustafa AS, Kralheim G, Degre M, Godal T. *Mycobacterium bovis* BCG-induced human T-cell clones from BCG-vaccinated healthy subjects: Antigen specificity and lymphokine production. Infect Immun. 1986; 53: 491.
40. Shevach EM, Rosenthal AS. Function of macrophages in antigen recognition by guinea pig T lymphocytes. II. Role of the macrophage in the regulation of genetic control of the immune response. J Exp Med. 1973; 138: 123.
41. Zinkernagel RM, Doherty PC. Restriction of in vitro T cell mediated cytotoxicity in lymphocytic choriomeningitis rising within a syngeneic or semi-allogeneic system. Nature. 1974; 248: 701.
42. Hurwitz JL, Heber-Katz E, Hackett C, Gerhard W. Characterisation of the murine TH response to influenza virus haemagglutinin: evidence for three major specificities. J Immunol. 1984; 133: 3371.
43. Towbin H, Gordon J. Immunoblotting and dot immunobinding – current status and outlook. J Immunol Methods. 1984; 72: 313.
44. Adorini L, Harvey MA, Miller A, Secarz EE. Fine specificity of regulatory T cells II. Suppressor and helper T cells are induced by different regions of hen egg lysozyme in a genetically non-responder mouse strain. J Exp Med. 1979; 150: 293.
45. Modlin RL, Kato H, Mehra V. Genetically restricted suppressor T cell clones derived from lepromatous leprosy lesions. Nature. 1986; 322: 459.
46. Mendez-Samperio P, Lamb J, Bothamley G, Stanley P, Ellis C, Ivanyi J. Molecular study of the T cell repertoire in family contacts and patients with leprosy. J Immunol. 1989; 142: 3599.
47. Converse PJ, Ottenhoff THM, Gebre N, Ehrenberg JP, Kiessing R. Cellular hormonal and yIFN responses to *Mycobacterium leprae* and BCG antigens in healthy individuals exposed to leprosy. Scand J Immunol. 1988; 27: 515.
48. Young DB. Structure of mycobacterial antigens. Br Med Bull. 1988; 44: 562–582.
49. Munk ME, Schoel B, Kaufmann SHE. T cell responses of normal individuals towards recombinant protein antigens of *Mycobacterium tuberculosis*. Eur J Immunol. 1988; 17: 351.
50. Oftung F, Mustafa AS, Shinnick TM, Houghten RA, Kvalheim G, Degre M, Lundin KEA, Godal T. Epitopes of the mycobacterium tuberculosis 65-kilodalton protein antigen as recognised by human T cells. J Immunol. 1988; 141: 2749.
51. Young DB, Kent L, Rees A, Lamb J, Ivanyi J. Immunological activity of a 38 kilodalton protein purified from *Mycobacterium tuberculosis*. Infect Immun. 1986; 54: 177.
52. Dockerell HM, Stoker NG, Lee SP, Jackson M, Grant KA, Joye NF, Lucas SB, Hasan R, Hussain R, McAdam KPW. T cell recognition of the18-kilodalton antigen of *Mycobacterium leprae*. Infect Immun. 1989; 57: 1979.
53. Munk ME, Schoel B, Modrow S, Karr RW, Young RA, Kaufmann SHE. T lymphocytes from healthy individuals with specificity to self epitopes shared by the mycobacterial and human 65-kilodalton heat shock protein. J Immunol. 1989; 143: 2844.
54. Faith A, Moreno C, Lathigra R, Roman E, Fernandez M, Brett S, Mitchell DM, Ivanyi J, Rees ADM. Analysis of human T cell epitopes in the 19,000 MW antigen of *Mycobacterium tuberculosis*: influence of HLA-DR. Immunology. 1991; 74: 1.
55. Mathews R, Scoging A, Rees ADM. Mycobacterial antigen specific human T-cell clones secreting macrophage activating factors. Immunology. 1985; 54: 17.
56. Emmrich F, Thole J, van Embden J, Kaufmann SHE. A recombinant 64 kilodalton protein of *Mycobacterium bovis* Bacillus Calmette-Guèrin specifically stimulates human T4 clones reactive to mycobacterial antigens. J Exp Med. 1985; 163: 1024.
57. Ottenhoff TAM, Klatser PR, Ivanyi J, Elfernik DG, de Wit MYL, de Vries RRP. Mycobacterium leprae-specific protein antigens defined by cloned human helper T-cells. Nature. 1986; 319: 66.
58. Rees ADM, Praputpittaya K, Scoging A, Dobson N, Ivanyi J, Young D, Lamb JR. T cell

activation by anti-idiotypic antibody: evidence for the internal image. Immunology. 1987; 60: 389.

59. Lamb JR, Rees ADM, Bal V, Ikeda H, Wilkinson D, de Vries RRP, Rothbard JB. Prediction and identification of an HLA-DR restricted determinant in the 19 kD protein of Mycobacterium tuberculosis. Eur J Immunol. 1988; 18: 973.

60. Van Schooten WCA, Ottenhoff THM, Klatser PR, Thole J, de Vries RRP, Kolk AHJ. T cell epitopes on the 36K and 65K *Mycobacterium leprae* antigens defined by human T cell clones. Eur J Immunol. 1988; 18: 849.

61. Rees ADM, Faith A, Roman E, Ivanyi J, Wiesmuller K-H, Moreno C. The effect of lipoylation on CD4 T-cell recognition of the 19 kDa mycobacterial antigen. Immunology. 1993; 80: 407.

62. Kaufmann SHE, Vath U, Thole JER, van Emden JDA, Emmrich F. Enumeration of T cells reactive with *Mycobacterium tuberculosis* organisms and specific for the recombinant 65 kDa protein. Eur J Immunol. 1987; 17: 351.

63. Ottenhoff TAM, Birhane Kale AB, Van Embden JDA, Thole JER, Kiessling R. The recombinant 65-Kd heat shock protein of *Mycobacterium bovis* bacillus Calmette-Guèrin/*M. tuberculosis* is a target molecule for CD4$^+$ cytotoxic T lymphocytes that lyse human monocytes. J Exp Med. 1988; 168: 1947.

64. Rees ADM, Scoging A, Mehlert A, Young DB, Ivanyi J. Specificity of proliferative response of human CD8 T cell clones to mycobacterial antigens. Eur J Immunol. 1987; 17: 197.

65. Van Eden W, de Vries RRP. Occasional review – HLA and leprosy: a reevaluation. Leprosy Rev. 1984; 55: 89.

66. de Vries RRP, Ottenhoff THM, van Schooten WCA. Human leukocyte antigens (HLA) and mycobacterial disease. Sem Immunopathol. 1988; 10: 305.

67. Bothamley GH, Swanson Beck J, Schreuder G, D'Amaro J, de Vries RRP, Kardjito T, Ivanyi J. Association of *M. tuberculosis* specific antibody levels with HLA. J Infect Dis. 1988; (in press).

68. McMichael AJ, Gotch FM, Rothbard JB. HLA-B37 determines an influenza A virus nucleoprotein epitopes recognised by cytotoxic T lymphocytes. J Exp Med. 1986; 164: 137.

69. Mustafa AS, Gill HK, Nerland A, Britton WJ, Mehra V, Bloom BR, Young RA, Godal T. Human T cell clones recognise a major *M. leprae* protein antigen expressed in *E. coli.* Nature. 1986; 319: 63.

70. Lamb JR, Ivanyi J, Rees ADM, Rothbard JB, Howland K, Young RA, Young DB. Mapping of T cell epitopes using recombinant antigens and synthetic peptides. EMBO J. 1987; 6: 1245.

71. Lamb JR, Ivanyi J, Rees ADM, Young OB. The identification of T cell epitopes in *Mycobacterium tuberculosis* using human T cell clones. Lepr Rev. 1986; 57 (Suppl 2): 131.

72. Oftung F, Mustafa AS, Husson R, Young RA, Godal T. Human T cell clones recognise two abundant *Mycobacterium tuberculosis* protein antigens expressed in *Escherichia coli.* J Immunol. 1987; 138: 927.

73. Van Eden W, Thole JER, van der Zee R, Noordzji A, van Embden JDA, Hensen EJ, Cohen IR. Cloning of the mycobacterial epitope recognized by T lymphocyte in adjuvant arthritis. Nature. 1988; 331: 171.

74. Res PCM, Schaar CG, Breedveld FC, van Eden W, van Embden JDA, Cohen LR, de Gries RRP. Synovial fluid T cells reactivity against 65 kDa heatshock protein of mycobacteria in early chronic arthritis. Lancet. 1988; i: 478.

75. Gaston JSH, Life PF, Bailey LC, Bacon PA. In vitro responses to a 65kDa mycobacterial protein by synovial T cells from inflammatory arthritis patients. J Immunol. 1989; 143: 2492.

76. Graeffe-Meeder ER, van der Zee R, Rijkers GT, Schuurman H-J, Kuis W, Bijlsma JWJ, Zeger BJM, van Eden W. Recognition of human 60kD heat-shock protein by mononuclear cells from patients with juvenile chronic arthritis. Lancet. 1991; 337: 1368.

77. Gaston JSH, Life PF, Jenner PJ, Colston MJ, Bacon PA. Recognition of a mycobacteria-specific epitope in the 65kD heat-shock protein by synovial fluid-derived T cell clones. J Exp Med. 1990; 171: 831.

78. Res PCM, Orsini DLM, Van Laar JM, Janson AAM, Abou-Zeid C, de Vries RRP. Diversity in antigen recognition by *Mycobacterium tuberculosis*-reactive T cell clones from the synovial fluid of rheumatoid arthritis patients. Eur J Immunol. 1991; 21: 1297.

79. Hermann E, Lohse AW, Van der Zee R, Van Eden W, Mayet WJ, Probst P, Poralla T, Meyer zum Buschenfelde KH, Fleischer B. Synovial fluid-derived *Yesinia*-reactive T cells responding to human 65 kDa heat-shock protein and heat stressed antigen presenting cells. Eur J Immunol. 1991; 21: 2139.

80. Rothbard JB, Taylor WR. A sequence pattern common to T cell epitopes. EMBO J. 1988; 7: 93.

81. Lamb JR, Bal V, Mendez-Semperio P, Mehlert A, So A, Rothbard J, Jindal S, Young RA, Young DB. Stress proteins may provide a link between the immune response to infection and autoimmunity. Int Immunol. 1989; 1: 191.

82. Delisi C, Berzofsky J. T cell antigenic structures tend to be amphipathic structures. Proc Natl Acad Sci USA. 1985; 82: 7048–52.

83. Chicz RM, Urban RG, Iane WS, Gorga JC, Stern LJ, Vignali DAA, Strominger J. Predominant naturally processed peptides bound to HLA-DR1 are derived from MHC-related molecule and are heterogenous in size. Nature. 1992; 358: 764.

84. Rothbard JB, Geffer ML. Interactions between immunogenic peptides and MAC proteins. Annu Rev Immunol. 1991; 9: 527.

85. Berzosky JA, Bensussan A, Cease KB, Bourge JF, Cleynier R, Lurhuma Z, Salaun J-J, Gallor C, Shearer GM, Zagury D. Antigenic peptides recognised by T lymphocytes from AIDS viral envelope immune humans. Nature. 1988; 334: 706.

86. Sinigaglia I, Guttinger M, Kilgus J, Dorant DM, Matile H, Etlinger H, Trzeciak A, Gillessen D, Pink JRL. A malaria T cell epitope recognised in association with most mouse and human class II molecules. Nature. 1989; 336: 778.

87. Geluk A, Bloemhoff W, De Vries RRP, Ottenhoff THM. Binding of a major T cell epitope of mycobacteria to a specific pocket within HLA-DR217 (DR3) molecules. Eur J Immunol. 1992; 22: 107.

88. Takahashi H, Cease H, Berzofsky JA. Identification of proteases that process distinct epitopes on the same protein. J Immunol. 1989; 142: 2221.

89. Van Noort JM, Boon J, Vander Drift ACM, Wagenhaar PA, Boots AMH, Boog CJP. Antigen processing by endosomal proteases determines which sites of sperm whale myoglobin are eventually by T-cells. Eur J Immunol. 1991; 21: 1989.

90. Van Noort JM, van der Drift ACM. The selectivity of Cathepsin D suggests an involvement of the enzyme in the generation of T-cell epitopes. J Biol Chem. 1989; 254: 14159.

91. Moll H, Mitchell GI, McConville MJ, Handman E. Evidence for T-cell recognition in mice of a purified liphophosophoglycan from *Lieschmania major*. Infect Immun. 1989; 57: 3349.

92. Ishioka GY, Lamont AG, Thomson D, Burlow N, Gaeta FCA, Sette A, Grey HM. MCH interaction and T cell recognition of carbohydrates and glycopeptides. J Immunol. 1992; 148: 2446.

93. Kaplan G, Ghandi RR, Weinstein DE, Levis WR, Patarroyo ME, Brennan PJ, Cohn ZA. *Mycobacterium leprae* antigen-induced suppression of T cell proliferation *in vitro*. J Immunol. 1987; 139: 3028.

94. Moreno C, Mehlert A, Lamb JR. The inhibitory effects of mycobacterial lipoarabino mannan and polysaccharides upon polyclonal and monoclonal human T cell proliferation. Clin Exp Immunol. 1988; 74: 206.

95. Saito H, Krauz DM, Takagaki Y, Hayday A, Eisen H, Toregawa S. Complete primary structure of a heterodimeric T cell receptor deduced from cDNA sequences. Nature. 1984; 309: 757–762.

96. Triebel T, Hercend T. Subpopulations of human peripheral T gamma delta lymphocytes. Immunol Today. 1989; 10: 186.

97. Modlin RL, Pimez C, Hofman FM, Torigan V, Uye Mura K, Rea TH, Bloom BR, Brenner MB. Lymphocytes bearing antigen-specific $\gamma\delta$ T-cell receptors accumulate in human infectious disease lesions. Nature. 1989; 339: 544.

98. Raulet DH. Antigens for $\gamma\delta$ T cells. Nature. 1989; 339: 342.

99. Janeway C. Frontiers of the immune system. Nature. 1988; 333: 804.

100. Rajasekar R, Sim G-K, Augustin A. Self heat shock and $\gamma\delta$ T cell reactivity. Proc Natl Acad Sci USA. 1990; 87: 1767.

101. Rees ADM, Donati Y, Lombardi G, LLamb JR, Polla BS, Lechler R. Stress-induced modulation of antigen-presenting cell function. Immunology. 1991; 74: 386.

102. Selmas K, Brosnan CF, Raine CS. Colocalisation of lymphocytes bearing gamma $\gamma\delta$ T cell receptor and heat shock protein hsp65$^+$ oligodendrocytes in multiple sclerosis. Proc Natl Acad Sci USA. 1991; 88: 6452.

103. Kabelitz D, Bender A, Prospero T, Wesselborg S, Janssen D, Pechhold K. The primary response of human $\gamma\delta$ + T cells to *Mycobacterium tuberculosis* is restricted to Vγ9-bearing cells. J Exp Med. 1991; 173: 1331.

104. De Libero G, Casorati G, Giachino C, Carbonara C, Migone N, Matzinger P, Lanzavecchia A. Selection by two powerful antigens may account for the presence of the major population of human peripheral $\gamma\delta$ T cells. J Exp Med. 1991; 173: 1311.

105. Pfeifer K, Schoel B, Gulle H, Kaufmann SHE, Wagner H. Primary responses of human T cells to mycobacteria: a frequent set of $\gamma\delta$ T cells are stimulated by protease-resistant ligands. Eur J Immunol. 1990; 20: 1175.

106. Strominger JL. The $\gamma\delta$ T cell receptor and Class 1b MHC-related proteins: Enigmatic molecules of immune recognition. Cell. 1989; 57: 895.

107. Porcelli S, Brenner MB, Greenslein JL, Balk SP, Terhorst C, Bleicher PA. Recognition of a cluster of differentiation antigens by human CD4$^-$ CD8$^-$ cytolytic T lymphocytes. Nature. 1989; 341: 447.

108. Porcelli S, Morita CT, Brenner MB. CD1b restricts the response of human CD4$^-$CD8$^-$ T lymphocytes to a microbial antigen. Nature. 1992; 360: 593.

109. Kabelitz D, Bender A, Schondelmaier S, Schoel B, Kaufmann SHE. A large fraction of human peripheral blood $\gamma\delta^+$ T cells is activated by *Mycobacterium tuberculosis* but not by its 65-kd heat shock protein. J Exp Med. 1990; 171: 667.

110. Kosbor D, Trinchieri G, Monos DS, Isobe M, Russo G, Haney JA, Zmijewski C, Croce CM. Human TCR-γ? CD8$^+$ T lymphocytes recognize tetanus toxoid in an MHC-restricted fashion. J Exp Med. 1989; 169: 1847.

111. Born W, Happ MP, Dallas A, Reardon C, Kubo R, Shinnick T, Brennan P, O'Brien R. Recognition of heat shock proteins and $\gamma\delta$ T cell function. Immunol Today. 1990; 11: 40.

112. Lamb JR, Young DB. T cell recognition of stress proteins: A link between infections and autoimmune disease. Mol Biol Med. 1990; 7: 311.

113. Young DB. Chaperonins and the immune response. Semin Cell Biol. 1990; 1: 27.

114. Schwartz RH. T lymphocyte recognition of antigen in association with gene products of the major histocompatibility complex. Annu Rev Immunol. 1985; 3: 237.

115. Buus S, Sette A, Colon SM, Miles C, Grey HM. The relationship between major histocompatibility complex (MHC) restriction and the capacity of Ia to bind immunogenic peptides. Science. 1987; 235: 1353.

116. Harris DP, Douglas-Jones AG, Wade S, Krahenbukl JL, Gillis TP, Watson JD. Genetic control of immune T cell proliferative responses to *Mycobacterium leprae* V. Evidence for cross-reactivity between host antigens and *M. leprae*. J Immunol. 1988; 141: 1695.

117. Cohen IR, Young DB. Autoimmunity, microbial immunity and the immunological homunculus. Immunol Today. 1991; 12: 105.

118. Fischer HP, Sharrock CEM, Colston MJ, Panayi GS. Limiting dilution analysis of proliferative T cell responses to mycobacterial 65 kDa heat-shock protein fails to show significant frequency differences between synovial fluid and peripheral blood of patients with rheumatoid arthritis. Eur J Immunol. 1991; 21: 2937.

119. Röcken M, Urban JF, Shevach EM. Infection breaks T-cell tolerance. Nature. 1992; 359: 79.

120. Polla BS. A role for heat shock proteins in inflammation. Immunol Today. 1988; 9: 134.

121. Kanengawa S, Donati YRA, Clerget M, Haridonneau-Parini I, Sinclair F, Mariethoz E, Perin M, Rees ADM, Slosman DO, Polla BS. Heat shock proteins: an autoprotective mechanisms for inflammatory cells? Semin Immunol. 1991; 3: 49.

122. Koga T, Wand-Wurttenberger A, De Buryn J, Munk ME, Schoel B, Kaufmann SHE. T cells against a bacterial heat shock protein recognise stressed macrophages. Science. 1989; 245: 1112.

123. Braciale TJ, Braciale VL. Antigen presentation: Structural themes and functional variations. Immunol Today. 1991; 12: 124.

124. Kuperberg G, Ellis J, Marcinklewicz J, Chain BM. Eur J Immunol. 1991; 21: 2791.

125. Hahn H, Kaufmann SHE. The role of cell mediated immunity in bacterial infections. Rev Infect Dis. 1981; 3: 1222.

126. Modlin RL, Mehra V, Fujimiya WL, Chang W-C, Horwitz DA, Bloom BR, Rea TH, Pattengate PK. Suppressor T lymphocytes from lepromatous leprosy skin lesions. J Immunol. 1986; 137: 2831.

127. Naher H, Sperling U, Hahn H. H-2K restricted granuloma formation by Ly-2$^+$ T cells in anti-bacterial protection to facultative intracellular bacteria. J Immunol. 1985; 134: 569.

128. Muller L, Cobbald SP, Waldmann H, Kaufmann SHE. Impaired resistance to *Mycobacterium tuberculosis* infection after selective *in vivo* depletion of L3T4$^+$ and Lyt 2$^+$ T cells. Infect Immun. 1987; 55: 2037.

129. Kaufmann SHE. CD8+ T lymphocytes in intracellular microbial infections. Immunol Today. 1988; 9: 168.

130. Kaleab B, Ottenhof T, Converse P. *et al.* Mycobacterial-induced cytotoxic T-cells as well as non-specific killer cells derived from healthy individuals and leprosy patients. Eur J Immunol. 1990; 20: 2651.

131. Brunt LM, Portnon DA, Unanue ER. Presentation of Listeria monocytogenes to CD8– T cells requires secretion of hemolysui and intracellular bacterial growth. J Immunol. 1990; 145: 3540.

132. Pfeifer JD, Wick MJ, Roberts RL, Findlay K, Normark SJ, Harding CV. Phagocytic processing of bacterial antigens for class I MHC presentation to T cells. Nature. 1993; 361: 359.

133. Stover CK, de la Cruz VF, Fuerst JR, Burlein JE, Bensou LA, Bennett LT, Bansal GP, Young JF, Lee MH, Hatfull GF, Snapper SB, Barletta RG, Jacobs WR, Bloom BR. New use of BCG for recombinant vaccines. Nature. 1991; 351: 456.

134. Dalton DK, Pitts-Meek S, Keshav S, Figari I, Bradley A, Stewart TA. Multiple defects of immune cell function in mice with disrupted interferon γ genes. Science. 1993; 259: 739.

135. Huang S, Hendriks W, Althage A, Hemmi S, Bluethmann H, Kamijo R, Vilcek J, Zinkernagel RM, Ague M. Immune response in mice lacking interferon γ receptor. Science. 1993; 259: 1742.

136. Nathan CF, Murray HW, Wiebe ME, Rubin BY. Identification of interferon as the lymphokine that activates human macrophage oxidative metabolism and antimicrobial immunity. J Exp Med. 1983; 158: 670.

137. Liew FY, Cox. Non-specific defence mechanisms: The role of nitric oxide. Immunoparasitol Today. 1991: A17.

138. Lowrie DB. How macrophages kill tubercle bacilli. J Med Microbiol. 1983; 16: 1.

139. Andrews PW, Rees ADM, Scoging A, Dobson N, Mathews R, Trevor-Wittal J, Coates ARM, Lowrie DB. Secretion of a macrophage activating factor distinct from interferon γ. Eur J Immunol. 1981; 14: 962.

140. Kindler V, Sappino AP, Grau GE *et al.* The inducing role of tumor necrosis factor in the development of bactericidal granulomas during BCG infection. Cell. 1989; 56: 731.

141. Balkwill F. Improving on the formula. Nature. 1993; 361: 207.

142. Amiri P, Locksley RM, Parslow TG, Sadik M, Rector F, Ritter D, McKerrow JH. Tumour necrosis factor α restores granulomas and induces parasite egg laying in schistosome infected SCID mice. Nature. 1992; 356: 604.

143. Haanen JB, de Waal Maleft P, Res T, Kraakman EM, Ottenhof THM, de Vries RRP, Spits H. Selection of a human T helper type I-like subset by mycobacteria. J Exp Med. 1991; 174: 583.

144. Kaplan G, Laal S, Sheftel G, Nusrat A, Nath I, Mathur NK, Mishra RS, Cohn ZA. The nature and kinetics of a delayed immune response to purified protein derivative of tuberculin in the skin of lepromatous leprosy patients. J Exp Med. 1988; 168: 1811.

3
Immunology of Fungal Infections

K. BAYSTON, C. TANG and J. COHEN

INTRODUCTION

Fungi are widely distributed in the environment, yet systemic fungal infections occur infrequently in normal individuals. Recently there has been a significant rise in the incidence of opportunistic infections in patients with impaired host defences, in part due to the increasing use of antineoplastic and immunosuppressive agents, and more recently as a consequence of human immunodeficiency virus (HIV) infection. In this chapter we will summarize some general aspects of fungal immunology, and then give a more detailed account of host responses to the important opportunistic and primary pathogenic fungi. Tropical mycoses and dermatophytes have been excluded.

GENERAL IMMUNOLOGY

The outcome of any host–fungus relationship is determined by a number of factors some, such as dose, relating to the infecting organism, and others which are host related. Considerable structural, antigenic and chemical differences exist between the various classes of fungi, and indeed between the different life cycle phases of a single fungal organism. The host responds to these various forms in different ways, being better equipped to deal with some fungal structures than others[1]. For example, primary pathogenic fungi (*Histoplasma capsulatum, Coccidioides immitis, Paracoccidioides brasiliensis* and *Blastomyces dermatididis*) are relatively resistant to the intracellular killing mechanisms of unactivated macrophages, while the opportunistic fungi (including *Aspergillus fumigatus, Candida albicans* and *Rhizopus oryzae*) are more readily eradicated by such mechanisms[2]. Blastoconidia of *Candida* and the germinating spores of *Aspergillus* are readily phagocytosed by neutrophils and macrophages, whereas the larger hyphal (or pseudohyphal) forms of these fungi cannot be ingested, and killing is therefore achieved by

49

extracellular mechanisms[3-6]. Production of toxins or enzymes by fungi may also influence pathogenicity[7-9]. *C. albicans* and *A. fumigatus* are both reported to produce endotoxin-like substances; these may be the cause of the shock-like syndrome sometimes seen in these infections[10-12]. Secretion of proteinases by *C. albicans*[13,14], *R. oryzae*[15] and *C. immitis*[9] may aid in tissue invasion and destruction. However, it has been shown recently that the production of elastase by *A. fumigatus* is unlikely to be a determinant of virulence in invasive disease[16]. Gliotoxin, a compound produced by *A. fumigatus*, has potent antiphagocytic and immunosuppressive activity *in vitro* and may compromise defence mechanisms in patients with systemic aspergillosis[17,18]. Immunosuppressive activity of many other fungal antigens is well documented and is of possible significance in potentiating or exacerbating fungal infections[19-22].

NON-SPECIFIC HOST DEFENCE MECHANISMS

The primary line of defence against fungal infection is provided by non-specific innate mechanisms. These include the mechanical and chemical barriers of skin and mucous membranes, the presence of normal bacterial flora, and various factors present in non-immune serum. Mechanisms by which bacteria inhibit fungi are thought to include competition for nutrients and mucosal receptors, bacterial elaboration of antifungal metabolites and changes in redox potential. The importance of these mechanisms is best established for *Candida*: indeed, suppression of the normal bacterial flora by antibiotics is one of the major predispositions to invasive candidosis. Other local factors include excessive moisture and breaching of the skin by indwelling lines or burns, damage to mucosa of the gastrointestinal tract secondary to radiation or chemotherapy and changes in vaginal pH due to hormonal fluctuations. The primary portal of entrance for many other fungi is the respiratory tract where cilial clearance is an important additional mechanism of resistance.

NATURAL CELLULAR MECHANISMS

Neutrophils and bronchoalveolar macrophages are the most important components of the cellular defences that have antifungal activity, but circulating monocytes, eosinophils, other tissue macrophages and natural killer (NK) cells also play a part. The majority of these cells are phagocytic, although NK cells and sometimes neutrophils kill by extracellular mechanisms. The phagocyte has a number of antimicrobial systems available to it, some of which involve oxidative processes while others are non-oxidative[23-26]. Under aerobic conditions in normal cells oxygen-dependent microbial killing mechanisms are probably of primary importance. The contact between fungal cell and neutrophil triggers an increase in oxygen consumption (the respiratory burst) which results in the generation of a battery of oxidizing agents, the most toxic of which are hydrogen peroxide and hypochlorous acid. Superoxide, hydroxyl radical, singlet oxygen, chloramine and aldehydes are other toxic products of the respiratory burst with potential fungicidal activity. The inherited disorder chronic granulomatous disease results from a mutation in a gene encoding a subunit of the neutrophil NADPH oxidase system[27] and is characterized by failure of the respiratory burst mechanism in stimulated phagocytes[28-30]. It is associated with an increased incidence of severe fungal and bacterial infections[31,32]. A number of other substances present in phagocytic cells also inhibit or kill fungi[26,33]. Cationic proteins, lysozyme, lactoferrin, acid phosphatase, β-glucuronidase and elastase are contained within primary and secondary cytoplasmic granules, and following phagocytosis are discharged into the phagosome where they may act in concert with oxidizing agents[24].

Fungal elements too large to be phagocytosed and killed intracellularly may be exposed to the extracellular fungicidal systems of neutrophils. The cells surround and attach to large structures such as *Zygomycete* and *Aspergillus* hyphae[34], candidal pseudohyphae[35], *B. dermatididis* yeasts[36] and encapsulated cryptococci[37]. It is thought that attachment triggers the respiratory burst and that oxidizing agents and cationic proteins are subsequently released onto the fungal surface and into the surrounding milieu[4,38]. Effects on the organism analogous to those occurring in the phagolysosome are then produced.

NK cells and other natural effector cells are non-phagocytic cells of the defence system that are present in the circulation and in high concentration in lung, liver and spleen[39,40]. They possess as yet undefined receptors for glycosylated structures on target cell membranes. Following attachment, lysis of the target cell occurs. NK activity is enhanced by interleukin 2 (IL-2), interferon-γ (IFN-γ) and opsonizing antibody. The importance of such cells in resistance to fungal infection is best documented for cryptococcosis[41-45] and paracoccidioidomycosis[46].

HUMORAL FACTORS

The role of complement and specific antibody in defence against fungi has been investigated at length, but despite this the relative importance of these factors in many instances remains uncertain. While specific antibodies are frequently present in the serum of patients with fungal infection (see below) and many fungi are known to activate complement with the resulting generation of chemotactic factors and opsonins[47-52], deficiencies of immunoglobulin and complement are rarely associated with fungal infection. Evidence for a protective role of antibody is best documented for *Candida* and *Cryptococcus*. Even so there are still inconsistencies between *in vitro* and *in vivo* data. *In vitro* the presence of antibody and/or complement enhances cryptococcal phagocytosis and killing[50,53-57]. In animals, a beneficial effect of passive immunization is only seen in complement-deficient mice[58,59], suggesting a limited role of antibody, whereas in man the correlation between increasing antibody titres and improved prognosis of cryptococcal infections is suggestive of an overall beneficial effect of antibody[60]. Experimental studies also support a role for antibody in protection against *C. albicans* infection[61-63]. Until recently, these data conflicted with a negative correlation between rising titres of *Candida* agglutinins and precipitins and clinical outcome in patients with systemic candidosis (reviewed in ref. 64). An antibody to a 47 kD antigen has now been found in patients recovering from this infection, and may be of prognostic significance[65-67]. In contrast, a striking negative correlation between rising antibody titres and prognosis has been shown in coccidioidomycosis, and a similar trend is also apparent in histoplasmosis and paracoccidioidomycosis. The use of serological techniques for diagnosis of invasive fungal infection has recently been reviewed in depth[68,69].

Much interest has focused on the role of cytokines such as IFN-γ, tumour necrosis factor α (TNFα) and interleukin 1 (IL-1). These may be produced *in vitro* following stimulation of mononuclear cells by a variety of fungal antigens[70-72], and in some instances enhance not only monocyte activity but also neutrophil phagocytosis and killing of fungi[57,73-79]. Although most studies have been carried out *in vitro*, IL-1 and TNFα have been shown to enhance the survival of mice with systemic candidosis[80-82]. Further studies are required to determine the precise role of these and other cytokines in immunity to the different fungi.

Factors in serum other than those acting to enhance natural cellular defence mechanisms also have fungicidal activity: the presence of serum in culture media is inhibitory to the growth of many fungal species[83-87]. Transferrin is thought to be the most important of these factors[88,89]. Iron, which is necessary for fungal nutrition, binds to transferrin and is rendered unavailable to the fungi. The resulting fungistasis is reversible upon addition of excess iron to the system[90].

ACQUIRED CELLULAR DEFENCES

Patients with defective T lymphocyte function are at greatly increased risk of developing a variety of fungal infections. This is particularly apparent in patients with HIV infection (reviewed in ref. 91), in whome a high incidence of mucocutaneous candidosis[92], cryptococcal meningitis[93-96] and disseminated histoplasmosis[97-99] has been reported. Coccidioidomycosis[100] and blastomycosis[101] have also been associated with AIDS, but fungal infections such as aspergillosis and mucormycosis, which depend primarily on innate defence mechanisms, are less common.

The mechanisms by which cellular immunity enhances fungal clearance are complex and poorly characterized. Macrophages, NK cells and neutrophils may be activated by lymphokines secreted by primed T cells, although proof of this is often lacking. Whether cytotoxic T cells have a role is uncertain. In patients with systemic mycoses and no known pre-existing immune defect, tests of cellular immunity are frequently abnormal. Absent delayed-type hypersensitivity (DTH) skin responses to an array of antigens is common, and the ability of T cells to transform and produce lymphokines is depressed. Suppressor cell populations stimulated by fungal antigens are thought to be the principal contributors to this effect[20-22,102-106]. Resolution of infection is often, but by no means always, associated with recovery of normal suppressor to helper T cell ratios and improvement in *in vitro* tests of T cell function[107]. Whether these defects in cellular immunity predispose to the development of infection or arise as a consequence of infection is often difficult to assess.

ASPERGILLOSIS

Aspergillus species are ubiquitous: soil, decomposing plant and animal matter, ventilation systems and building construction materials are common sources[108-110]. Spores are released into the air and are constantly inhaled[111]. Disease due to *Aspergillus* may be caused by a number of mechanisms (reviewed in ref. 7), including allergy to inhaled spores (asthma, allergic bronchopulmonary aspergillosis, extrinsic allergic alveolitis), colonization of abnormal pulmonary tissue (aspergilloma) and active fungal invasion (chronic necrotizing aspergillosis, invasive aspergillosis). Only about 20 of the 260 or so species in the genus *Aspergillus* have been linked conclusively with invasive disease, and less than 10 of these with any degree of regularity[110]. Of these *A. fumigatus* is by far the most important. Other thermotolerant and therefore potentially pathogenic species known to be associated with invasive disease in man are *A. flavus*, *A. niger*, *A. nidulans*, *A. terreus* and *A. glaucus*. Hypersensitivity to inhaled *Aspergillus* conidia is generally not species specific.

The association between *Apsergillus* lung disease and asthma is well documented. *Aspergillus* spores are found in the sputum of about 8% of asthmatics[112]. Around 10% of these patients show weak serum precipitin reactions and 20–40% have positive immediate skin tests to *Aspergillus* antigens[113,114]. *Aspergillus* species may also be isolated from the sputum of patients with cystic fibrosis[115,116] and other chronic pulmonary disorders[112], all of whom share with asthmatics the tendency to produce viscid secretions, with impaired mucociliary clearance and bronchospasm – factors which enhance respiratory tract colonization by aspergilli. Sensitization to inhaled *Aspergillus* spores and production of IgE antibodies occur in a manner analogous to sensitization by other inhaled allergens.

Allergic bronchopulmonary aspergillosis (ABPA) occurs in approximately 1% of asthmatics and is rare in the absence of documented asthma[117]. Factors determining susceptibility within the asthmatic population are unclear. Younger individuals tend to have asthma for many years before developing ABPA; the converse is true in adults over 30 years of age[118]. Although increased exposure to *Aspergillus* spores prior to development of ABPA has been reported[119] there is no consistent relationship with levels of exposure[118,120]. ABPA develops when inhaled spores (usually *A. fumigatus*) colonize the bronchial mucous membranes of asthmatics and elicit both IgE and immune complex-mediated tissue injury[108,117]. This induces bronchospasm and an inflammatory reaction in surrounding tissue. Bronchial damage is common and may lead to proximal bronchiectasis. Clinical features include episodic bronchospasm, pulmonary infiltrates (which may be transient or fixed) and pulmonary and peripheral eosinophilia[118]. A positive immediate skin test to *Aspergillus* antigen is characteristic. In addition, 85% of patients with ABPA have specific IgE antibodies to an antigen with a molecular weight of 18 kD[121]. This antigen has also been found in the serum and urine of patients with invasive aspergillosis[122] and has been shown to be a potent cellular toxin, restrictocin[123,124]. *Aspergillus* precipitins are present in the majority of cases[125,126], in up to one-third of patients with cystic fibrosis[115] and in about 10% of those with uncomplicated asthma[127]. Positive reactions are uncommon in non-atopic individuals.

Extrinsic allergic alveolitis results from an immune response to inhaled *Aspergillus* antigens in non-atopic individuals and usually occurs following repeated exposure to organic dust containing high numbers of spores. 'Malt workers' lung' is seen in brewery workers exposed to mouldy barley containing *A. clavatus*[128]; there is considerable debate regarding the pathogenic mechanisms underlying this disorder. Patients have elevated levels of specific IgG and an Arthus reaction to skin testing. This suggested that extrinic allergic alevolitis was primarily an immune complex disease. It now seems, however, that a lymphocyte-directed hypersensitivity reaction may also be involved[110]. Characteristic clinical features are cough, fever and dyspnoea, with radiographic evidence of diffuse pulmonary infiltration occurring some 4–5 h following inhalation of dusts. A restrictive defect is usual in pulmonary function tests.

Aspergilloma is a condition in which devitalized and poorly draining areas of lung (such as old tuberculous cavities and healed lesions of sarcoidosis or histoplasmosis) are colonized by *Aspergillus* species[129–132]. Hyphal proliferation leads to formation of a fungus ball within the cavity. Local invasion may lead to erosion of vascular structures and episodes of haemoptysis. The high antigen load is a strong immunostimulant, resulting in positive serum precipitin reactions in over 90% of patients[133].

Chronic necrotizing aspergillosis is characterized by indolent invasion, and later cavity formation, in previously abnormal pulmonary tissue[134]. Dissemination is unusual. Patients tend to be middle-aged, have pre-existing pulmonary pathology, and frequently also have some degree of immunosuppression (e.g. low-dose steroid therapy, connective tissue disease or diabetes mellitus).

The two major risk factors for invasive aspergillosis are prolonged neutropenia and treatment with high-dose steroids. Patients most at risk are bone marrow and organ transplant recipients and patients receiving intensive chemotherapy for acute leukaemia or high-dose steroids. Patients with chronic granulomatous disease are also susceptible, but invasive aspergillosis is often less fulminant in these individuals, whose non-oxidative killing mechanisms are enhanced[32,135]. Although invasive aspergillosis has not been a feature of AIDS, there has been an increase in the number of reported cases[136,137], particularly in association with end-stage disease. It has also been reported in otherwise healthy individuals, but is rare[138]. The most frequent site of infection is the lungs: over 90% of patients present with one or more pulmonary lesions[139–141]. Dissemination occurs in up to 25% of patients[140,141] and most commonly involves the gastrointestinal tract, CNS, kidney, liver and thyroid gland. Resolution of the underlying immunological disorder is usually necessary for any prospect of cure[142].

Aspergillus spores (conidia) are small (3–5 μm) and readily enter the terminal bronchioles or alveoli after inhalation. To cause invasive disease these resting conidia must become metabolically active and swell, then germinate to form hyphae. The immunocompetent host has highly efficient natural defence mechanisms which can prevent aspergillosis. As the first line of defence, inhaled conidia are phagocytosed by bronchoalveolar macrophages via lectin-like receptors[143]. Up to 92% of ingested conidia are killed under aerobic and anaerobic conditions[3,144,145], suggesting that bronchoalveolar macrophages have the capacity to kill conidia by both oxidative and non-oxidative mechanisms[144]. Neither activation by T lymphocytes, nor complement nor antibody is required for bronchoalveolar macrophages to kill spores[144]. Neutrophils and other tissue macrophages are relatively ineffective against resting conidia and are unable to inhibit germination[19,144,146,147]; ingestion is defective, stimulation of the respiratory burst is suboptimal and killing is poor. Two reasons for this have been postulated. Robertson et al.[19] found that resting spores released a low molecular weight substance from their surface that interfered with the triggering of the respiratory burst and production of reactive oxygen intermediates. Others have suggested that an amorphous hydrophobic layer composed of rodlets[148] which surrounds the cell wall of *Aspergillus* is protective[149,150].

Conidial morphology changes during transformation from the resting to the metabolically active, germinating state; the protective layer is lost and underlying cell wall antigens are exposed. Although phagocytosed resting conidia are not killed by neutrophils, germinating spores stimulate the generation of more oxidative products and up to 30% of ingested spores are killed[146]. A 3–6 h lag period between ingestion and killing of spores by bronchoalveolar macrophages suggests that conidial activation is also required for effective intracellular killing by these cells[144]. Those conidia which escape killing by bronchoalveolar macrophages and neutrophils germinate and proceed to grow as hyphae (the tissue-invasive form of *Aspergillus*). These structures are too large to undergo phagocytosis but are susceptible to extracellular killing by neutrophils and monocytes[5,34,135]. In summary, bronchoalveolar macrophages kill inhaled *Aspergillus* conidia, and neutrophils provide defence against germinating conidia and hyphae.

Although resistance to *Aspergillus* is primarily dependent on innate immunity, animal studies suggest that acquired immunity, and in particular cell-mediated immunity, may also play a role (reviewed in ref. 7). The results of several studies in mice support this. First, resistance to experimental infection with *A. fumigatus* increases with age. This resistance is significantly reduced following the administration of anti-lymphocyte globulin[151]. Second, New Zealand Black mice, which develop defective cell-mediated immunity with age, succumb more readily to *Aspergillus* infection than do CBA control mice[152]. Lastly, when athymic (nu/nu) and imunocompetent (nu/+) mice are immunized subcutaneously with *Aspergillus* conidia, only nu/+ mice are protected from subsequent challenge[153]. Depletion of B cells does not alter the resistance of mice to infection[154], and no protection is afforded by passive transfer of rabbit antiserum to *A. fumigatus*[153]. In man, neutropenic patients are at significantly greater risk of invasive aspergillosis than are AIDS patients, suggesting that classical cell-mediated immune mechanisms do not play a dominant role in resistance to this fungus.

Although double immunodiffusion and counterimmunoelectrophoresis have been widely used to detect *Aspergillus* precipitins for the serodiagnosis of ABPA and aspergilloma, these methods have proved disappointing in the diagnosis of invasive aspergillosis in immunocompromised individuals, largely because patients are unable to produce detectable levels of antibody. Analysis of the serological response by immunoblot has demonstrated antibody against a 40 kD immunodominant antigen in patients with invasive aspergillosis. Its presence has been linked to survival by some but a protective role for this antibody has not been proven[155,156].

More recently, interest has focused on the detection of circulating antigens for diagnosing invasive aspergillosis. Galactomannan, a cell wall glycoprotein, has been found in the serum of patients by both radioimmunoassay and enzyme-linked immunosorbent assay[157,158]. Regular testing of serum and urine from patients at risk of invasive aspergillosis showed antigenaemia to be the first indicator of invasive disease in 16 of 19 patients[159].

MUCORMYCOSIS

The causative agents of mucormycosis are Zygomycete fungi of the order Mucorales. The three species that commonly produce disease in man are *Rhizopus oryzae*, *Rhizomucor (Mucor) pusillus* and *Absidia corymbifera*. These fungi are widely found in nature on decaying vegetation and other organic material[160]. In common with aspergillosis, most infections occur in immuno-compromised individuals. The usual portal of entry is the respiratory tract, although primary gastrointestinal and cutaneous mucormycosis are well recognized entities. Typically, mucormycosis is characterized by deep tissue invasion with a predilection for vascular structures and subsequent haemorrhage, necrosis and infarction of infected tissues. Characteristic patterns of tissue involvement have led to classification of mucormycosis as rhinocerebral, pulmonary, gastrointestinal and cutaneous[161]. Dissemination may occur from any of these primary sites but most commonly arises from pulmonary infection. Certain underlying host disorders are associated with particular patterns of infection: diabetic ketoacidosis and steroid therapy with the rhinocerebral form, neutropenia with pulmonary infection, malnutrition with gastrointestinal disease and burns with cutaneous mucormycosis.

Host defences against mucormycosis are poorly understood. Since most infections follow inhalation of spores, experimental work has centred on resistance mechanisms within the respiratory tract. Bronchoalveolar macrophages and neutrophils appear to be of paramount importance. They provide a sequential defence system by preventing spore germination (alveolar macrophages) and exerting fungicidal activity against hyphae (neutrophils). Serum factors which are as yet poorly characterized play a synergistic role in resistance[162-164]. Whether acquired immunity is important remains to be determined.

Bronchoalveolar macrophages phagocytose inhaled spores avidly and inhibit their germination; unlike phagocytosed *Aspergillus* conidia, however, *Mucorales* spores remain viable[145]. Although *A. fumigatus* conidia are all removed from lungs of normal mice within 2 days of intranasal inoculation, resting spores of *R. oryzae* may still be found within alveolar macrophages at 10 days. Bronchoalveolar macrophages of diabetic or steroid-treated mice are unable to prevent spore germination[145]. Steroid treatment of experimental aspergillosis appears to modify macrophage function directly by preventing macrophage phagolysosome fusion[165,166]; the same mechanism is thought to be involved in mucormycosis. In cells from diabetic mice neither phagolysosome fusion nor respiratory burst activity is defective[165]. Rather, impaired macrophage phagocytosis combined with favourable tissue conditions promote growth of the organism. Reduced attachment of macrophages to *Mucorales* spores occurs in diabetic serum[165]: this effect is specific for mucormycosis. Hydrogen peroxide production in response to opsonized *Rhizopus* spores is also impaired in macrophages from diabetic mice, and acid phosphatase and lysozyme activity is decreased[15].

Ketoacidosis may also enhance spore germination and hyphal growth by a number of other mechanisms. Growth of *Rhizopus*, for instance, is optimal at an acid pH and high glucose concentration, and *Mucor* species have a ketoreductase which allows them to utilize ketone bodies for their metabolism[167]. It has been postulated that the reduced affinity of transferrin for iron as pH falls means that more free iron is available for fungal utilization[88]. Recent reports of an increased incidence of mucormycosis in patients receiving desferrioxamine during long-term dialysis are of interest in this regard; it is suggested that iron bound to desferrioxamine acts as a growth factor[168]. Finally, levels of a non-antibody, non-complement, heat-stable, dialysable factor which is present in normal serum and has an inhibitory effect on spore germination are reduced in diabetic ketoacidosis[162].

Once spore germination has occurred neutrophils are central to containing hyphal growth. Histological specimens from patients with mucormycosis demonstrate a predominantly neutrophil infiltrate surrounding invading hyphae. Neutrophils attach to and swarm over the surface of hyphae that are too large to be ingested and release fungicidal substances into the surrounding milieu that cause hyphal death[34]. Hyphae of *R. oryzae* generate chemotactic factors for neutrophils both directly and indirectly by activating the alternative pathway of complement[169]. Although the generation of chemotactic factors is not impaired by diabetes, neutrophil chemotaxis is reduced in ketoacidotic serum.

The importance of acquired immunity in host resistance to mucormycosis is not well established. Murine experiments have produced data both supporting and refuting a role for antibodies in resistance (reviewed in ref. 7). The role of cell-mediated immunity is also unclear. Athymic mice are no more susceptible than immunocompetent mice to lethal infection with *Absidia*[170], and lymphocyte depletion does not increase susceptibility to infection[171]. In clinical practice, patients with disorders of acquired cellular immunity rarely develop mucormycosis.

Standardized serological tests for the diagnosis of mucormycosis are not available. One study has reported the identification of five immunodominant antigens by immunoblotting. Using an enzyme immunoassay, antibody was detected in sera from all five patients with mucormycosis who were studied, with titres ranging from 1:64 to 1:32000[172]. More recently, an enzyme-linked immunosorbent assay which detects antibody to homogenates of R. arrhizus and R. pulsillus has been evaluated in 43 patients with mucormycosis. The test had a sensitivity of 87% and specificity of 94%[173].

CANDIDOSIS

The genus *Candida* includes many species of yeast-like fungi, the most extensively studied of which is *C. albicans*. The species of *Candida* that are capable of producing disease in man normally live commensally as part of the indigenous flora of mucosal surfaces, in particular the gastrointestinal tract and vagina. Alterations in the host flora, composition of body fluids (as occurs in diabetes, pregnancy or during hyperalimentation) or cellular defence systems may predispose to the development of candidosis. *C. albicans* is the most pathogenic of *Candida* species and the most common cause of human candidosis, but *C. tropicalis*, *C. stellatoidea*, *C. parapsilosis*, *C. krusei*, *C. pseudotropicalis*, *C. guilliermondi* and *C. (Torulopsis) glabrata* may also cause invasive disease. *C. tropicalis* is an increasingly important cause of invasive candidosis in immunosuppressed patients[174,175].

Candida are dimorphic fungi: they exist in yeast form as saprophytes, and as yeast cells and pseudohyphae (or hyphae) in tissue-invasive stages. Important steps in the pathogenesis of candidosis are adherence and germination. Adherence is thought to be mediated principally by a cell-surface adhesin, probably a mannoprotein[176,177]. Other factors affecting adherence include cell-surface hydrophobicity and the secretion of acid proteinase[14,178-180]. Avirulent species of *Candida* adhere poorly to epithelial cells, endothelial cells or fibrin-platelet matrices compared with pathogenic species[13,176]. *C. albicans* and *C. tropicalis* have the highest rate of adherence. Germination is associated with enhanced adherence and the capacity to invade tissues. Strains of *Candida* unable to germinate display reduced pathogenicity[181].

The spectrum of disease caused by *Candida* is wide. Candidiasis can take the form of superficial infection of skin or mucous membranes, a chronic infection of nails, a chronic disease of skin and mucous membranes, sometimes associated with endocrine failure (chronic mucocutaneous candidosis) or a severe and often fatal systemic disease.

Factors associated with the development of acute mucocutaneous candidosis are broad-spectrum antibiotic therapy, diabetes, pregnacy, use of the oral contraceptive, steroid therapy and obesity. The most common sites of infection are the mouth (thrush) and vagina. Other manifestations include oesophagitis, balanitis, folliculitis, nappy rash, perianal candidosis, paronychia and uncommonly, a generalized cutaneous eruption.

Chronic mucocutaneous candidosis (CMCC) is characterized by persistent and recurrent candidal infections affecting the skin, nails and mucous membranes to a variable degree. There is considerable heterogeneity in its aetiology[182-184]. Congenital thymic abnormalities such as the Di George syndrome, immunodeficiency disorders associated with T cell dysfunction (e.g. severe combined immunodeficiency syndrome, Wiskott–Aldrich syndrome) and polyendocrinopathies associated with an autosomal recessive pattern of inheritance are associated with CMCC, but most patients have no such underlying disorder. The most consistent abnormality is a selective defect in DTH skin responses and in tests of lymphocyte proliferation and lymphokine production in response to candidal antigens. Mucocutaneous candidosis similar to that seen in patients with CMCC is now frequently seen in patients with HIV infection[91].

The previously rare problem of systemic candidosis is becoming increasingly common. Individuals most at risk are those with severe neutropenia or defective neutrophil function. The presence of indwelling venous catheters, prolonged use of antibiotics, parenteral feeding, high-dose steroid therapy and damage to mucosal surfaces arising from radiotherapy and chemotherapy are common additional factors[174,185]. Systemic candidosis may present as single or multiple organ disease, with or without candidaemia: the kidney is frequently affected[186]. Candidaemia may also occur following surgery and during invasive procedures such as urinary catheterization, intravenous infusions and haemodialysis[187].

In the last decade a new syndrome of systemic *Candida* infection has been recognized[188-190]. This was initially termed hepatosplenic candidosis but the term 'chronic systemic candidosis' has recently been coined in recognition of the multiple organ involvement and the chronicity of the disease[190]. The most common underlying condition is acute leukaemia. Patients characteristically develop a fever of unknown origin during a period of neutropenia. The fever persists following recovery of the white cell count and is associated with abnormal liver function tests. Imaging studies demonstrate multiple abscesses in the liver and spleen. It has been suggested that antileukaemic drugs which are toxic to the gastrointestinal tract facilitate local invasion by *Candida* organisms which then migrate to the liver and spleen via the portal circulation.

Many factors are involved in resistance to candidal infection. Natural resistance mechanisms include intact skin and mucous membranes, presence of normal bacterial flora, hormones, undefined serum factors, complement, and cells of the phagocytic system (reviewed in refs. 6, 191). A mannoprotein from *C. albicans* has recently been shown to stimulate the release of lactoferrin from neutrophils: this inhibits candidal growth[192]. In addition, a peptide with anti-candidal activity has been isolated from bovine ciliated respiratory mucosa. This peptide is related to the defensin family of antimicrobial peptides[193,194], although the extent to which it contributes to the defence of the airway is not clear. Once surface defence mechanisms have been breached neutrophils are thought to provide the major defence against *Candida*. In man, neutropenia is one of the major risk factors for systemic candidosis[174]. Patients with defective neutrophil function are also at risk, as is illustrated by the increased incidence of systemic candidosis in patients with chronic granulomatous disease[32]. Reported rates of candidacidal activity *in vitro* vary considerably, largely due to differences in experimental conditions such as phagocyte to yeast ratios and length of incubation. Some generalizations may be made, however. Neutrophils readily phagocytose candidal blastospores and kill up to 80% of those ingested. Tissue macrophages, peripheral blood monocytes and eosinophils also display anticandidal activity *in vitro*, although killing is generally less effective than that by neutrophils[195-197]. Killing occurs principally by oxidative mechanisms[195,196] although non-oxidative mechanisms may be important in some circumstances[26].

Candidacidal activity of neutrophils, monocytes and bronchoalveolar macrophages may be significantly enhanced in the presence of cytokines such as TNFα, IFN-γ and IL-1[74-76,201-203]. Evidence that cytokines may be important modulators of anticandidal activity *in vivo* comes from several studies. Secretion of TNFα is a normal response of monocytes and NK cells to stimulation with *C. albicans*[72]. In mice, intraperitoneal administration of *C. albicans* induces endogenous TNFα, levels of which continue to rise for at least 24 h[204]. Both recombinant TNFα[80] and IL-1[81,82] protect mice from systemic *Candida* infection. In contrast, Garner *et al.*[205] could not show a protective role for IFN-γ *in vivo*. Mycelial forms of *Candida* cannot be ingested by phagocytic cells but appear to be sensitive to extracellular killing mechanisms[4,206].

Glucan, chitin and mannan are the principal components of the cell wall of *Candida*. Mannan activates the alternative pathway of complement and indirectly stimulates the production of chemotactic factors[207] and opsonins. These and other humoral factors contribute to host defences against candidosis, although they are less important on their own than are the primary cellular defences. Neutrophils can attach to receptors on the surface of blastospores and pseudohyphae in the absence of opsonins, but for optimal phagocytosis complement is also required[195,208,209]. Specific antibodies against *Candida* are present in the majority of normal individuals[64]. Systemic infection can be prevented by passive immunization of mice[62], and neutrophil phagocytosis of *Candida in vitro* is enhanced in the presence of antibody and complement[61]. These findings appear to conflict with the observation that increasing antibody titres are associated with an unfavourable outcome[64], although a more detailed analysis of antibody responses in systemic candidosis has revealed that in some patients increased levels of a specific antibody directed against a 47 kD antigen is associated with an improved prognosis[65-67].

Substances other than antibody and complement present in normal serum also have anticandidal activity. A factor that is present in the majority of children (95%) and adults under the age of 50 years (98%) but which is absent or in reduced levels in the serum of patients with diabetic ketoacidosis, leukaemia, CMCC and systemic candidosis, causes clumping of *Candida* and inhibits growth[83]. The relationship between host iron status and fungal disease is complex. Binding of free iron to transferrin reduces candidal growth rates and impedes transformation from yeast to pseudohyphal state[88]. It has recently been shown that the enhanced anti-candidal activity of human neutrophils seen after treatment with IL-2 is mediated by the release of transferrin[210]. However, *C. albicans* possesses a homologue of the human complement receptor CR-3, which mediates rosette formation by complement-coated red blood cells *in vitro*, and which may facilitate the acquisition of iron by *Candida* in the host[211]. In contrast, iron deficiency may reduce the integrity of mucosal and cutaneous epithelial surfaces and impair cellular defence mechanisms[212]. Copper and vitamins A and C may also influence virulence of *Candida* and host susceptibility to infection (reviewed in ref. 6).

Most normal individuals have demonstrable cell-mediated immunity to candidal antigens as a result of exposure to colonizing *Candida* species; the principal role of this in man appears to be in protection against mucocutaneous candidosis. Individuals with disorders predominantly of T cell function, such as CMCC and AIDS, often suffer from severe mucocutaneous candidiasis, but rarely develop systemic candidosis. Some experimental animal studies have shown a role for cellular immunity, but many have not[6,191]. Activated macrophages and activated multinucleated giant cells[213] phagocytose and kill *Candida in vitro* more effectively than non-activated cells.

Modulation of the immune response by *Candida* has been shown both *in vitro* and *in vivo*. Mannan, which may be found in the circulation of patients with systemic candidosis, has both immunostimulatory and immunosuppressive properties[4,214,215], and glucan is involved in reducing the adherence of neutrophils following exposure to *C. albicans in vitro*[216]. The CR3-like receptors on the surface of *C. albicans* can bind to iC3b or C3d[217,218] and iC3b receptor inhibits phagocytosis by non-covalently binding iC3b and masking the recognition site for neutrophil CR3[219]. Upregulation of iC3b receptors occurs following mycelial transformation and in high concentrations of glucose. Hyphal forms of *Candida* may impair phagocyte candidacidal activity by secreting substances which slow granulocyte chemotaxis, prevent further contact between neutrophil and hyphal surfaces and inhibit activation of the respiratory burst[220]. *In vivo*, both whole *C. albicans* cells and cell extracts increase susceptibility of mice to subsequent infection by *Candida* and/or bacteria (reviewed in ref. 6). T cell suppression has been shown *in vitro* and *in vivo* and may account for these findings[21,221]. More studies are required to determine the relevance of immunomodulation by *Candida* in man.

CRYPTOCOCCOSIS

Cryptococcosis is a systemic fungal disease of man and animals caused by *C. neoformans*, a yeast with worldwide distribution, the life cycle of which is not fully understood. In man, *C. neoformans* exists as a large encapsulated yeast. In nature, isolates are most commonly poorly or non-encapsulated yeast cells. A sexual (mycelial) form has been recognized but this has never been found in nature. Yeast isolates may be divided into four serotypes A, B, C and D based on differences in capsular polysaccharide[222,223]. Mating of A and D (*C. neoformans* var *neoformans*), and B and C strains (*C. neoformans* var *gatti*) gives rise to the two different mycelial forms of

Cryptococcus, Filobasidiella neoformans var *neoformans* and *F. neoformans* var *bacillispora*[224]. A/D are the most common serotypes isolated from clinical specimens or the environment[109]. Soil, particularly that enriched with pigeon droppings, is the most common environmental source. Prior to the AIDS epidemic, serotypes B/C accounted for the majority of cases of cryptococcosis in central Africa and many in Southern California, Australasia, southern Asia and South America[109]. The only known environmental source of this serotype is the Eucalyptus tree, *E. camaldulensis*[225]. Unlike individuals infected with *C. neoformans* var *neoformans*, those with disease due to *C. neoformans* var *gatti* rarely have an obvious underlying immunodeficiency[226]. Serotypes A/D and B/C differ antigenically and biochemically, and there is some evidence to suggest that this is associated with differences in virulence.

Clinical disease due to infection with *C. neoformans* var *neoformans* occurs infrequently in the immunocompetent host, even when levels of exposure are high[227]. Systemic cryptococcal infection in the West is primarily a disease of the immunosuppressed patient. High-dose steroid therapy, Hodgkin's disease, sarcoidosis, organ transplantation and AIDS are major underlying predispositions[60,93]. The initial focus of infection is usually the lung, although this is frequently asymptomatic. Dissemination occurs in over 80% of compromised patients but in only 14% of immunocompetent individuals[228]. Although organisms may disseminate to virtually any organ there is a particular predilection for the central nervous system. The absence of soluble anticryptococcal factors in cerebrospinal fluid along with the ability of cryptococci to use brain dopamine for melanogenesis may favour local proliferation[229-231]. Responses to the infection vary from no tissue reaction (as is commonly seen in AIDS patients), to a diffuse inflammatory reaction or granuloma formation. Meningitis is the most commonly diagnosed form of cryptococcosis. The clinical presentation is often insidious and the course chronic; untreated cryptococcal meningitis is invariably fatal.

Cryptococcosis is generally thought to be acquired by the pulmonary route. Infectious particles are inhaled and, if they are small enough, escape pulmonary clearance mechanisms and enter the terminal alveoli. It is not known whether these infectious particles are small unencapsulated yeasts or the basidiospores of the sexual (mycelial) form. Whatever the case, within a few hours of inhalation, conditions within the lung promote the synthesis of capsular polysaccharide, a substance which binds to and surrounds the yeast cell. It seems that the high CO_2 concentration present in lung tissue along with the presence of thiamine, glutamate and neutral pH promotes the activity of an enzyme system essential to capsular polysaccharide synthesis[232].

Cryptococcal polysaccharide inhibits binding and ingestion of yeast cells by unactivated phagocytes. A number of mechanisms have been proposed, including the increase in organism size[233], creation of a barrier that prevents contact between ligands on the yeast cell wall and their receptor on the phagocyte[234], masking of opsonins which may be situated on the cell wall beneath the capsular surface[235] and physicochemical properties of the capsule surface itself[235]. The capsular polysaccharide also induces the production of suppressor cell populations which further impair host cellular defence mechanisms[20]. Acapsular mutants are typically avirulent in animals[235].

The immune response to *C. neoformans* is complex. Although clinical data suggest that cell-mediated immunity is principally involved in protection, natural defence mechanisms and humoral immunity are probably also important. A neutrophil response characterizes the initial host reaction in experimental pulmonary cryptococcosis and leads to clearance of most inhaled organisms[236]. A mononuclear infiltrate develops later. Neutrophils can phagocytose and kill cryptococci *in vitro*, principally by oxidative mechanisms[233]. Lysosomal cationic proteins as well as other non-oxidative components of neutrophils are cryptococcidal *in vitro* and may supplement oxygen-dependent mechanisms *in vivo*[237]. Although unactivated neutrophils will only ingest weakly encapsulated yeast cells, in the presence of lymphocyte supernatants, anticryptococcal activity is significantly increased and even quite heavily encapsulated cryptococci are phagocytosed and killed[238]. This is related to the increased expression of CR3 receptors on the surface of activated neutrophils. Resting monocytes and macrophages may also ingest poorly encapsulated *C. neoformans* yeasts, but fungicidal activity is poor[239]. Interferon-γ-activated murine macrophages demonstrate enhanced extra-cellular and intracellular killing of *C. neoformans*; the latter is particularly evident in the presence of specific anticapsular antibody[57,79]. Studies with human macrophages have so far failed to show an influence of cytokines[240] on macrophage anticryptococcal activity which is independent of nitric oxide production[241].

There is evidence that NK cells, which are particularly numerous in lung and lymphoid tissue, are also important in defence against cryptococci[42,45] and that this activity is primarily antibody-dependent[43,44] and independent of capsule size[41].

The capsule is a relatively immunologically inert structure which is unrecognized by phagocytes unless it is opsonized by either complement or capsule-specific antibody[56]. C3 generated from activation of the classical (and more importantly alternative) pathways of complement binds avidly to the capsule surface of *C. neoformans* and can be shown significantly to enhance phagocytosis[50,55,242]. Activation of the alternative pathway also induces chemotaxis, a response which can be ablated by administration of anti-C5[243] IgG in normal serum is deposited at low density throughout the capsule, whereas capsule-specific antibody binds to the surface and is available for opsonization[56]. Circulating immune complexes of anti-capsule antibody and free capsular polysaccharide may modify phagocytosis[51,56]. It has been suggested that immune complexes bind to the Fc receptors of macrophages and influence phagocytosis in two ways[57]. First, bound immune complexes block Fc receptors, reducing the number of available binding sites to which antibody-coated yeast cells may attach. Second, binding induces macrophage activation and subsequently augments the interaction of opsonized yeast cells with complement receptor sites.

The relative significance of humoral factors in resistance to *C. neoformans* is unknown. Complement is probably most important, but specific anti-capsule antibody seems to be necessary for optimal phagocytosis. This may explain the clinical finding that increasing antibody titres correlate with improved prognosis, while disseminated cryptococcosis is associated with low or absent antibody titres[60]. The role of passive immunization in experimental cryptococcosis is not established however[59], and hypogamma-globulinaemia is not a risk factor for cryptococcosis in man. However, the systemic administration of a murine monoclonal antibody directed against the capsular polysaccharide ameliorates the course of intracerebral crypto-coccosis in immunocompetent mice[244], and it will be of interest to see if this approach to therapy is of benefit in the clinical setting. Other serum factors such as transferrin have anticryptococcal activity *in vitro*, but their role *in vivo* is unknown.

The importance of T cell-mediated immunity is well established, although the mechanism is unknown. The unifying factor in the various disease states known to predispose to cryptococcosis in man is defective T cell function. In experimental cryptococcosis, athymic mice succumb to invasive disease more readily than do normal mice[245]. Interestingly, the increased numbers of activated macrophages and NK cells present in athymic mice lead to rapid initial clearance of injected cryptococci, but these mechanisms are subsequently overwhelmed. In normal mice heightened clearance of yeast cells from 2 weeks onwards coincides with the acquisition of cellular immunity, as demonstrated by the development of positive DTH responses. Transfer of immune T lymphocytes confers immunity on recipient mice, whereas treatment with anti-lymphocyte serum decreases survival of *C. neoformans*-infected mice[246,247]. Karaoui et al.[248] showed that alveolar macrophages of mice were fungistatic 14 days following airborne exposure to *C. neoformans* and peritoneal macrophages were fungicidal after 21–28 days. These effects were transient however; during progressive infection intracellular killing became defective as a result of an acquired 'immunosup-pressive state'. Disseminated cryptococcosis in man is also associated with depressed cellular immune mechanisms[249]. Anergy, and absent or blunted T cell responses to both specific and non-specific antigens are common findings, probably caused by the effect of T cell suppressor populations induced by intact yeast cells and free capsular polysaccharide[104,250].

DIMORPHIC FUNGI

Most potentially pathogenic fungi are opportunists, and cause serious infections only in immunocompromised individuals. A few fungi, however, can produce serious systemic infection in seemingly normal hosts. These virulent fungi share the property of thermal dimorphism, growing as mycelia in the saprophytic soil phase at 22°C but as yeasts in tissues at 37°C. This is in contrast with opportunistic fungi, which tend to grow as hyphae within human tissue. The yeast forms of pathogenic dimorphic fungi are especially adapted to resist the natural defences that normally prevent fungal invasion. Acquired immunity is thus of major importance in limiting and eliminating infection with such organisms. *H. capsulatum, B. dermatitidis, C. immitis* and *P. brasiliensis* are the most commonly encountered dimorphic fungi.

HISTOPLASMOSIS

H. capsulatum is a soil organism which grows abundantly in the presence of bird droppings or bat guano. The organism is widely distributed throughout the USA (particularly in the mid-west), Central and South America and a number of African and Asian countries, but is rare in Europe and absent in Australasia. Infection occurs when microconidia are inhaled following the disruption of contaminated soil. These small spores can elude non-specific defence mechanisms in the respiratory tract and enter the alveoli, where germination occurs. Transition to the yeast phase results from the activation of temperature-dependent yeast-specific genes and is essential for virulence[251,252]. Following germination, the yeast phase of the organism invades locally and may disseminate via the lymphatic system to organs of the reticuloendothelial system. Almost all individuals living in an endemic area have been infected by adulthood, but in the majority this infection is subclinical: a positive skin test to histoplasmin or characteristic radiological changes are the only evidence of past infection. The spectrum of clinically apparent disease includes symptomatic acute pulmonary histoplasmosis (an acute febrile illness which may occur in normal individuals exposed to a heavy inoculum), chronic pulmonary histoplasmosis, and disseminated histoplasmosis, a potentially fatal complication of primary exposure that occurs in infants, immunosuppressed patients and occasionally in otherwise normal adults[253,254]. The incidence of disseminated histoplasmosis has risen dramatically in recent years due to the increased incidence in patients with HIV infection[98,99]. Reports of disseminated histoplasmosis in AIDS patients resident in non-endemic areas indicates that this can arise from reactivation of latent infection.

In experimental pulmonary histoplasmosis the earliest host tissue response to *H. capsulatum* consists of an infiltrate of neutrophils[255]. An influx of mononuclear cells soon follows, and later dominates the mixed inflammatory reaction. Despite this brisk inflammatory response significant numbers of *H. capsulatum* can be cultured from the lung 1 week after infection. By day 14, large numbers of lymphocytes appear within granulomas and this is associated with clearance of the organism. Although neutrophils may ingest and kill *H. capsulatum in vitro*[256,257], their role *in vivo* appears limited. In contrast, there is abundant evidence that acquired cellular immunity is the major form of defence against *H. capsulatum*. Individuals with defective cell-mediated immunity are particularly at risk of disseminated disease[98,99], whereas healthy individuals exposed to *H. capsulatum* develop positive histoplasmin skin-test reactions and active lymphocyte transformation responses to *Histoplasma* antigens *in vitro*, in the absence of symptoms[253,258]. Experimentally, immunity to histoplasmosis can be transferred by lymphoid cells from immunized animals[259], an effect which is abrogated by T cell depletion[260]. Transient protective immunity can also be conferred by administration of a CD4$^+$ T cell clone to athymic or irradiated mice[261]. The mechanisms of cell-mediated immunity are not fully understood, but the activated macrophage is thought to be the principal effector cell.

The fate of *H. capsulatum* within resting and activated macrophages has been studied in detail. In the early phases of infection macrophages bind to and phagocytose *H. capsulatum* yeasts but fail to kill them, providing a highly permissive intracellular environment for their multiplication[262]. Binding occurs via the CR3/LFA-1/p150,90 (CD18) family of leukocyte adherence-promoting glycoproteins, a mechanism that is independent of serum opsonins[263]. Once internalized, unactivated macrophages fail to develop fungicidal mechanisms as a result of the failure of *H. capsulatum* yeast cells to trigger superoxide release[264,265]. This may be due to the triggering of a specific phagocytic signal by the binding of *H. capsulatum* to CD18[263]. In contrast, macrophages from immune animals restrict the intracellular growth of *H. capsulatum*[266–268]. Recent studies indicate that lymphokines released from immune lymphocytes may mediate this effect[269]. In mice, IFN-γ activates macrophages and suppresses the intracellular growth of *H. capsulatum*[270]: this is associated with the stimulation of both oxidative and non-oxidative antifungal mechanisms[271,272]. In contrast, human macrophages activated with recombinant IFN-γ fail to affect intracellular *H. capsulatum*[273], although synergism with other cytokines was not evaluated in this study. Recent work suggests that TNF-α may also be important in the host response to *H. capsulatum*[71,271,272]: antibody against TNFα can accelerate the course of experimental histoplasmosis and increase the fungal load[274].

Specific antibody and complement appear not to play a major role in defence against *H. capsulatum*. Neither B cells[275] nor serum[276] from immune donors protect naive mice from infection. In man, disease progression has been associated with increasing complement-fixing antibody titres[277].

Suppression of cellular immunity by *H. capsulatum* has been documented in man and in animals. Anergy and reduced T cell responses to histoplasmin are common in individuals with disseminated disease, even where there is no pre-existing impairment of cellular immunity[22,102,258]. This is thought to arise primarily from the stimulation of populations of suppressor cells which down-regulate cellular immune responses[102,278]. Successful treatment is associated with a shift from dominant suppressor to helper T cell activity and recovery of T cell function[22].

Coccidioidomycosis

C. immitis is endemic in Southwestern USA, Mexico and parts of Central and South America. Most infections with this organism are benign and self-limited, but dissemination may occur and lead to serious disease. A higher incidence of invasive disease has been reported in members of dark-skinned races (in particular Filipino's, Hispanics and Blacks), in pregnant women, in individuals receiving corticosteroids or cytotoxic drugs, in patients undergoing haemodialysis and, recently, in AIDS patients[279–281]. Much of the information on the incidence of disseminated coccidioidomycosis comes from large surveys carred out in endemic areas in the first half of this century. From these data, the respective contributions of environmental exposure and inherent racial predisposition to the observed 175-fold greater incidence of dissemination in Filipinos over that observed in white Americans are unclear. Exposure to soil containing high concentrations of *C. immitis* certainly increases the risk of symptomatic and severe coccidioidomycosis independent of race[282]. The development of severe disease in pregnancy may be linked to a general suppression of cell-mediated immunity and changes in sex hormones that stimulate the growth of *C. immitis*[283].

C. immitis is a complex soil fungus that exists as arthroconidia-forming mycelia in its saprophytic state and as spherules and endospores in the parasitic tissue phase[281]. The immune response to *C. immitis* is similar to that against other virulent dimorphic fungi. An early neutrophil response fails to limit growth of the organism, and acquired cell-mediated immunity is needed to contain or eradicate foci of infection. The primary portal of entry of *C. immitis* is the lung. Inhaled arthroconidia enter alveoli, where they undergo multiple nuclear divisions to form large spherules containing many infective endospores. Rupture of the spherule leads to seeding of other areas, where the cycle is repeated. Each spherule has the potential to release hundreds of endospores, in contrast to most other yeast-like fungi infecting humans, which divide by budding to form single daughter cells.

Susceptibility to phagocytosis and phagocyte-killing mechanisms differs considerably between the various life cycle stages of *C. immitis*[284,285]. The initial polymorphonuclear infiltrate is probably attributable to the activation of complement by both the inhaled saprophytic form and the tissue invasive form of *C. immitis*[52,286]. The inhaled arthroconidia are small (2–5 μm) and can be ingested by phagocytic cells. Ingestion is limited, however, by the antiphagocytic properties of the hyphal outer wall layer, a sleeve of hydrophobic material (a remnant of the original hyphal wall) which partially encompasses arthroconidia[281]. Opsonization by immune serum enhances neutrophil phagocytosis but only marginally increases intracellular killing, despite activation of the respiratory burst[281,284]. In the absence of lymphokines macrophages ingest but are unable to kill arthroconidia due to defective phagolysosome fusion[287]. As natural defence mechanisms are only partially effective in suppressing germination of arthroconidia, spherule formation occurs.

Spherules are remarkably resistant to the effects of phagocytic cells. Not only is the 30–80 μm spherule too large to be engulfed, but its cell wall is thick and surrounded by a glycoprotein matrix that both resists intimate contact with neutrophils and protects against inhibitory or fungicidal substances[284]. The rupture of mature spherules and release of endospores, which may be facilitated by the production of proteinases[9], is associated with an intense neutrophilic response[288]. Newly released endospores are held together in packets by fibrillar material derived from the spherule cell wall[281]. These packets are resistant to phagocytosis due to their size and fibrillar coating. Later, when the endospores separate and the fibrillar material dissipates, susceptibility to phagocytosis increases. Levels of intracellular killing by unactivated cells are no greater than for arthroconidia, however. In one study, immunologically activated neutrophils were found to have enhanced antifungal activity against endospores but not against other forms of *C. immitis*[289]. Of interest in this regard is the recent demonstration that spherules are potent inducers of TNFα, a cytokine with known neutrophil activating properties[70].

C. immitis is highly immunogenic and induces a range of cellular and humoral immune responses, only some of which are protective. Although antibodies have opsonic activity *in vitro* there is no evidence that they have significant survival value to the host. Immune serum confers no protection against lethal infection by *C. immitis* in mice[290]. Moreover, progressive coccidioidomycosis in humans is strongly associated with increasing humoral responses, and recovery with diminishing complement fixation titres[291,292].

Primary asymptomatic infection is associated with the development of specific cellular immunity, while patients with disseminated disease often have absent or diminished T cell-mediated responses. Studies in experimental animals provide further evidence for a protective role of immune lymphocytes. Transfer of T cell-enriched lymphocyte populations from immune mice prevents lethal disease in non-immune recipients[290] and congenitally athymic mice are more susceptible than normal mice to infection[293]. The mechanism of protection by immune T cells has been investigated *in vitro*. Beaman and co-workers[294] showed that lymphocytes from immune mice enhance the activity of macrophages against endospores and arthroconidia by promoting phagolysosome fusion. Subsequently, this effect was shown to be mediated by a lymphokine(s) produced by Lyt-1$^+$Lyt-2$^-$ lymphocytes[287], and a similar increase in fungicidal activity has been observed in human monocytes activated with either IFN-γ or TNFα[295]. Incubation of murine peritoneal or alevolar macrophages with recombinant IFN-γ reproduces this effect[74].

Anergy is common in human and experimental disseminated coccidioidomycosis. One explanation is that exposure to high levels of coccidioidal antigens leads to predominant suppressor cell activity, and consequent depressed lymphocyte responses to *C. immitis*[296]. It is likely that macrophages as well as T cell populations are involved in this activity[297]. Serum mediated suppression has also been shown but the mechanism is not understood. Recovery from infection is associated with reversal of anergy.

Blastomycosis

B. dermatididis is the causative agent of blastomycosis, a fungal infection primarily involving the lungs but with a propensity for widespread dissemination, particularly to bone, skin and prostate[298]. Infection may be asymptomatic but how frequently this occurs is unknown. Distant involvement has been reported as a result of late reactivation, but this is controversial. Studies of the epidemiology and pathogenesis of blastomycosis have been hampered by difficulties in culturing the organism from the environment and by the poor sensitivity and specificity of skin testing with blastomycin. Areas of endemicity have largely been recognized by the incidence of reported cases of infection: most of these have been in rural North America.

The mechanisms of resistance to *B. dermatididis* are not clearly understood. The lesions of blastomycosis are characterized initially by a massive neutrophil influx, and later by suppurative necrosis and granuloma formation[299].

Non-specific defence mechanisms of neutrophils and alveolar macrophages appear to play an active, but limited role in containing infection. Intracellular and extracellular killing by human phagocytes has been studied in depth by Drutz and Frey[36]. Conidia, the infective particles of *B. dermatididis*, were found to be dramatically susceptible to non-specific host defences, a finding that may explain the relative rarity of blastomycosis as a clinical problem. They were readily phagocytosed by neutrophils, peripheral blood monocytes and monocyte-derived macrophages. In the presence of serum, divalent cations and complement, neutrophils killed approximately 50% of those ingested, predominantly by oxidative mechanisms. Peripheral blood monocytes were less active but macrophages killed 90% of ingested conidia: this killing can be enhanced by prior stimulation with lymphokines[300]. Conversion to the yeast form was associated with increased resistance to killing, possibly related to altered composition of the cell wall[301]. *B. dermatididis* yeasts are strongly chemotactic, a finding which accounts for the dense infiltrate of neutrophils in the initial tissue reaction. Two chemotactic factors have been identified: a soluble chemotaxin which directly stimulates the migration of neutrophils and monocytes[302], and an alkali-soluble cell wall fraction obtained from virulent strains of *B. dermatididis*[303]. *B. dermatididis* yeasts are generally too large to be ingested by neutrophils. However resistance to killing does not appear to be related to size, as strains of *B. dermatididis* small enough to be ingested generally survive despite evidence that phagocyte metabolic pathways are activated[36,304]. Yeasts too large to be ingested may be killed by external neutrophil attachment and degranulation, although most (80%) are not. Yeasts are also resistant to intracellular killing by monocytes and macrophages.

Ultimately, control of infection appears to require acquired cell-mediated immune mechanisms. Although patients with disseminated blastomycosis usually have no underlying immunodeficiency there is some evidence that immunosuppression by corticosteroids, haematological malignancy or HIV infection may increase susceptibility[101,298]. Athymic mice are more susceptible to infection with both conidia and yeasts than are immunocompetent animals[305]: reduced susceptibility to infection correlates with the development of cellular immune responses[306] and resistance can be transferred by T lymphocytes[307]. In man, macrophages from immune subjects have enhanced activity against *B. dermatididis* compared with those from non-immune subjects[308]. Concanavalin A-stimulated lymph node cells, supernatants from concanavalin A-stimulated spleen cells and recombinant IFN-γ activate tissue macrophages to kill *B. dermatididis in vitro*[309]. IFN-γ also activates neutrophils, producing increased antifungal activity[73]. Activated macrophages appear to kill *B. dermatididis* by a mechanism independent of products of the oxidative burst[309], whereas the enhanced capacity of activated neutrophils is due at least in part to increased oxidative killing mechanisms[73]. Untreated patients with severe blastomycosis are often anergic and their lymphocytes non-reactive, while treated patients generally have active T cell responses to *Blastomyces* antigens for up to 2 years following exposure[310-312]: induction of suppressor cell populations is thought to be the explanation[299].

Production of antibody is not thought to be an important aspect in immunity to this fungus. Experimental studies in mice fail to show a positive effect of antibody[306]. In man, serological testing has until recently been hampered by poor sensitivity and specificity. A newly developed, highly specific and sensitive enzyme immunoassay[313] has shown that active disease is associated with elevated antibody levels while recovery from infection is associated with falling titres[314].

Paracoccidioidomycosis

Paracoccidioidomycosis is a granulomatous disease caused by the dimorphic fungus *P. brasiliensis*, an organism limited in distribution to humid areas of Latin America. Within endemic areas skin test surveys suggest that exposure to *P. brasiliensis* is frequent, and that subclinical infection is the most common manifestation[315,316]. Clinical disease is found most frequently in adults, particularly in agricultural workers, and there is a pronounced predilection for males, despite an equal rate of skin positivity between the sexes[110,316]. These data suggest that hormonal factors play a significant role in the pathogenesis of paracoccidioidomycosis, and this is supported by the finding that an oestrogen, 17β-oestradiol, binds to a cytosolic receptor that inhibits mycelium-to-yeast transformation[317].

The lungs are the site of primary infection, although pulmonary disease is frequently inapparent. Dissemination may then occur to skin, mucous membranes, lymph nodes and other organs. Clinical infection is classified[318] as the chronic isolated organic form, which predominantly affects adult males and has a good prognosis, a chronic mixed form, with progressive involvement of two or more organs, and an acute or subacute progressive form, associated with rapid dissemination and a poor outcome and which generally affects younger individuals. Paracoccidioidomycosis has only rarely been reported in immunocompromised individuals, but in rats, malignancy has been shown to result in dissemination[319]. The organism may remain latent for long periods of time and only become clinically manifest many years after an infected individual has left an endemic area[320].

Infection is thought to arise following inhalation of spores which then germinate to form yeast cells. The initial tissue reaction is an alveolitis dominated by alveolar macrophages[321]. This is followed by a striking infiltrate of neutrophils and later by granuloma formation[49,322]. Reasons for the unusual neutrophil influx have been investigated. Activation of the alternative complement pathway by *P. brasiliensis* yeasts has been demonstrated, but this is not the only factor: mice deficient in complement still produce a neutrophilic tissue response to *P. brasiliensis*[49]. More importantly, macrophages exposed to *P. brasiliensis* secrete a low molecular weight protein (possibly interleukin 8) which induces an active chemotaxis of neutrophils *in vivo*[323]. Natural defence mechanisms are probably able to eradicate small numbers of inhaled spores, but fungicidal activity against the yeast form of *P. brasiliensis* is poor[2,324]. Although neutrophils phagocytose *P. brasiliensis* yeasts and trigger a respiratory burst, most ingested yeasts remain viable[325]. This intrinsic resistance of yeast cells to neutrophil killing mechanisms may be related to the high concentration of α1-3 glucan in the cell wall[326]. Mutant strains containing 1,3-mannan instead of α1-3 glucan are less resistant to killing by neutrophils *in vitro* and are unable to produce disease in experimentally infected animals.

Macrophages also ingest *P. brasiliensis* (particularly in the presence of opsonins) but again killing mechanisms fail: the organism survives and multiplies intracellularly[327]. This has been linked to a failure of phagolyso-some fusion, a mechanism of resistance found in other virulent fungi[328]. Exposure of macrophages to lymphocyte supernatants or to recombinant IFN-γ significantly enhances killing[324,327] by a mechanism which is apparently independent of the oxidative burst. NK cells may also play a role in limiting disease to the lung. Data are limited but in one study murine splenic cells with characteristics of NK cells inhibited the *in vitro* growth of *P. brasiliensis*[46].

The role of acquired immune mechanisms has not been fully determined. Both positive and negative effects of antibodies on host defence can be demonstrated. Although specific antibody has been shown to have opsonic properties *in vitro*[49], immune complexes containing specific antibody are postulated to be immunosuppressive[329]. Specific antibodies are preset in patients with paracoccidioidomycosis but they do not appear to have protective value[330]. In contrast, a correlation between cellular immune responses and resistance to infection has been established and possible mechanisms have been identified. Athymic mice are more susceptible than normal mice to infection with *P. brasiliensis*[322]. Human patients with acute progressive forms of paracoccidioidomycosis tend to have impaired cell-mediated immunity, as indicated by poorly reactive skin tests and impaired *in vitro* lymphocyte transformation to paracoccidioidin, whereas recovery from infection is generally associated with restoration of T cell function[107,318,331]. Patients with less severe forms of disease demonstrate a range of immunological reactivity. Altered ratios of T-helper to T-suppressor cells are associated with disseminated disease, a finding which may explain in part the immune depression exhibited by patients (reviewed in ref. 328).

References

1. Diamond RD. Fungal surfaces: Effects of interactions with phagocytic cells. Rev Infect Dis. 1988; 10: S428–S431.
2. Schaffner A, Davis CE, Schaffner T, Markert M, Douglas H, Braude AI. *In vitro* susceptibility of fungi to killing by neutrophil granulocytes discriminates between primary pathogenicity and opportunism. J Clin Invest. 1986; 78: 511–524.
3. Schaffner A, Douglas H, Braude AI. Selective protection against conidia by mononuclear and against mycelia by polymorphonuclear phagocytes in resistance to *Aspergillus*. J Clin Invest. 1982; 69: 617–631.
4. Diamond RD, Krzesicki R. Mechanisms of attachment of neutrophils to *Candida albicans* pseudohyphae in the absence of serum, and of subsequent damage to pseudohyphae by microbicidal processes of neutrophils *in vitro*. J Clin Invest. 1978; 61: 360–369.
5. Diamond RD, Clark RA. Damage to *Aspergillus fumigatus* and *Rhizopus oryzae* hyphae by oxidative and non-oxidative microbicidal products of human neutrophils *in vitro*. Infect Immun. 1982; 38: 487–495.
6. Rogers TJ, Balish E. Immunity to *Candida albicans*. Microbiol Rev. 1980; 44: 660–682.

7. Waldorf AR. Host-parasite relationship in opportunistic mycoses. *CRC Crit Rev Microbiol.* 1986; 13: 133–172.

8. Cole GT, Zhu S, Pan S, Yuan L, Kruse D, Sun SH. Isolation of antigens with proteolytic activity from *Coccidioides immitis.* Infect Immun. 1989; 57: 1524–1534.

9. Resnick S, Pappagianis D, McKerrow JH. Proteinase production by the parasitic cycle of the pathogenic fungus *Coccidioides immitis.* Infect Immun. 1987; 55: 2807–2815.

10. Salvin SB. Endotoxin in pathogenic fungi. J Immunol. 1952; 69: 89–99.

11. Tilden EB, Hatton EH, Freeman S, Williamson WM, Koenig VL. Preparation and properties of the endotoxins of *Aspergillus fumigatus* and *Aspergillus flavus.* Mycopathol Mycol Appl. 1961; 4: 325–346.

12. Chaudhary B, Singh B. Role of endotoxin of *Aspergillus fumigatus* in its pathogenicity. Mycosen. 1982; 26: 430–434.

13. Ray TL, Payne CD. Scanning electron microscopy of epidermal adherence and cavitation in murine candidiasis: a role for *Candida* acid proteinase. Infect Immun. 1988; 56: 1942–1949.

14. Borg M, Ruchel R. Expression of extracellular acid proteinase by proteolytic *Candida* spp. during experimental infection of oral mucosa. Infect Immun. 1988; 56: 626–631.

15. Waldorf AR, Diamond DR. Aspergillosis and mucormycosis. In: Cox RA, ed. Immunology of the Fungal Diseases. Boca Raton, Florida: CRC Press, 1989; 29–55.

16. Tang CM, Cohen J, Van Noorden S, Krausz T, Holden DW. The alkaline protease of *Aspergillus fumigatus* is not a virulence determinant in two murine models of invasive pulmonary aspergillosis. Infect Immun. 1993; 61: 1650–1656.

17. Müllbacher A, Waring P, Eichner RD. Identification of an agent in cultures of *Aspergillus fumigatus* displaying anti-phagocytic and immunomodulating activity *in vitro.* J Gen Microbiol. 1985; 131: 1251–1258.

18. Eichner RD, Al Salami M, Wood PR, Müllbacher A. The effect of gliotoxin upon macrophage function. Int J Immunopharmacol. 1986; 8: 789–797.

19. Robertson MD, Seaton A, Milne LJR, Raeburn JA. Suppression of host defences by *Aspergillus fumigatus.* Thorax. 1987; 42: 19–25.

20. Blackstock R, McCormack J, Hall NK. Induction of a macrophage-suppressive lymphokine by soluble cryptococcal antigens and its association with models of immunologic tolerance. Infect Immun. 1987; 55: 233–239.

21. Piccolella E, Lombardi G, Morelli R. Generation of suppressor cells in the response of human lymphocytes to a polysaccharide from *Candida albicans.* J Immunol. 1981; 126: 2151–2155.

22. Artz RP, Bullock WE. Immunoregulatory responses in experimental disseminated histoplasmosis: depression of T cell dependent and T effector responses by activation of splenic suppressor cells. Infect Immun. 1979; 23: 893–902.

23. Babior BM. Oxygen-dependent microbial killing by phagocytes (first of two parts). N Engl J Med. 1978; 298: 659–725.

24. Spitznagel JK, Shafer WM. Neutrophil killing of bacteria by oxygen-independent mechanisms: A historical summary. Rev Infect Dis. 1985; 7: 398–403.

25. Clark RA. The human neutrophil respiratory burst oxidase. J Infect Dis. 1990; 161: 1140–1147.

26. Lehrer RI, Ladra KM, Hake RB. Nonoxidative fungicidal mechanisms of mammalian granulocytes: demonstration of components with candidacidal activity in human, rabbit, and guinea pig leukocytes. Infect Immun. 1975; 11: 1226–1234.

27. Clarke RA. The human neutrophil respiratory burst. J Infect Dis. 1990; 161: 1140–1147.

28. Curnutte JT, Whitten DM, Babior BM. Defective superoxide production by granulocytes from patients with chronic granulomatous disease. N Engl J Med. 1974; 290: 593–597.

29. Segal AW. Absence of both cytochrome b_{245} subunits from neutrophils in X-linked chronic granulomatous disease. Nature. 1987; 326: 88–91.

30. Segal AW, Cross AR, Garcia RC, Borregaard N, Valerius NH, Soothill JF, Jones OTG. Absence of cytochrome b_{245} in chronic granulomatous disease. A multicenter European evaluation of its incidence and relevance. N Engl J Med. 1983; 308: 245–251.

31. Johnston RB, Newman SL. Chronic granulomatous disease. Pediatr Clin N Am. 1977; 24: 365–376.

32. Cohen MS, Isturiz RE, Malech HL, Root RK, Wilfert CM, Gutman L, Buckley RH. Fungal

infection in chronic granulomatous disease. The importance of the phagocyte in defense against fungi. Am J Med. 1981; 71: 59–66.

33. Levitz SM, Selsted ME, Ganz T, Lehrer RI, Diamond RD. *In vitro* killing of spores and hyphae of *Aspergillus fumigatus* and *Rhizopus oryzae* by rabbit neutrophil cationic peptides and bronchoalveolar macrophages. J Infect Dis. 1986; 154: 483–489.

34. Waldorf AR. Pulmonary defense mechanisms against opportunistic fungal pathogens. Immunol Ser. 1989; 47: 243–271.

35. Diamond RD, Krzesicki R, Jao W. Damage to pseudohyphal forms of *Candida albicans* neutrophils in the absence of serum in vitro. J Clin Invest. 1978; 61: 349–359.

36. Drutz DJ, Frey CL. Intracellular and extracellular defenses of human phagocytes against *Blastomyces dermatididis* conidia and yeasts. J Lab Clin Med. 1985; 105: 737–750.

37. Kalina M, Kletter Y, Shahar A, Arouson M. Acid phosphatase release from intact phagocytic cells surrounding a large size parasite. Proc Soc Exp Biol Med. 1971; 136: 407–410.

38. Howard DH. Mechanisms of resistance in the systemic mycoses. In: Nahmia AJ, O'Reilly RJ, eds. Comprehensive Immunology. Immunology of Human Infection Part 1. Bacteria, Mycoplasmae, Chlamydiae and Fungi. New York: Plenum, 1981: 475–494.

39. Cambridge G. Licensed to kill. Br Med J. 1986; 293: 904–905.

40. Jondal M. The human NK cell – a short overview and an hypothesis on NK recognition. Clin Exp Immunol. 1987; 70: 255–262.

41. Murphy JW, McDaniel DO. *In vitro* reactivity of natural killer (NK) cells against *Cryptococcus neoformans*. J Immunol. 1982; 128: 1577–1583.

42. Hidore MR, Murphy JW. Correlation of natural killer cell activity and clearance of *Cryptococcus neoformans* from mice after adoptive transfer of splenic nylon wool non-adherent cells. Infect Immun. 1986; 51: 547–555.

43. Nabavi N, Murphy JW. Antibody-dependent natural killer cell-mediated growth inhibition of *Cryptococcus neoformans*. Infect Immun. 1986; 51: 556–562.

44. Miller MF, Mitchell TG, Storkus WJ, Dawson JR. Human natural killer cells do not inhibit growth of *Cryptococcus neoformans* in the absence of antibody. Infect Immun. 1990; 58: 639–645.

45. Hidore MR, Murphy JW. Natural cellular resistance of beige mice against *Cryptococcus neoformans*. J Immunol. 1986; 137: 3624–3631.

46. Jimenez BE, Murphy JW. *In vitro* effects of natural killer cells against *Paracoccidioides brasiliensis* yeast phase. Infect Immun. 1984; 46: 552–558.

47. Kozel TR, Brown RR Pfrommer GST. Activation and binding of C3 by *Candida albicans*. Infect Immun. 1987; 55: 1890–1894.

48. Kozel TR, Wilson MA, Farrell TP, Levitz SM. Activation of C3 and binding to *Aspergillus fumigatus* conidia and hyphae. Infect Immun. 1989; 57: 3412–3417.

49. Calich VLG, Kipnis TL, Mariano M, Neto CF, Da Silva WD. The activation of the complement system by *Paracoccidioides brasilensis in vitro*; its opsonic effect and possible significance for an *in vivo* model of infection. Clin Immunol Immunopathol. 1979; 12: 20–30.

50. Kozel TR, Pfrommer GST. Activation of the complement system by *Cryptococcus neoformans* leads to binding of iC3b to the yeast. Infect Immun. 1986; 52: 1–5.

51. Griffin FM Jr. Roles of macrophage Fc and C3b receptors in phagocytosis of immunologically coated *Cryptococcus neoformans*. Proc Natl Acad Sci USA. 1981; 78: 3853–3857.

52. Galgiani JN, Yam P, Pretz LD, Williams PL, Stevens DA. Complement activation by *Coccidioides immitis*: *in vitro* and clinical studies. Infect Immun. 1980; 28: 944–949.

53. Kozel TR, McGaw TG. Opsonization of *Cryptococcus neoformans* by human immunoglobulin G: role of immunoglobulin G in phagocytosis by macrophages. Infect Immun. 1979; 25: 255–261.

54. Diamond RD, May JE, Kane M, Frank MM, Bennett JE. The role of late complement components and the alternate complement pathway in experimental cryptococcosis. Proc Soc Exp Biol Med. 1973; 144: 312–315.

55. Diamond RD, May JE, Kane M, Frank MM, Bennett JE. The role of classical and alternate pathways in host defenses against *Cryptococcus neoformans* infection. J Immunol. 1974; 112: 2260–2270.

56. Kozel TR, Highison B, Stratton C. Localisation on encapsulated *Cryptococcus neoformans* of serum components opsonic for phagocytosis by macrophages and neutrophils. Infect

Immun. 1984; 43: 574–579.
57. Levitz SM, Dibenedetto DJ. Differential stimulation of murine resident peritoneal cells by selectively opsonized encapsulated and acapsular *Cryptococcus neoformans*. Infect Immun. 1988; 56: 2544–2551.
58. Dromer F, Charreire J, Contrepois A, Carbon C, Yeni P. Protection of mice against experimental cryptococcosis by anti-*Cryptococcus neoformans* monoclonal antibody. Infect Immun. 1987; 55: 749–752.
59. Sanford JE, Lupan DM, Schlageter AM, Kozel TR. Passive immunization against *Cryptococcus neoformans* with an isotype-switch family of monoclonal antibodies reactive with cryptococcal polysaccharide. Infect Immun. 1990; 58: 1919–1923.
60. Diamond RD, Bennett JE. Prognostic factors in cryptococcal meningitis. A study in 111 cases. Ann Intern Med. 1974; 80: 176–181.
61. Pereira HA, Hosking CS. The role of complement and antibody in opsonization and intracellular killing of *Candida albicans*. Clin Exp Immunol. 1984; 57: 307–314.
62. Mourad S, Friedman L. Passive immunization of mice against *Candida albicans*. Sabouraudia. 1968; 6: 103–105.
63. Matthews RC, Burnie JP, Howat D, Rowland T, Walton F. Autoantibody to heat-shock protein 90 can mediate protection against systemic candidosis. Immuology. 1991; 74: 20–24.
64. Taschdjian CL, Seelig MS, Kozinn PJ. Serological diagnosis of candidal infections. CRC Crit Rev Clin Lab Sci. 1973; 4: 19–59.
65. Matthews RC, Burnie JP, Tabaqchali S. Immunoblot analysis of the serological response in systemic candidiasis. Lancet. 1984; ii: 1415–1418.
66. Matthews R, Burnie J, Smith D, Clark I, Midgley J, Conolly M, Gazzard B. *Candida* and AIDS: evidence for protective antibody. Lancet. 1988; ii: 263–266.
67. Matthews RC, Burnie JP, Tabaqchali S. Isolation of immunodominant antigens from sera of patients with systemic candidiasis and characterization of serological response to *Candida albicans*. J Clin Microbiol. 1987; 25: 230–237.
68. de Repentigny L. Serological techniques for diagnosis of fungal infection. Eur J Clin Microbiol Infect Dis. 1989; 8: 362–375.
69. de Repentigny LS. Serodiagnosis of candidiasis, aspergillosis, and cryptococcosis. Clin Infect Dis. 1992; 14: S11–22.
70. Slagle DC, Cox RA, Kuruganti U. Induction of tumor necrosis factor alpha by spherules of *Coccidioides immitis*. Infect Immun. 1989; 57: 1916–1921.
71. Smith JG, Graybill JR, Williams DM, Ahrens J. A role for tumor necrosis factor (TNF) in murine histoplasmosis? In: Twenty-ninth Interscience Conference on Antimicrobial Agents and Chemotherapy, 1989; 307.
72. Djeu JY, Blanchard DK, Richards AL, Friedman H. Tumor necrosis factor induction by *Candida albicans* from human natural killer cells and monocytes. J Immunol. 1988; 141: 4047–4052.
73. Morrison CJ, Brummer E, Stevens DA. *In vivo* activation of peripheral blood polymorphonuclear neutrophils by gamma interferon results in enhanced fungal killing. Infect Immun. 1989; 57: 2953–2958.
74. Beaman L. Fungicidal activation of murine macrophages by recombinant gamma interferon. Infect Immun. 1987; 55: 2951–2955.
75. Ferrante A. Tumor necrosis factor alpha potentiates neutrophil antimicrobial activity: increased fungicidal activity against Torulopsis glabrata and *Candida albicans* and associated increases in oxygen radical production and lysosomal enzyme release. Infect Immun. 1989; 57: 2115–2122.
76. Vecchiarelli A, Todisco T, Puliti M, dottorini M, Bistoni F. Modulation of anti-*Candida* activity of human alveolar macrophages by interferon-gamma or interleukin-1-alpha. Am J Resp Cell Mol Biol. 1989; 1; 49–55.
77. Djeu JY, Blanchard DK, Halkias D, Friedman H. Growth inhibition of *Candida albicans* by human polymorphonuclear neutrophils: activation by interferon-gamma and tumor necrosis factor. J Immunol. 1986; 137: 2980–2984.
78. Sugar AM, Field KG. Cytotoxic and cytostatic effects of recombinant tumor necrosis factor (rTNF) and *Blastomyces dermatididis*. Clin Res. 1986; 34: 534A.
79. Flesch IEA, Schwamberger G, Kaufmann SHE. Fungicidal activity of IFN-gamma-activated

macrophages. Extracellular killing of *Cryptococcus neoformans*. J Immunol. 1989; 142: 3219–3224.

80. Parant M, Parant F, Vinit M-A, Chedid L. Action protectrice du 'tumor necrosis factor' (TNF) obtenu par recombinaison genetique contre l'infection experimentale bacterienne ou fongique. C R Acad Sci Paris. 1987; 304: 1–4.

81. Van't Wout JW, Van der Meer JWM, Barza M, Dinarello CA. Protection of neutropenic mice from lethal *Candida albicans* infection by recombinant interleukin 1. Eur J Immunol. 1988; 18: 1143–1146.

82. Pecyk RA, Fraser-Smith EB, Matthews TR. Efficacy of interleukin-1B against systemic *Candida albicans* infection in normal and immunosuppressed mice. Infect Immun. 1989; 57: 3257–3258.

83. Roth FJ Jr., Goldstein MI. Inhibition of growth of pathogenic yeasts by human serum. J Invest Dermatol. 1961; 36: 383–387.

84. Louria DB, Smith JK, Brayton RG, Buse M. Anti-*Candida* factors in serum and their inhibitors. 1. Clinical and laboratory observations. J Infect Dis. 1972; 125: 102–114.

85. Baum GL, Artis D. Growth inhibition of *Cryptococcus neoformans* by cell free human serum. Am J Med Sci. 1961; 241: 613–616.

86. Gale GR, Welch AM. Studies of opportunistic fungi. 1. Inhibition of *Rhizopus oryzae* by human serum. Am J Med Sci. 1961; 241: 604–612.

87. Diamond RD. Immunology of invasive fungal infections. In: Nahmias AJ, O'Reilly RJ, eds. Comprehensive Immunology. Immunology of Human Infection Part 1. Bacteria, Mycoplasmae, Chlamydiae and Fungi. New York: Plenum; 1981: 585–633.

88. Elin RJ, Wolff SM. Effect of pH and iron concentration on growth of *Candida albicans* in human serum. J Infect Dis. 1973; 127: 705–712.

89. Artis WM, Fountain JA, Delcher HK, Jones HE. A mechanism of susceptibility to mucormycosis in diabetic ketoacidosis: transferrin and iron availability. Diabetes. 1982; 31: 1109–1111.

90. Caroline L, Taschdjian CL, Kozinn PJ, Schade AL. Reversal of serum fungistasis by the addition of iron. J Invest Dermatol. 1964; 42: 415–419.

91. Mandal B. AIDS and fungal infections. J Infect. 1989; 19: 199–205.

92. Editorial. Oral candidosis in HIV infection. Lancet. 1989; ii: 1491–1492.

93. Chuck SL, Sande MA. Infections with *Cryptococcus neoformans* in the acquired immuno-deficiency syndrome. N Engl J Med. 1989; 321: 794–799.

94. Zuger A, Louie E, Holzman RS, Simberkoff MS, Rahal JJ. Cryptococcal disease in patients with the acquired immunodeficiency syndrome. Diagnostic features and outcome of treatment. Ann Intern Med. 1986; 104: 234–240.

95. Kovacs JA, Kovacs AA, Polis M, Wright WC, Gill VJ, Tuazon CU, Gelmann ER, Lane HC, Longfield R, Overturf G, Macher AM, FAuci AS, Parillo JE, Bennett JE, Masur H. Cryptococcosis in the acquired immunodeficiency syndrome. Ann Intern Med. 1985; 103: 533–538.

96. Eng RHK, Bishburg E, Smith SM. Cryptococcal infections in patients with the acquired immune deficiency syndrome. Am J Med. 1986; 81: 19–23.

97. Wheat LJ, Connolly-Stringfield P, Kohler RB, Frame PT, Gupta MR. *Histoplasma capsulatum* polysaccharide antigen detection in diagnosis and management of disseminated histoplasmosis in patients with acquired immunodeficiency syndrome. Am J Med. 1989; 87: 396–145.

98. Johnson PC, Khardori N, Najjar AF, Butt F, Mansell PWA, Sarosi GA. Progressive disseminated histoplasmosis in patients with acquired immunodeficiency syndrome. Am J Med. 1988; 85: 152–158.

99. Huang CT, McGarry T, Cooper S, Saunders R, Andavolu R. Disseminated histoplasmosis in the acquired immunodeficiency syndrome. Report of five cases from a nonendemic area. Arch Intern Med. 1987; 147: 1181–1184.

100. Bronnimann DA, Adam RD, Galgiani JN, Habib MP, Petersen EA, Porter B, Bloom JW. Cociccidoidomycosis in the acquired immunodeficiency syndrome. Ann Intern Med. 1987; 106: 372–379.

101. Chiu J, Berman S, Tan G, Tilles J. Disseminated blastomycosis in HIV infected patients. Fourth International Conference on AIDS, 430.

102. Stobo JD, Paul S, Van Scoy RE, Hermans PE. Suppressor thymus-derived lymphocytes

in fungal infection. J Clin Invest. 1976; 57: 319–328.

103. Breen JF, Lee IC, Vogel FR, Friedman H. Cryptococcal capsular polysaccharide-induced modulation of murine immune responses. Infect Immun. 1982; 36: 47–51.

104. Blackstock R, Hall NK. Non-specific immunosuppression by *Cryptococcus neoformans* infection. Mycopathologia. 1984; 86: 35–43.

105. Murphy JW. Effects of first-order *Cryptococcus*-specific T-suppressor cells on induction of cells responsible for delayed-type hypersensitivity. Infect Immun. 1985; 48: 439–445.

106. Khakpour FR, Murphy JW. Characterization of a third-order suppressor T cell (Ts3) induced by cryptococcal antigen(s). Infect Immun. 1987; 55: 1657–1662.

107. Mok PWY, Greer DL. Cell-mediated immune responses in patients with paracoccidioido-mycosis. Clin Exp Immunol. 1977; 28: 89–98.

108. Gordon IJ, Evans CC. *Aspergillus* lung disease. J R Coll Physicians Lond. 1986; 20: 206–211.

109. Opal SM, Asp AA, Cannady PB Jr, Morse PL, Burton LJ, Hammer PG II. Efficacy of infection control measures during a nosocomial outbreak of disseminated aspergillosis associated with hospital construction. J Infect Dis. 1986; 153: 634–637.

110. Rippon JW. Medical Mycology. The Pathogenic Fungi and the Pathogenic Actinomycetes. 3rd Edn. Philadelphia: W.B. SAunders Co.

111. Warren RE, Warnock DW. Clinical manifestations and management of aspergillosis in the compromised patient. In: Warnock DW, Richardson MD, eds. Fungal Infection in the Compromised Patient. Chichester: John Wiley and Sons, 1982: 119–153.

112. Pepys J, Riddell RW, Citron KM, Clayton YM, Short EI. Clinical and immunological significance of *Aspergillus fumigatus* in the sputum. Am Rev Resp Dis. 1959; 80: 167–180.

113. Longbottom JL, Pepys J. Pulmonary aspergillosis: Diagnostic and immunological significance of antigens and C-substance in *Aspergillus fumigatus*. J Pathol Bacteriol. 1964; 88: 141–151.

114. Malo JL, Paquin R. Incidence of immediate sensitivity to *Aspergillus fumigatus* in a North American asthmatic population. Clin Allergy. 1979; 9: 377–384.

115. Mearns M, Longbottom J, Batten J. Precipitating antibodies to *Aspergillus fumigatus* in cystic fibrosis. Lancet. 1967; 1: 538–539.

116. Zeaske R, Bruns WT, Fink JN, Greenberger PA, Colby H, Liotta JL, Roberts M. Immune responses to *Aspergillus* in cystic fibrosis. J Allergy Clin Immunol. 1988; 82: 73–77.

117. Pepys J. Fungi in pulmonary allergic diseases. In: Nahmias AJ, O'Reilly RJ, eds. Comprehensive Immunology. Immunology of Human Infection Part 1. Bacteria, Mycoplasmae, Chlamydiae and Fungi. New York: Plenum. 1981: 561–584.

118. McCarthy DS, Pepys J. Allergic broncho-pulmonary aspergillosis. Clinical immunology: (1) Clinical features. Clin Allergy. 1971; 1: 261–286.

119. Henderson AH. Allergic aspergillosis: review of 32 cases. Thorax. 1968; 23: 501–512.

120. Vernon DRH, Allan F. Environmental factors in allergic bronchopulmonary aspergillosis. Clin Allergy. 1980; 10: 217–227.

121. Arruda LK, Platts-Mills TA, Longbottom JL, el-Dahr JM, Chapman MD. *Aspergillus fumigatus*: identification of 16, 18 and 45 kD antigens recognized by human IgG and IgE antibodies and murine monoclonal antibodies. J Allergy Clin Immunol. 1992; 89: 1166–76.

122. Latgé JP, Moutaouakil M, Debeaupuis JP, Bouchara JP, Haynes K, Prevost MC. The 18-kilodalton antigen secreted by *Aspergillus fumigatus*. Infect Immun. 1991; 59: 2586–2594.

123. Arruda LK, Platts-Mills TA, Fox JW, Chapman MD. *Aspergillus fumigatus* allergen I, a major IgE-binding protein, is a member of the mitogillin family of cytotoxins. J Exp Med. 1990; 172: 1529–1532.

124. Lamy B, Moutaouakil M, Latgé J-P, Davies J. Secretion of a potential virulence factor, a fungal ribonucleotoxin, during human aspergillosis infections. Mol Microbiol. 1991; 5: 1811–1815.

125. Wang JL, Patterson R, Rosenberg M, Roberts M, Cooper BJ. Serum IgE and IgG antibody activity against *Aspergillus fumigatus* as a diagnostic aid in allergic bronchopulmonary aspergillosis. Am Rev Resp Dis. 1978; 117: 917–927.

126. Malo JL, Longbottom J, Mitchell J, Hawkins R, Pepys J. Studies in chronic allergic bronchopulmonary aspergillosis: 3 Immunological findings. Thorax. 1977; 32: 269–274.

127. Schwartz HJ, Citron KM, Chester EH, Kaimal J, Barlow PB, Baum GL, Schuyler MR. A comparison of the prevalence of sensitization to *Aspergillus* antigens among asthmatics in Cleveland and London. J Allergy Clin Immunol. 1978; 62: 9–14.

128. Riddle HFV, Channell S, Blyth W, Weir DM, Lloyd M, Amos WMG, Grant IWB. Allergic alveolitis in a maltworker. Thorax. 1968; 23: 271–280.

129. British Tuberculosis Association. *Aspergillus* in persistent lung cavities after tuberculosis. Tubercle. 1968; 49: 1–11.

130. Karas A, Hankins JR, Attar S, Miller JE, McLaughlin JS. Pulmonary aspergillosis: an analysis of 41 patients. Ann Thorac Surg. 1976; 22: 1–7.

131. Eastridge CE, Young JM, Cole F, Gourley R, Pate JW. Pulmonary aspergillosis. Ann Thorac Surg. 1972; 13: 397–403.

132. Battaglini JW, Murray GF, Keagy BA, Starek PJK, Wilcox BR. Surgical management of pulmonary aspergilloma. Ann Thorac Surg. 1985; 39: 512–516.

133. Longbottom JL, Clive FT. Diagnostic precipitin test in aspergillus pulmonary mycetoma. Lancet. 1964; i: 588–589.

134. Binder RE, Faling J, Pugatch RD, Mahasaen C, Snider GL. Chronic necrotizing pulmonary aspergillosis: a discrete clinical entity. Medicine. 1982; 61: 109–124.

135. Diamond RD, Huber E, Haudenschild CC. Mechanisms of destruction of *Aspergillus fumigatus* hyphae mediated by human monocytes. J Infect Dis. 1983; 147: 474–483.

136. Denning DW, Follansbee SE, Scolaro M, Norris S, Edelstein H, Stevens DA. Pulmonary aspergillosis in the acquired immunodeficiency syndrome. New Engl J Med. 1991; 324: 654–662.

137. Minamoto GY, Barlam TF, Van der Els NJ. Invasive aspergillosis in patients with AIDS. Clin Infect Dis. 1992; 14: 66–74.

138. Karam GH, Griffin FM Jr. Invasive pulmonary aspergillosis in nonimmunocompromised, nonneutropenic hosts. Rev Infect Dis. 1986; 8: 357–363.

139. Fisher BD, Armstrong D, Yu B, Gold JWM. Invasive aspergillosis. Progress in early diagnosis and treatment. Am J Med. 1981; 71: 571–577.

140. Meyer RD, Young LS, Armstrong D, Yu B. Aspergillosis complicating neoplastic disease. Am J Med. 1973; 54: 6–15.

141. Young RC, Bennett JE, Vogel CL, Carbone PP, DeVita VT. Aspergillosis: the spectrum of the disease in 98 patients. Medicine. 1970; 49: 147–173.

142. Aisner J, Schimpff SC, Wiernik PH. Treatment of invasive aspergillosis: relation of early diagnosis and treatment to response. Ann Intern Med. 977; 86: 539–543.

143. Kan VL, Bennett JE. Lectin-like attachment sites on murine pulmonary alveolar macrophages bind *Aspergillus fumigatus* conidia. J Infect Dis. 1988; 158: 407–414.

144. Schaffner A, Douglas H, Braude AI, Davis CE. Killing of *Aspergillus* spores depends on the anatomical source of the macrophage. Infect Immun. 1983; 42: 1109–1115.

145. Waldorf AR, Levitz SM, Diamond RD. In vivo bronchoalveolar macrophage defense against *Rhizopus oryzae* and *Aspergillus fumigatus*. J Infect Dis. 1984; 150: 752–760.

146. Levitz SM, Diamond RD. Mechanisms of resistance of *Aspergillus fumigatus* conidia to killing by neutrophils *in vitro*. J Infect Dis. 1985; 152: 33–42.

147. Robertson MD, Raeburn JA, Gormley IP, Seaton A. Do phagocytic cells ingest spores of *Aspergillus fumigatus*? Thorax. 1985; 40: 237.

148. Stringer ML, Dean RA, Sewall TC, Timberlake WE. *Rodletless*, a new Aspergillus developmental mutant induced by directed gene inactivation. Genes Dev. 1991; 5: 1161–1171.

149. Cole GT, Sekiya T, Kasai R, Yokoyama T, Nozawa Y. Surface ultrastructure and chemical composition of the cell walls of conidial fungi. Exp Mycol. 1979; 3: 132–156.

150. Diamond RD. Fungal surfaces: effects of interactions with phagocytic cells. Rev Infect Dis. 1989; 10: S428–431.

151. Corbel MJ, Eades SM. Examination of the effect of age and acquired immunity on the susceptibility of mice to infection with *Aspergillus fumigatus*. Mycopathologia. 1977; 60: 79–85.

152. Corbel MJ, Eades SM. The relative susceptibility of New Zealand Black and CBA mice to infection with opportunistic fungal pathogens. Sabouraudia. 1976; 14: 17–32.

153. Williams DM, Weiner MH, Drutz DJ. Immunologic studies of disseminated infection with *A. fumigatus* in the nude mouse. J Infect Dis. 1981; 143: 726–733.

154. Monga DP. Studies on experimental aspergillosis in immunodeficient mice. Zentralbl Bakteriol Mikrobiol Hyg (A). 1983; 254: 552–560.
155. Matthews R, Burnie JP, Fox A, Tabaqchali S. Immunoblot analysis of serological responses in invasive aspergillosis. J Clin Pathol. 1985; 38: 1300–1303.
156. Burnie JP, Matthews RC. Recent laboratory observations in the diagnosis of systemic fungal infection: Candida and Aspergillus. In: Holmberg K, Meyer RD, eds. Diagnosis and Therapy of Systemic Fungal Infections. New York: Raven Press, 1989: 101–113.
157. Talbot GH, Weiner MH, Gerson SL, Provencher M, Hurwitz S. Serodiagnosis of invasive aspergillosis: validation of the Aspergillus fumigatus antigen radioimmunoassay. J Infect Dis. 1987; 155: 12–27.
158. Sabetta JR, Miniter P, Andriole VT. The diagnosis of invasive aspergillosis by an enzyme-linked immunosorbent assay for circulating antigen. J Infect Dis. 1985; 152: 946–953.
159. Rogers TR, Haynes KA, Barnes RA. Value of antigen detection in predicting invasive pulmonary aspergillosis. Lancet. 1990; 336: 1210–1213.
160. Benbow EW, Stoddart RW. Systemic zygomycosis. Postgrad Med J. 1986; 62: 985–996.
161. Lehrer RI, Howard DH, Sypherd PS, Edwards JE, Segal GP, Winston DJ. Mucormycosis. Ann Intern Med. 93: 93–108.
162. Gale GR, Welch AM. Studies of opportunistic fungi. I. Inhibition of Rhizopus oryzae by human serum. Am J Med Sci. 1961; 45: 604–612.
163. Eng RHK, Corrado M, Chin E. Susceptibility of zygomycetes to human serum. Sabouraudia. 1981; 19: 111–115.
164. Waldorf AR, Ruderman N, Diamond RD. Specific susceptibility to mucormycosis in murine diabetes and bronchoalveolar macrophage defense against Rhizopus. J Clin Invest. 1984; 74: 150–160.
165. Merkow L, Pardo M, Epstein SM, Verney E, Sidransky H. Lysosomal stability during phagocytosis of Aspergillus flavus spores by alveolar macrophages of cortisone-treated mice. Science. 1968; 160: 79–81.
166. Merkow LP, Epstein SM, Sidransky H, Verney E, Pardo M. The pathogenesis of experimental pulmonary aspergillosis. Am J Pathol. 1971; 62: 57–74.
167. Polli VC, Diekmann H, Kis Z, Ettlinger L. Uber das vorkommen ketonreduktasen bei mikroorganismen. Pathol Microbiol. 1965; 28: 93–98.
168. Goodill JJ, Abuelo JG. Mucormycosis – a new risk of deferoxamine therapy in dialysis patients with aluminium or iron overload. N Engl J Med. 1988; 317: 54.
169. Chinn RYW, Diamond RD. Generation of chemotactic factors by Rhizopus oryzae in the presence and absence of serum: relationship to hyphal damage mediated by human neutrophils and effects of hyperglycaemia and ketoacidosis. Infect Immun. 1982; 38: 1123–1129.
170. Corbel MJ, Eades SM. Experimental mucormycosis in congenitally athymic (nude) mice. Mycopathologia. 1977; 62: 117–120.
171. Corbel MJ, Eades SM. Factors determining the susceptibility of mice to experimental phycomycosis. J Med Microbiol. 1975; 8: 551–564.
172. Wysong DR, Waldorf AR. Electrophoretic and immunoblot analysis of Rhizopus arrhizus antigens. J Clin Microbiol. 1987; 25: 358–363.
173. Kaufman L, Turner LF, McLaughlin DW. Indirect enzyme-linked immunosorbent assay for zygomycosis. J Clin Microbiol. 1991; 27: 1979–1982.
174. Maksymiuk AW, Thongprasert S, Hopfer R, Luna M, Fainstein V, Bodey GP. Systemic candidiasis in cancer patients. Am J Med. 1984; 77: 20–27.
175. Wingard JR, Merz WG, Saral R. Candida tropicalis: a major pathogen in immunocompromised patients. Ann Intern Med. 1979; 91: 539–543.
176. Calderone RA, Scheld WM. Role of fibronectin in the pathogenesis of candidal infection. Rev Infect Dis. 1987; 9: S400–S403.
177. Sawyer RT, Horst MN, Garner RE, Hudson J, Jenkins PR, Richardson AL. Altered hepatic clearance and killing of Candida albicans in the isolated perfused mouse liver model. Infect Immun. 1990; 58: 2869–2874.
178. Hazen KC. Participation of yeast cell surface hydrophobicity in adherence of Candida albicans to human epithelial cells. Infect Immun. 1989; 57: 1894–1900.
179. Rotrosen D, Calderone RA, Edwards JE Jr. Adherence of Candida species to host tissues and plastic surfaces. Rev Infect Dis. 1986; 8: 73–85.

180. Magee BM, Hube B, Wright RJ, Sullivan PJ, Magee PT. The genes encoding the secreted aspartyl proteinases of *Candida albicans* constitute a family with at least three members. Infect Immun. 1993; 61: 3240–3243.

181. Sobel JD, Muller G, Buckley HB. Critical role of germ tube formation in the pathogenesis of candidal vaginitis. Infect Immun. 1984; 44: 576–580.

182. Kirkpatrick CH. Host factors in defense against fungal infections. Am J Med. 1984; 77: 1–12.

183. Lehner T, Wilton JMA, Ivanyi L. Immunodeficiencies in chronic muco-cutaneous candidosis. Immunology. 1972; 22: 775–787.

184. Ahonen P, Myllarniemi S, Sipila I, Perheentupa J. Clinical variation of autoimmune polyendocrinopathy–candidiasis–ectodermal dystrophy (APECED) in a series of 68 patients. N Engl J Med. 1990; 322: 1829–1836.

185. Edwards JE Jr. Candidaemia and *Candida* catheter-associated sepsis. In: Holmberg K, Meyer RD, eds. Diagnosis and Therapy of Systemic Fungal Infections. New York: Raven Press, 1989: 39–46.

186. Parker JC Jr, McCloskey JJ, Knauer KA. Pathobiologic features of human candidiasis. A common deep mycosis of the brain, heart and kidney in the altered host. Am J Clin Pathol. 1976; 65: 991–1000.

187. Bross J, Talbot GH, Maislin G, Hurwitz S, Strom BL. Risk factors for nosocomial candidaemia: a case-control study in adults without leukaemia. Am J Med. 1989; 87: 614–620.

188. Tashjian LS, Abramson JS, Peacock JE. Focal hepatic candidiasis: a distinct clinical variant of candidiasis in immunocompromised patients. Rev Infect Dis. 1984; 6: 689–703.

189. Thaler M, Pastakia B, Shawker TH, O'Leary T, Pizzo PA. Hepatic candidiasis in cancer patients: the evolving picture of the syndrome. Ann Intern Med. 1988; 108: 88–100.

190. Bodey GP, Anaissie EJ. Chronic systemic candidiasis. Eur J Clin Microbiol Infect Dis. 1989; 8: 855–857.

191. Domer JE, Carrow EW. Candidiasis. In: Cox RA, ed. Immunology of the Fungal Diseases. Boca Raton, Florida: CRC Press, 1989: 57–92.

192. Palma C, Serbousek D, Torosantucci A, Cassone A, Djeu JY. Identification of a mannoprotein fraction from *Candida albicans* that enhances human polymorphonuclear leukocyte (PMNL) functions and stimulates lactoferrin in PMNL inhibition of candidal growth. J Infect Dis. 1992; 166: 1103–1112.

193. Diamond G, Zasloff M, Eck H, Brasseur M, Lee Maloy W, Bevins CL. Tracheal antimicrobial peptide, a cysteine-rich peptide from mammalian tracheal mucosa: peptide isolation and cloning of a cDNA. Proc Natl Acad Sci USA. 1991; 88: 3952–3956.

194. Diamond G, Jones DE, Bevins CL. Airway epithelial cells are the site of expression of a mammalian antimicrobial peptide gene. Proc Natl Acad Sci USA. 1993; 90: 4596–4600.

195. Lehrer RI, Cline MJ. Interaction of *Candida albicans* with human leukocytes and serum. J Bacteriol. 1969; 98: 996–1004.

196. Lehrer RI. Measurement of candidacidal activity of specific leukocyte types in mixed cell populations. I. Normal, myeloperoxidase-deficient, and chronic granulomatous disease neutrophils. Infect Immun. 1970; 2: 42–47.

197. Lehrer RI. Measurement of candidacidal activity of specific leukocyte types in mixed cell populations. II. Normal and chronic granulomatous disease eosinophils. Infect Immun. 1971; 3: 800–802.

198. Wagner DK, Collins-Lech C, Sohnle PG. Inhibition of neutrophil killing of *Candida albicans* pseudohyphae by substances which quench hypochlorous acid and chloramines. Infect Immun. 1986; 51: 731–735.

199. Lehrer RI. The fungicidal activity of human monocytes: a myeloperoxidase-linked mechanism. Clin Res. 1971; 18: 408.

200. Marodi L, Korchak HM, Johnston RB Jr. Mechanisms of host defense against *Candida* species. I. Phagocytosis by monocytes and monocyte-derived macrophages. J Immunol. 1991; 146: 2783–2789.

201. Jupin C, Parant M, Chedid L. Involvement of reactive oxygen intermediates in the candidacidal activity of human neutrophils stimulated by muramyl dipeptide or tumor necrosis factor. Immunobiology. 1989; 180: 68–79.

202. Kullberg BJ, van't Wout HWM, van Furth R. Role of granulocytes in increased host

resistance to *Candida albicans* induced by recombinant interleukin-1. Infect Immun. 1990; 58: 3319–3324.

203. Stevenhagen A, van Furth R. Interferon-gamma activates the oxidative killing of *Candida albicans* by human granulocytes. Clin Exp Immunol. 1993; 91: 170–175.

204. Riipi L, Carlson E. Tumor necrosis factor (TNF) is induced in mice by *Candida albicans*: role of TNF in fibrinogen increase. Infect Immun. 1990; 58: 2750–2754.

205. Garner RE, Kuruganti U, Czarniecki CW, Chiu HH, Domer JE. In vivo immune responses to *Candida albicans* modified by treatment with recombinant murine gamma interferon. Infect Immun. 1989; 57: 1800–1808.

206. Diamond RD, Haudenschild CC. Monocyte-mediated serum-independent damage to hyphal and pseudohyphal forms of *Candida albicans in vitro*. J Clin Invest. 1981; 67: 173–182.

207. Denning TJV, Davies RR. *Candida albicans* and the chemotaxis of polymorphonuclear neutrophils. Sabouraudia. 1973; 11: 210–221.

208. Ferrante A, Thong YH. Requirement of heat-labile opsonins for maximal phagocytosis of *Candida albicans*. Sabouraudia. 1979; 17: 293–297.

209. Wilton JMA. The role of Fc and C3b receptors in phagocytosis by inflammatory polymorphonuclear leukocytes in man. Immunology. 1977; 32: 955–961.

210. Djeu JY, Liu JH, Wei S, Rui H, Pearson CA, Leonard WJ, Blanchard DK. Function associated with IL-2 receptor-beta on human neutrophils. Mechanism of activation of antifungal activity against *Candida albicans* by IL-2. J Immunol. 1993; 150: 960–970.

211. Moors MA, Stull TL, Blank KJ, Buckley HR, Mosser DM. A role for complement receptor-like molecules in iron acquisition by *Candida albicans*. J Exp Med. 1992; 175: 1643–1651.

212. Macdougall LG, Anderson R, McNab GM, Katz J. The immune response in iron-deficient children: impaired cellular defense mechanisms with altered humoral components. J Pediatr. 1975; 86: 833–843.

213. Enelow RI, Sullivan GW, Carper HT, Mandell GL. Cytokine-induced human multinucleated giant cells have enhanced candidacidal activity and oxidative capacity compared with macrophages. J Infect Dis. 1992; 166: 664–668.

214. Domer J, Elkins K, Ennist D, Baker P. Modulation of immune responses by surface polysaccharides of *Candida albicans*. Rev Infect Dis. 1988; 10: S419–S422.

215. Smail EH, Cronstein BN, Meshulam T, Esposito AL, Diamond RD. In vitro, *Candida albicans* releases the immune modulator adenosine and a second, high molecular weight agent that blocks neutrophil killing. J Immunol. 1992; 148: 3588–3595.

216. Vuddhakul K, Seow WK, McCormack JG, Thong YH. Direct modulation of human neutrophil behaviour by *Candida albicans*. Int Arch Allergy Appl Immunol. 1989; 90: 291–296.

217. Saxena A, Calderone R. Purification and characterization of the extracellular C3d-binding protein of *Candida albicans*. Infect Immun. 1990; 58: 309–314.

218. Eigentler A, Schulz TF, Larcher C, Breitwieser E-M, Myones BL, Petzer AL, Dierich MP. C3bi-binding protein on *Candida albicans*: temperature-dependent expression and relationship to human complement receptor type 3. Infect Immun. 1989; 57: 616–622.

219. Gilmore BJ, Retsinas EM, Lorenz JS, Hostetter MK. An iC3b receptor on *Candida albicans*: structure, function and correlates for pathogenicity. J Infect Dis. 1988; 157: 38–46.

220. Diamond RD, Oppenheim F, Nakagawa Y, Krzesicki R, Haudenschild CC. Properties of a product of *Candida albicans* hyphae and pseudohyphae that inhibits contact between the fungi and human neutrophils *in vitro*. J Immunol. 1980; 125: 2797–2804.

221. Rogers TJ, Balish E. Effect of systemic candidiasis on blastogenesis of lymphocytes from germfree and conventional rats. Infect Immun. 1978; 20: 142–150.

222. Wilson DE, Bennett JE, Bailey JW. Serologic grouping of *Cryptococcus neoformans*. Proc Soc Exp Biol Med. 1968; 127: 820–823.

223. Ikeda R, Shinoda T, Fukazawa Y, Kaufman L. Antigenic characterization of *Cryptococcus neoformans* serotypes and its application to serotyping of clinical isolates. J Clin Microbiol. 1982; 16: 22–29.

224. Kwon-Chung KJ, Bennett JE, Rhodes JC. Taxonomic studies on *Filobasidiella* species and their anamorphs. Antonie van Leeuwenhoek. 1982; 48: 25–38.

225. Ellis DH, Pfeiffer TJ. Natural habitat of *Cryptococcus neoformans* var *gatti*. J Clin Microbiol. 1990; 28: 1642–1644.
226. Kwon-Chung KJ, Bennett JE. Epidemiologic differences between the two varieties of *Cryptococcus neoformans*. Am J Epidemiol. 1984; 120: 123–130.
227. Atkinson AJ Jr, Bennett JE. Experience with a new skin test antigen prepared from *Cryptococcus neoformans*. Am Rev Resp Dis. 1968; 97: 637–643.
228. Kerkering TM, Duma RJ, Shadomy S. The evolution of pulmonary cryptococcosis. Clinical implications from a study of 41 patients with and without compromising host factors. Ann Intern Med. 1981; 94: 611–616.
229. Igel HJ, Bolande RP. Humoral defense mechanisms in cryptococcosis: substances in normal human serum, saliva, and cerebrospinal fluid affecting the growth of *Cryptococcus neoformans*. J Infect Dis. 1966; 116: 75–83.
230. Kwon-Chung KJ, Rhodes JC. Encapsulation and melanin formation as indicators of virulence in *Cryptococcus neoformans*. Infect Immun. 1986; 51: 218–223.
231. Polacheck I, Platt Y, Aronovitch J. Catecholamines and virulence of *Cryptococcus neoformans*. Infect Immun. 1990; 58: 2919–2922.
232. Granger DL, Perfect JR, Durack DT. Virulence of *Cryptococcus neoformans*. Regulation of capsule synthesis by carbon dioxide. J Clin Invest. 1985; 76: 508–516.
233. Diamond RD, Root RK, Bennett JE. Factors influencing killing of *Cryptococcus neoformans* by human leukocytes *in vitro*. J Infect Dis. 1972; 125: 367–376.
234. Kozel TR, Gotschlich EC. The capsule of *Cryptococcus neoformans* passively inhibits phagocytosis of the yeast by macrophages. J Immunol. 1982; 129: 1675–1680.
235. Kozel TR, Hermerath CA. Binding of cryptococcal polysaccharide to *Cryptococcus neoformans*. Infect Immun. 1984; 43: 879–886.
236. Gadebusch HH. Mechanisms of native and acquired resistance to infection with *Cryptococcus neoformans*. CRC Crit Rev Microbiol. 1972; 1: 311–320.
237. Lehrer RI, Ladra KM. Fungicidal components of mammalian granulocytes active against *Cryptococcus neoformans*. J Infect Dis. 1977; 136: 96–99.
238. Kozel TR, Pfrommer GST, Redelman D. Activated neutrophils exhibit enhanced phagocytosis of *Cryptococcus neoformans* opsonized with normal human serum. Clin Exp Immunol. 1987; 70: 238–246.
239. Mitchell TG, Friedman L. In vitro phagocytosis and intracellular fate of variously encapsulated strains of *Cryptococcus neoformans*. Infect Immun. 1972; 5: 491–498.
240. Levitz SM, Farrell TP. Growth inhibition of *Cryptococcus neoformans* by cultured human monocytes: role of the capsule, opsonins, the culture surface and cytokines. Infect Immun. 1990; 58: 1201–1209.
241. Cameron ML, Granger DL, Weinnberg JB, Kozumbo WJ, Koren HS. Human alveolar and peritoneal macrophages mediate fungistasis independently of L-arginine oxidation to nitrite or nitrate. Am Rev Resp Dis. 1990; 142: 1313–1319.
242. Davies SF, Clifford DP, Hoidal JR, Repine JE. Opsonic requirements for the uptake of *Cryptococcus neoformans* by human polymorphonuclear leukocytes and monocytes. J Infect Dis. 1982; 145: 870–874.
243. Diamond RD, Erickson NF III. Chemotaxis of human neutrophils and monocytes induced by *Cryptococcus neoformans*. Infect Immun. 1982; 38: 380–382.
244. Mukherjee J, Pirofski LA, Scharff MD, Casadevall A. Antibody-mediated protection in mice with lethal intracerebral *Cryptococcus neoformans* infection. Proc Natl Acad Sci USA. 1993; 90: 3636–3640.
245. Cauley LK, Murphy JW. Response of congenitally athymic (nude) and phenotypically normal mice to *Cryptococcus neoformans* infection. Infect Immun. 1979; 23: 644–651.
246. Lim TS, Murphy JW. Transfer of immunity to cryptococcosis by T-enriched splenic lymphocytes from *Cryptococcus neoformans* sensitized mice. Infect Immun. 1980; 30: 5–11.
247. Fung PYS, Murphy JW. In vitro interactions of immune lymphocytes and *Cryptococcus neoformans*. Infect Immun. 1982; 36: 1128–1138.
248. Karaoui RM, Hall NK, Larsh HW. Role of macrophages in immunity and pathogenesis of experimental cryptococcosis induced by the airborne route – Part II: Phagocytosis and intracellular fate of *Cryptococcus neoformans*. Mycosen. 1977; 20: 409–422.
249. Diamond RD, Bennett JE. Disseminated cryptococcosis in man: decreased lymphocyte transformation in response to *Cryptococcus neoformans*. J Infect Dis. 1973; 127: 694–697.

250. Murphy JW. Influence of cryptococcal antigens on cell-mediated immunity. Rev Infect Dis. 1988; 10: S432–S435.
251. Medoff G, Kobayashi GS, Painter A, Travis S. Morphogenesis and pathogenicity of *Histoplasma capsulatum*. Infect Immun. 1987; 55: 1355–1358.
252. Keath EJ, Painter AA, Kobayashi GS, Medoff G. Variable expression of a yeast-phase-specific gene in *Histoplasma capsulatum* strains differing in thermotolerance and virulence. Infect Immun. 1989; 57: 1384–1390.
253. Goodwin RA Jr, Des Prez RM. Histoplasmosis. Am Rev Resp Dis. 1978; 117: 929–956.
254. Sathapatayavongs B, Batteiger BE, Wheat J, Slama TG, Wass JL. Clinical and laboratory features of disseminated histoplasmosis during two large urban outbreaks. Medicine. 1983; 62: 263–270.
255. Baughman RP, Kim CK, Vinegar A, Hendricks DE, Schmidt DJ, Bullock WE. The pathogenesis of experimental pulmonary histoplasmosis. Correlative studies of histopathology, bronchoalveolar lavage, and respiratory function. Am Rev Resp Dis. 1986; 134: 771–776.
256. Howard DH. Fate of *Histoplasma capsulatum* in guinea pig polymorphonuclear leukocytes. Infect Immun. 1973; 8: 412–419.
257. Schnur RA, Newman SL. The respiratory burst response to *Histoplasma capsulatum* by human neutrophils. Evidence for intracellular trapping of superoxide anion. J Immunol. 1990; 144: 4765–4772.
258. Cox RA. Immunologic studies of patients with histoplasmosis. Am Rev Resp Dis. 1979; 120: 143–149.
259. Tewari RP, Sharma D, Solotorovsky M, Lafemina R, Balint J. Adoptive transfer of immunity from mice immunized with ribosomes or live yeast cells of *Histoplasma capsulatum*. Infect Immun. 1977; 15: 789–795.
260. Tewari RP, Sharma DK, Mathur A. Significance of thymus-derived lymphocytes in immunity elicited by immunization with ribosomes or live yeast cells of *Histoplasma capsulatum*. J Infect Dis. 1978; 138: 605–613.
261. Allendoerfer R, Magee DM, Deepe GS Jr, Graybill JR. Transfer of protective immunity in murine histoplasmosis by a CD4+ T-cell clone. Infect Immun. 1993; 61: 714–718.
262. Howard DH. Intracellular behaviour of *Histoplasma capsulatum*. J Bacteriol. 1964; 87: 33–38.
263. Newman SL, Bucher C, Rhodes J, Bullock WE. Phagocytosis of *Histoplasma capsulatum* yeasts and microconidia by human cultured macrophages and alveolar macrophages. J Clin Invest. 1990; 85: 223–230.
264. Eissenberg LG, Goldman WE. *Histoplasma capsulatum* fails to trigger release of superoxide from macrophages. Infect Immun. 1987; 55: 29–34.
265. Kurita N, Terao K, Brummer E, Ito E, Nishimura K, Miyaji M. Resistance of *Histoplasma capsulatum* to killing by human neutrophils. Evasion of oxidative burst and lysosomal-fusion products. Mycopathologia. 1991; 115: 207–213.
266. Hill GA, Marcus S. Study of cellular mechanisms in resistance to systemic *Histoplasma capsulatum* infection. J Immunol. 1960; 85: 6–13.
267. Howard DH. Further studies on the inhibition of *Histoplasma capsulatum* within macrophages from immunized animals. Infect Immun. 1973; 8: 577–581.
268. Howard DH, Otto V, Gupta RK. Lymphocyte-mediated cellular immunity in histoplasmosis. Infect Immun. 1971; 4: 605–610.
269. Wu-Hsieh B, Zlotnik A, Howard DH. T-cell hybridoma-produced lymphokine that activates macrophages to suppress intracellular growth of *Histoplasma capsulatum*. Infect Immun. 1984; 43: 380–385.
270. Wu-Hsieh B, Howard DH. Inhibition of the intracellular growth of *Histoplasma capsulatum* by recombinant murine gamma interferon. Infect Immun. 1987; 55: 1014–1016.
271. Wolf JE, Massof SE. *In vivo* activation of macrophage oxidative burst activity by cytokines and amphotericin B. Infect Immun. 1990; 58: 1296–1300.
272. Wolf JE, Abegg AL, Travis SJ, Kobayashi GS, Littli JR. Effects of *Histoplasma capsulatum* on murine macrophage functions: inhibition of macrophage priming, oxidative burst, and antifungal activities. Infect Immun. 1989; 57: 513–519.
273. Fleischman J, Wu-Hsieh B, Howard DH. The intracellular fate of *Histoplasma capsulatum* in human macrophages is unaffected by recombinant human inteferon-gamma. J Infect

Dis. 1990; 161: 143–145.

274. Wu-Hsieh BA, Lee GS, Franco M, Hofman FM. Early activation of splenic macrophages by tumor necrosis factor alpha is important in determining the outcome of experimental histoplasmosis in mice. Infect Immun. 1992; 60: 4230–4238.

275. Khardori N, Chaudhary S, McConnachie P, Tewari RP. Characterization of lymphocytes responsible for protective immunity to histoplasmosis in mice. Mycosen. 1983; 26: 523–532.

276. Taylor ML, Diaz S, Gonzalez PA, Sosa AC, Toriello C. Relationship between pathogenesis and immune regulation mechanisms in histoplasmosis: a hypothetical approach. Rev Infect Dis. 1984; 6: 775–782.

277. Wheat LJ, French MLV, Kohler RB, Zimmerman SE, Smith WR, Norton JA, Eitzen HE, Smith CD, Slama TG. The diagnostic laboratory tests for histoplasmosis. Analysis of experience in a large urban outbreak. Ann Intern Med. 1982; 97: 680–685.

278. Nickerson DA, Havens RA, Bullock WE. Immunoregulation in disseminated histo-plasmosis: characterization of splenic suppressor cell populations. Cell Immunol. 1981; 60: 287–297.

279. Drutz DJ, Catanzaro A. Coccidioidomycosis. Part II. Am Rev Resp Dis. 1978; 117: 727–771.

280. Ampel NM, Wieden MA, Galgiani JN. Coccidioidomycosis: Clinical update. Rev Infect Dis. 1989; 11: 897–911.

281. Drutz DJ, Huppert M. Coccidioidomycosis: factors affecting the host-parasite interaction. J Infect Dis. 1983; 147: 372–390.

282. Larsen RA, Jacobson JA, Morris AH, Benowitz BA. Acute respiratory failure caused by primary pulmonary coccidioidomycosis. Two case reports and review of the literature. Am Rev Resp Dis. 1988; 131: 797–799.

283. Drutz DJ, Huppert M, Sun SH, McGuire WL. Human sex hormones stimulate the growth and maturation of Coccidioides immitis. Infect Immun. 1981; 32: 897–907.

284. Frey CL, Drutz DJ. Influence of fungal surface components on the interaction of Coccidioides immitis with polymorphonuclear neutrophils. J Infect Dis. 1986; 153: 933–943.

285. Galgiani JN. Inhibition of different phases of Coccidioides immitis by human neutrophils or hydrogen peroxide. J Infect Dis. 1986; 153: 217–222.

286. Galgiani JN, Isenberg RA, Stevens DA. Chemotaxigenic activity of extracts from the mycelial and spherule phases of Coccidioides immitis for human polymorphonuclear leukocytes. Infect Immun. 1978; 21: 862–865.

287. Beaman L, Benjamini E, Pappagianis D. Activation of macrophages by lymphokines: enhancement of phagosome-lysosome fusion and killing of Coccidioides immitis. Infect Immun. 1983; 39: 1201–1207.

288. Huppert M, Sun SH, Gleason-Jordan I, Vukovich KR. Lung weight parallels disease severity in experimental coccidioidomycosis. Infect Immun. 1976; 14: 1356–1368.

289. Brummer E, Beaman L, Stevens DA. Killing of endospores, but not arthroconidia, of Coccidioides immitis by immunologically activated polymorphonuclear neutrophils. In: Einstein HE, Catanzaro A, eds. Coccidioidomycosis – Proceedings of the 4th International Conference. Washington DC: National Foundation for Infectious Diseases, 1985: 201–213.

290. Beaman L, Pappagianis D, Benjamini E. Mechanisms of resistance to infection with Coccidioides immitis in mice. Infect Immun. 1979; 23: 681–685.

291. Forbus WD, Besterbreurtje AM. Coccidioidomycosis: a study of 95 cases of the disseminated type with special reference to the pathogenesis of the disease. Mil Surg. 1946; 99: 653–719.

292. Drutz DJ, Catanzaro A. Coccidioidomycosis. Part 1. Am Rev Resp Dis. 1978; 117: 559–585.

293. Beaman L, Pappagianis D, Benjamini E. Significance of T cells in resistance to experimental coccidioidomycosis. Infect Immun. 1977; 17: 580–585.

294. Beaman L, Benjamini E, Pappagianis D. Role of lymphocytes in macrophage-induced killing of Coccidioides immitis in vitro. Infect Immun. 1981; 34: 347–353.

295. Beaman L. Effects of recombinant gamma-interferon and tumor necrosis factor on in vitro interactions of human mononuclear phagocytes with Coccidioides immitis. Infect Immun. 1991; 59: 4227–4229.

296. Cox RA. Immunosuppression by cell wall antigens of *Coccidioides immitis*. Rev Infect Dis. 1988; 120: S415–S418.

297. Catanzaro A. Suppressor cells in coccidioidomycosis. Cell Immunol. 1981; 64: 235–245.

298. Sarosi GA, Davies SF. Blastomycosis. Am Rev Resp Dis. 1979; 120: 911–938.

299. Deepe GS Jr, Taylor CL, Bullock WE. Evolution of inflammatory response and cellular immune responses in a murine model of disseminated blastomycosis. Infect Immun. 1985; 50: 183–189.

300. Brummer E, Hanson LH, Stevens DA. Kinetics and requirements for activation of macrophages for fungicidal activity: effect of protein synthesis inhibitors and immunosuppressants on activation and fungicidal mechanism. Cell Immunol. 1991; 132: 236–245.

301. Kanetsuna F, Carbonell LM. Cell wall composition of the yeastlike and mycelial forms of *Blastomyces dermatitidis*. J Bacteriol. 1971; 106: 946–948.

302. Thurmond LM, Mitchell TG. *Blastomyces dermatididis* chemotactic factor: kinetics of production and biological characterization evaluated by a modified neutrophil chemotaxis assay. Infect Immun. 1984; 46: 87–93.

303. Cox RA, Mills LR, Best GK, Denton JF. Histologic reactions to cell walls of an avirulent and a virulent strain of *Blstomyces dermatididis*. J Infect Dis. 1974; 129: 179–186.

304. Sixbey JW, Fields BT, Sun CN, Clark RA, Nolan CM. Interactions between human granulocytes and *Blastomyces dermatididis*. Infect Immun. 1979; 23: 41–44.

305. Frey CL, DeMarsh PL, Drutz DJ. Divergent patterns of pulmonary blastomycosis induced by conidia and yeasts in athymic and euthymic mice. Am Rev Resp Dis. 1989; 140: 118–124.

306. Morozumi PA, Brummer E, Stevens DA. Protection against pulmonary blastomycosis: correlation with cellular and humoral immunity in mice after subcutaneous nonlethal infection. Infect Immun. 1982; 37: 670–678.

307. Brummer E, Morozumi PA, Vo PT, Stevens DA. Protection against pulmonary blastomycosis: adoptive transfer with T lymphocytes, but not serum, from resistant mice. Cell Immunol. 1982; 73: 349–359.

308. Bradsher RW, Ulmer WC, Marmer DJ, Townsend JM, Jacobs RF. Intracellular growth and phagocytosis of *Blastomyces dermatididis* by monocyte-derived macrophages from previously infected and normal subjects. J Infect Dis. 1985; 151: 57–64.

309. Brummer E, Stevens DA. Fungicidal mechanisms of activated macrophages: evidence for nonoxidative mechanisms for killing of *Blastomyces dermatididis*. Infect Imun. 1987; 55: 3221–3224.

310. Smith DT. Immunologic types of blastomycosis: a report on 40 cases. Ann Intern Med. 1949; 31: 463–469.

311. Bradsher RW. Development of specific immunity in patients with pulmonary or extrapulmonary blastomycosis. Am Rev Resp Dis. 1984; 129: 430–434.

312. Klein BS, Bradsher RW, Vergeront JM, Davis JP. Development of long-term specific cellular immunity after acute *Blastomyces dermatitidis* infection: assessments following a large point-source outbreak in Wisconsin. J Infect Dis. 1990; 161: 97–101.

313. Klein BS, Kuritsky JN, Chappell WA, Kaufman L, Green J, Davies SF, Williams JE, Sarosi GA. Comparison of the enzyme immunoassay, immunodiffusion and complement fixation tests in detecting antibody in human serum to the A antigen of *Blastomyces dermatididis*. Am Rev Resp Dis. 1986; 133: 144–148.

314. Klein BS, Vergeront JM, Kaufman L, Bradsher RW, Kumar UN, Mathai G, Varkey B, Davis GP. Serological tests for blastomycosis: assessment during a large point-source outbreak in Wisconsin. J Infect Dis. 1987; 155: 262–268.

315. Restrepo MA. The ecology of *Paracoccidioides brasiliensis*: a puzzle still unsolved. Sabouraudia. 1985; 23: 323–334.

316. Restrepo MA, Robledo VM, Ospina CA, Restrepo IM, Correa LA. Distribution of paracoccidioidin sensitivity in Colombia. Am J Trop Med Hyg. 1968; 17: 25–37.

317. Restrepo A, Salazar ME, Cano LE, Stover EP, Feldman D, Stevens DA. Estrogens inhibit mycelium-to-yeast transformation in the fungus *Paracoccidioides brasiliensis*: implications for resistance of females to paracoccidioidomycosis. Infect Immun. 1984; 46: 346–353.

318. Mota NGS, Rezkallah-Iwasso MT, Peracoli MTS, Audi RC, Mendes RP, Marcondes J, Marques SA, Dillon NL, Franco MF. Correlation between cell-mediated immunity and clinical forms of paracoccidioidomycosis. Trans R Soc Trop Med Hyg. 1988; 79: 765–772.

319. Sugar AM, Restrepo A, Stevens DA. Paracoccidioidomycosis in the immunosuppressed host: report of a case and review of the literature. Am Rev Resp Dis. 1984; 129: 340–342.
320. Ajello L, Polonelli L. Imported paracoccidioidomycosis: a public health problem in non-endemic areas. Eur J Epidemiol. 1988; 1: 160–165.
321. Mackinnon JE. Pathogenesis of South American blastomycosis. Trans R Soc Trop Med Hyg. 1959; 53: 487–494.
322. Robledo MA, Graybill JR, Ahrens J, Restrepo A, Drutz DJ, Robledo M. Host defense against experimental paracoccidioidomycosis. Am Rev Resp Dis. 1982; 125: 563–567.
323. Calich VLG, Coppi Vaz CA, Burger E. PMN chemotactic factor produced by glass-adherent cells in the acute inflammation caused by *Paracoccidioides brasiliensis*. Br J Exp Pathol. 1985; 66: 57–65.
324. Brummer E, Hanson LH, Restrepo A, Stevens DA. *In vivo* and *in vitro* activation of pulmonary macrophages by IFN-gamma for enhanced killing of *Paracoccidioides brasiliensis* or *Blastomyces dermatididis*. J Immunol. 1988; 140: 2786–2789.
325. Goihman-Yahr M, Essenfeld-Yahr E, De Albornoz MC, Varzabal L, De Gomez MH, San Martin B, Ocanto A, Gil F, Convit J. Defect of *in vitro* digestive ability of polymorpho-nuclear leukocytes in paracoccidioidomycosis. Infect Immun. 1980; 28: 557–566.
326. San-Blas G, San-Blas F, Serrano LE. Host–parasite relationships in the yeastlike form of *Paracoccidioides brasiliensis* strain IVIC Pb9. Infect Immun. 1971; 15: 343–346.
327. Brummer E, Hanson LH, Restrepo A, Stevens DA. Intracellular multiplication of *Paracoccidioides brasiliensis* in macrophages: killing and restriction of multiplication by activated macrophages. Infect Immun. 1989; 57: 2289–2294.
328. Jimenez-Finkel B, Restrepo-Moreno A. Paracoccidioidomycosis. In: Cox RA, ed. Immunology of the Fungal Diseases. Boca Raton, Florida: CRC Press, 1989: 227–247.
329. Arango M, Oropeza F, Anderson O, Contreras C, Bianco N, Yarzabal L. Circulating immune complexes and *in vitro* cell reactivity in paracoccidioidomycosis. Mycopathologia. 1982; 79: 153–158.
330. Correa LA, Giraldo MR. Study of immune mechanisms in paracoccidioidomycosis I. Changes in immunoglobulins (IgG, IgM and IgA). Proc First Pan Am Symp. 1972; 254: 245–250.
331. Restrepo A, Restrepo M, de Restrepo F, Aristizabal LH, Moncada LH, Velez H. Immune responses in paracoccidioidomycosis. A controlled study of 16 patients before and after treatment. Sabouraudia. 1978; 16: 151–163.

4
The Immune Response to Virus Infection

A. A. NASH and J. G. P. SISSONS

INTRODUCTION

Viruses are obligate intracellular pathogens and the capacity to resist them is critically important to all multicellular organisms. This requirement to resist intracellular pathogens has been a particular force in the evolution of the vertebrate immune system: equally the study of the immune response to viruses has led to many advances in understanding basic mechanisms of the immune response.

The host response to virus infection can be considered under the headings of natural or non-specific and innate resistance, and specific inducible immunity (Table 1).

NATURAL AND NON-SPECIFIC RESISTANCE

A number of mechanisms operate within the first few hours of a virus infection, before the induction of specific immunity, which do not depend

Table 1 Host defence against viral infection – three phases

Phase	Characteristics	Mechanisms
Immediate ($<4\,h$)	Non-specific, innate No memory No specific T cells	Natural killer cells Lack of cell receptors
Early (4–96 h)	Non-specific, inducible No memory No specific T cells	Interferons (IFN) α and β IFN-activated NK cells
Late ($>96\,h$)	Specific, inducible Memory Specific T cells	Specific antibody Cytotoxic T cells

on conventional immunological memory or display particular specificity. Although most attention has centred on the specific immune response, it is now recognized that these non-specific types of resistance to virus infection are probably of considerable importance, at least for certain virus infections.

Natural killer (NK) cells may affect resistance to certain viruses. This class of cytotoxic lymphocyte binds to and kills virus-infected and tumour-derived cells *in vitro*. They are spontaneously cytotoxic and do not show immunological memory, nor do they have surface T cell markers or rearranged T cell receptor genes. NK cells express CD16 (the CD16 molecule is an Fc receptor – FcγRIII) and are derived from bone marrow (it should however be noted that some CD3$^+$ T cells can also mediate non-MHC restricted cytotoxicity, particularly when treated *in vitro* with interleukin-2 (IL-2). These are sometimes called lymphokine activated killer (LAK) cells. The cytotoxicity of NK cells is enhanced by interferons (IFN) and IL-2; they thus not only participate in immediate, innate resistance but also in early non-specific inducible (by IFN) resistance. The receptor through which NK cells recognize their targets and the ligand on their target cells for any such receptor are not yet fully defined. Although virus-infected cells show increased susceptibility to lysis by NK cells there is no evidence that virally encoded proteins themselves are target structures. There is evidence for an inverse correlation between expression of Class I major histocompatibility complex (MHC) molecule expression on cells and their susceptibility to lysis by NK cells – in this context it is noteworthy that an increasing number of viruses are being reported to decrease expression of surface Class I MHC molecules by a variety of mechanisms. In addition to their role in enhancing the cytotoxicity of NK cells, IFNs can also protect uninfected cells from NK-mediated lysis: this may possibly be mediated by the ability of IFN to increase the expression of Class I MHC antigens by a direct effect on their transcription. All these observations have led to the hypothesis that there are two types of receptor on NK cells capable of mediating activation and recognition, and that these have opposite functions when bound to their ligands on target cells. The candidate molecules have been identified in the mouse, both encoded in a gene complex on mouse chromosome 6 (the NK gene complex). These are the NKR-P1 molecule which may activate NK cells through recognition of the target cell ligand, and the Ly-49 molecule which may recognize target cell MHC molecules and transmit negative signals which inhibit NK cytotoxicity. Both are integral membrane proteins, and sequence analysis has shown them to be members of the C-type lectin supergene family. It thus seems likely we will soon know more of the mechanism of NK cell recognition in mice and humans[1]. It should be noted that this same class of CD16$^+$ cells is also the principal effector cell mediating antibody-dependent cellular cytotoxicity (ADCC), but in this case the NK cells recognize their target cells by virtue of their Fc receptor engaging with antibody bound to viral determinants on the cell surface.

The role of NK cells in experimental virus infections has been studied by depletion and adoptive transfer, and by using the beige strain of mice which have a genetic defect resulting in diminished function of NK but not T cells, although only a limited number of virus infections have been studied in this model. Depletion of NK cells in neonatal mice by administration of antibody to the glycolipid asialo-GM1, or infection of the beige strain, results in increased susceptibility to murine cytomegalovirus (CMV) infection but not infection with other viruses, such as lymphocytic choriomeningitis virus. The adoptive transfer of cloned NK cells reverses this increased susceptibility[2]. In humans, a single NK cell-deficient patient with recurrent severe herpes virus infections (including CMV) has been reported[3]; however the fact that there is only this single case report, and that this subject did not apparently suffer any problems until her teens makes it doubtful whether true genetic deficiency of NK cells in humans has yet been described.

It is surmised that NK cells may represent a primitive type of cellular immunity, and be an evolutionary forerunner of specific cytotoxic T cells[4].

Interferons are also involved in non-immunologically specific resistance to virus infection[5]. There are three types of IFN: α ('leukocyte') IFN is encoded by a family of some 20 genes on human chromosome 9; β ('fibroblast') IFN is encoded by a single gene also on chromosome 9; and γ ('immune' or Type II) IFN is encoded by a single gene on chromosome 12. Transcription of IFN is induced by virus infections – viruses probably interfere with the synthesis of labile repressors of IFN gene transcription. When released from virus-infected cells IFN confers an antiviral state on other cells by a process involving new protein synthesis. In addition to being induced by viruses, double-stranded RNA also induces IFN release and IFNγ is produced by T cells whenever they are activated by antigens or mitogens.

The exact mechanism by which IFNs induce the antiviral state remains uncertain, but is usually associated with the inhibition of virus mRNA translation and involves the induction of cellular gene expression by turning on transcription. IFN-inducible genes contain specific IFN response sequences (IRS) in their promoter/regulatory regions; there are different IRS for IFNα and β and for IFNγ. Transcription of IFN-inducible genes is mediated by DNA binding proteins ('IFN regulatory factors') which are themselves IFN inducible. Specific candidate mechanisms for the induction of the antiviral state include the induction of the enzyme 2'5'-oligoadenylate synthetase and production of an RNAse, and induction of a 67 kD protein kinase which inhibits protein initiation factor. A rather special case is the Mx gene, which was first identified in strains of mice resistant to influenza virus. Transcription of this gene is induced by IFNα and β, but not γ, and directly by virus infection. The Mx protein inhibits primary transcription of influenza virus genes, but confers no resistance against other viruses.

IFN have many other biological effects, besides the antiviral action for which they were first described and named, particularly growth regulatory actions. It is now recognized that IFNγ is more properly regarded as an interleukin or cytokine[6]: it is a product of activated T cells and is the major macrophage activating factor, besides having effects on terminal B and T cell differentiation. It also induces Class II MHC expression on many cell types (all IFNs increase Class I MHC expression). Another cytokine, tumour necrosis factor α (TNFα), has also recently been described as having an antiviral effect which is synergistic with that of IFNs.

IFNs have found limited therapeutic use in humans as antivirals – they

Table 2 Possible mechanisms of antibody and complement mediated neutralization of viruses

---

1. Antibody inhibits binding to a cellular receptor.
   Antibody allows attachment but blocks penetration.
   Antibody allows penetration but inhibits uncoating.
   Antibody allows uncoating but inhibits a later function.

2. Antibody mediates agglutination/aggregation of virus particles.

3. Antibody and complement inhibits binding to cell receptors.
   Antibody and complement mediates lysis of enveloped viruses–virolysis.

---

have dose-related and limiting side-effects of malaise and fatigue. IFNα is used to treat chronic hepatitis B infection and may lead to viral clearance: however it is uncertain how much of its effect is due to a direct action and how much T cell mediated through induction of MHC expression on hepatocytes. IFN are also used in humans for cancer therapy, particularly treatment of hairy cell leukaemia.

Macrophages also show 'innate resistance'. For some viruses certain mouse strains display resistance *in vivo* which correlates with susceptibility of their macrophages and other cells to infection *in vitro* (e.g. mouse hepatitis virus, murine cytomegalovirus). This resistance maps to non-H2 genes and, in the case of murine CMV, to a gene on chromosome 6 designated CMV1, which interestingly is linked to the NK gene complex[7]. Resistance due to the genetically determined absence of virus receptors has also been postulated but not convincingly shown. Most genetic resistance to virus infection operates through genes which regulate the immune response, in particular the MHC genes (see below).

ROLE OF ANTIBODY AND COMPLEMENT IN VIRUS INFECTIONS

Antibodies play an important role in protection against virus infection. Generally speaking, their main contribution is in prevention of reinfection. However, even during the primary infection, where viruses may spread locally from one cell type to another, or during viraemia, antibody can play a decisive role in the control and resolution of the infection.

Antibody molecules produced in response to virus infection display a variety of effector functions, including neutralization of infectious virions and the destruction of virus-infected cells via complement-mediated lysis and ADCC. Macrophages are also involved in opsonizing virus particles via Fc receptors and restricting virus replication. However, this mode of entry into a cell can prove advantageous to some viruses, notably the flaviviruses and lentiviruses, whose infectivity is enhanced by low, sub-neutralizing, concentrations of specific antibody – a process known as antibody-dependent enhancement (ADE) of virus infection[8].

One of the most effective functions of antibody is neutralization of virus infectivity. This process can occur in a variety of ways (Table 2). Neutralization by blocking the binding of the virus to specific cell receptors is possibly the most important mechanism. The inactivation of picornaviruses, orthomyxoviruses and retroviruses has been widely studied. In the case of rhinoviruses (members of the picornaviruses) or poliovirus, major neutralization epitopes map to the rim of canyons or pits on the viral capsid, which are the sites for binding to cellular receptors, such as ICAM-1 for rhinovirus and the poliovirus receptor (members of the immunoglobulin super gene family)[11]. Antibodies binding to the rim will therefore inhibit this process. The same principle holds for glycoproteins on enveloped viruses, such as gP-120 of human immunodeficiency virus (HIV)[12] or haemagglutinin of influenza A[13]; antibodies to these block binding to CD4 or sialic acid residues on cell membranes respectively. Neutralization via this mechanism is highly effective, although there are pitfalls. The highly selective nature of antibodies for these regions on the virus, can lead to selection for viruses that escape neutralization. This process is seen in nature with antigenic drift in influenza A viruses and the lentiviruses – HIV, visna and equine infectious anaemia[14,15]. Similar strategies are employed by rhinoviruses and coxsackieviruses, where multiserotypes exist that vary in their antigenicity at regions on the rim of canyons or pits[16].

In another form of antibody-mediated neutralization, the virus–antibody complex may bind to the cell membrane but fail to become internalized; penetration is therefore blocked. In this instance the antibody would interfere with the 'zipper' mechanism, thus preventing endocytosis. Examples include poliovirus and influenza. In other circumstances the virus–antibody complex may become internalized but uncoating, which is required in order to release nucleic acid, is blocked. An example of this mechanism is West Nile virus (a flavivirus), whose normal uncoating by fusion with the vesicle is blocked[17]. These and other processes have been reviewed elsewhere[18,19].

Neutralization is clearly the most effective mechanism operating on the mucosal surfaces, where local IgA is observed to be an important outer defence system. Local immunity is activated in respiratory and gut infections and correlates with prevention of reinfection with viruses such as influenza, polio and rotavirus.

The Fc region of immunoglobulin molecules increases the effector activity of antibodies to include complement and Fc receptor-bearing (FcR) cells. Initially, antibodies may be of low affinity and have weak neutralizing activity. The activation of the complement system can act in synergy with such antibodies to bring about the neutralization of viruses. This process is best illustrated using monoclonal antibodies which will only neutralize virus in the presence of complement. One mechanism involves the activation of complement which rapidly coats the virion surface and thus blocks attachment to cellular receptors. In the case of some enveloped viruses, such as Sindbis virus, Sendai virus and rubella, activation of the membrane attack complex of complement can lead to perforation of the virion membrane, a process known as virolysis (reviewed in ref. 20). In some experimental situations, complement alone, in the absence of antibody, may become activated by viral glycoproteins, resulting in neutralization. An example is the activation of human complement by p15E of murine leukaemia virus[21]. This viral protein activates the classical pathway of complement via C1q, which progresses to virolysis. Sindbis virus is an example of a virus that can activate either the classical or alternative complement pathways[22].

The significance of these events *in vivo* are sometimes difficult to evaluate. Administration of cobra venom factor to mice, in order to exhaust endogenous C3 activity, has little effect on the resolution of many virus infections studied. One exception is Sindbis virus infection: increased viraemia is observed in C3-depleted mice compared to undepleted animals[22]. However, this is only a transient affect. Other evidence from natural complement deficiency states in man and animals has indicated that such individuals are not prone to severe virus infections[23].

So far we have considered the action of antibodies and complement on the virion. As obligate intracellular pathogens, virus-infected cells clearly become a major target for attack by antibody and complement. In general, antibodies are less effective against infected cells, although they can interfere with the egress of virus from an infected cell and can also block virus-induced cell fusion. A high density of membrane-bound antibody (approximately 5×10^6 IgG molecules/cell) is required for complement-mediated lysis of measles virus-infected cells. Interestingly, lysis occurred following the activation of the alternative complement pathway[24]. Such a mechanism is likely to be effective late in the virus life cycle in a cell, and therefore may not influence the spread of virus locally. ADCC is more efficient, requiring relatively small amounts of antigen: a concentration of 10^3 viral antigen molecules on the membrane is required to mediate cell killing. NK or K cell recognition of IgG (via the FcγRIII (CD16) receptor) mediates lysis of infected cells by a perforin-dependent mechanism[25]. Macrophages and neutrophils are also highly efficient in killing virus infected cells in the presence of antibody.

The relative contribution of each mechanism to protection against or recovery from virus infection *in vivo* has to some extent been dissected using monoclonal antibodies. Antibodies that neutralize viruses *in vitro* are also protective when administered experimentally to mice. The fact that neutralization is a major mechanism in protection is demonstrated using F(ab)$_2$ or F(ab) fragments directed against the F protein of respiratory syncytial virus, which are able to block ongoing virus infection in the lung by inhibiting the fusogenic properties of the F protein[26]. Non-neutralizing monoclonal antibodies against some viruses, such as herpes simplex, can also protect against infection when passively injected into mice. The mechanism of protection is not attributed to complement, since protection is seen in C5-deficient animals, but implicates ADCC (reviewed in ref. 27).

In Sindbus virus infection of the nervous system, both neutralizing and non-neutralizing antibodies can dramatically inhibit growth of the neurone-tropic virus in neurones. The mechanism of recovery *in vivo* does not correlate with levels of complement or ADCC, and evidence from infection of neurone cultures *in vitro* suggests that antibody interaction with viral glycoprotein on the plasma membrane is sufficient to induce a protective response in the neurone[28]. Precisely what effect this interaction has on intracellular virus replication is far from clear.

Not all encounters between virus and antibody necessarily lead to protection: some may eventually favour the persistence of virus or an increased viral pathogenicity.

The fluidity of viral protein in a cell membrane can lead to capping when antibody is present. This phenomenon has been well studied with measles-infected HeLa cells, in which capping of the HN complex led to the persistence of virus intracellularly. Indeed, prolonged exposure of the infected cells to antibody leads to a reduction in measles virus matrix protein expression, leading to intracellular expression of viral antigens only[29]. This experimental system bears striking similarities to subacute sclerosing panencephalitis (SSPE), a disease in which measles-like virus persists in neurones, eventually destroying these cells and leading to the death of the infected individual.

As mentioned earlier, the uptake of virus–antibody complexes via Fc receptors on macrophages can lead to an enhanced infection of these cells by flaviviruses such as dengue virus. Experimental evidence from monkeys given subneutralizing doses of dengue-2 virus antisera and the virus showed increased viraemia compared with monkeys receiving the virus only (reviewed in ref. 30).

Such examples, clearly highlight the adaptive value of viruses in the face of the immune system. The more 'simple' RNA viruses rely on mutational changes at key antigenic sites to evade recognition by antibodies, whereas more complex DNA viruses, such as herpes simplex virus, encode glyco-proteins with Fc receptor (gE–gI) or complement (gC) binding activities, an activity that has probably evolved to interfere with the function of these host effector mechanisms.

T CELL IMMUNITY TO VIRUSES

Despite the obvious value of antibody in the immune response to viruses, the absence of antibody/immunoglobulin molecules in immunodeficiency states such as agammaglobulinaemia does not predispose the host to severe or life-threatening viral infections. Such individuals cope adequately with, for example, measles or herpes simplex virus infection. This contrasts with the situation in T cell immunodeficiency states such as Di George syndrome (congenital absence of the thymus) or in nude athymic mice, where infections are more severe and life-threatening. Cutaneous infection with herpes simplex virus in the nude mice results in a spreading lesion, with the virus travelling deep into the nervous system: the animals die by the second week after infection. Although passive neutralizing antibodies may delay this process, it is the adoptive transfer of HSV-specific T cells that protects the mice, resolving the infection[31].

T cells exhibit a variety of functions in virus infections. Most of the antibody response is thymus-dependent, requiring the presence of CD4[+] T cells for class switching and affinity maturation. CD4[+] T cells also act to help in the induction of cytotoxic T cell responses and in the recruitment and activation of macrophages at sites of virus production. CD4[+] T cells may also participate directly in cytolytic reactions if viral antigen is presented on MHC Class II molecules. Class II killers, as they are sometimes called, have been demonstrated during measles virus infection and efficiently kill measles virus-infected target cells *in vitro*[32]. Such killer cells have also been seen in infections with other viruses, including herpes simplex virus[33] and influenza virus[34].

The usual mechanism for presenting foreign antigens on MHC Class II molecules involves endocytosis and lysosomal degradation of proteins to generate peptides which can then associate with Class II molecules en route to the plasma membrane. Dendritic cells, macrophages and B lymphocytes are important in this process. The latter can select antigens specifically via antibody on the cell surface, leading to receptor-mediated endocytosis, with subsequent processing and presentation by MHC Class II. This process can offer the B lymphocyte distinct advantages in acquiring T cell help. For example, an antibody with specificity for the haemagglutinin of influenza virus can lead to the internalization of the whole virus, with degradation of haemagglutinin and other viral antigens such as matrix protein and neuraminidase. These proteins can all be presented by the B cell and may lead to interactions with T cells specific for any of these influenza virus proteins. Thus a B cell specific for haemagglutinin can receive help from a T cell specific for the M protein. This form of cognate interaction has been referred to as intermolecular–intrastructural help[35].

Clearly, some viruses are able to infect antigen-presenting cells directly, bypassing the exogenous antigen processing machinery. This raises the question whether other pathways exist for virus antigens to interact with MHC Class II molecules. Recent evidence from measles virus infection has suggested alternative pathways, where viral peptides may interact with Class II molecules en route to the cell surface[36,37].

CD4[+] T cell killing is clearly restricted to cell types expressing Class II molecules. A more efficient surveillance system involves the recognition of MHC Class I antigens by T cells. In recent years a great deal of knowledge has accumulated on the processes involved in the presentation of viral antigens via MHC Class I molecules. In brief, following a virus infection and the production of viral proteins, cytoplasmic catabolic processes, including levels of proteosomes, are increased, leading to degradation of viral proteins, predominantly to nonamer peptides. These enter the endoplasmic reticulum via peptide transporters (part of the ABC system of ATP-dependent peptide transport) and interact with the Class I heavy chain. This process stabilizes heavy and light chain (β_2-microglobulin) association. This remarkable process can involve any viral protein, provided there is selectivity by the MHC and to some extent by the peptide transporters. In this way it is easy to see how viral nuclear proteins, such as immediate early gene products of murine or human CMV, can be recognized[38,39]. Indeed, the ability of the T cell to recognize early viral antigens implies that an infected cell can be killed before new progeny are assembled. A feature of this T cell recognition system is the dominance of certain peptide–MHC combinations. For example, the dominant (80%) CD8[+] T cell response to murine CMV infection of Balb/c mice is directed to a pentapeptide in pp89 (an immediate early protein)[40]. This is quite remarkable when one considers the antigenic complexity of murine CMV, which has more than 100 potential gene products.

The importance of CD8[+] T cell–MHC Class I interaction in the immune response to virus infections has been illustrated in a number of ways and with a variety of viruses. Depletion of CD8[+] T cells can lead to more severe (sometimes lethal) infection; adoptive transfer of immune CD8[+] T cells accelerates recovery from a primary infection or protects the host from a lethal infection; and CD8[+] T cells isolated from infected tissues show lytic activity to virus-infected target cells *in vitro*. Virus infections in which these observations are particularly relevant, largely because they have been well studied, include influenza A, respiratory syncytial virus, cytomegalovirus and lymphocytic choriomeningitis virus (LCMV).

A wealth of evidence *in vitro* suggests that the anti-viral action of CD8[+] T cells is most probably exerted via cell killing. The lytic event probably involves perforin or the generation of lymphotoxin. Whether this accounts for the resolution of a viral infection *in vivo* is unclear; other factors, including cytokines such as IFNγ may also be involved.

In some viral infections the contribution of CD4[+] T cells to recovery is probably more significant than that of CD8[+] T cells. This is particularly true for some picornavirus infections and in cutaneous herpes simplex virus infection. In infection of mice with Theiler's virus (a murine picornavirus), depletion of CD4[+] cells leads to an overwhelming and fatal infection. The mechanism here almost certainly involves the generation of virus-specific antibodies which are involved in restricting the viral spread[41]. In contrast, the depletion of CD8[+] T cells in this virus–host system does not greatly affect the survival of the host[42]. In the case of cutaneous herpes simplex virus infections, CD4[+] T cells are also actively involved in virus clearance, even in the absence of antiviral antibodies or CD8[+] T cells. The mechanism of antiviral immunity probably involves the activation of macrophages by IFNγ[43]. Several experiments have shown that macrophages are potent inhibitors of herpes simplex virus function. This is achieved at various levels: direct killing of virus infected cells, the local production of IFNα and β, the production of arginase which depletes arginine, an essential amino acid for virus replication, and endocytosis and restriction of virus replication by intracellular killing mechanisms[44].

The significance of CD4[+] T cells in viral immunity was further highlighted in experiments on mice lacking the gene for β_2 microglobulin, which have no functional MHC Class I molecules, or those lacking CD8[+] cells (so called gene 'knock-out' mice), produced by a process involving homologous recombination. In both situations CD4[+] T cells substituted for the absent CD8[+] T cells and controlled influenza and Sendai infections, which are normally resolved by CD8[+] cytotoxic T cells[45]. This demonstrates the adaptive value of the T cell response and implies that a strict regulation of effector function is operating during normal immune responses.

Clearly, both the major subsets of $\alpha\beta$ T cells are involved in antiviral immunity to varying degrees. The nature of the virus, its route of entry and spread may determine the nature of the T cell response evoked and the magnitude of that response. This is highlighted in LCMV infection of the central nervous system, where CD8[+] T cells damage the brain, resulting in death[46]. Examples of CD4[+] T cell immunopathology include ocular damage following HSV infection and pneumonia following influenza or respiratory syncytial virus (RSV) infection.

γ/δ T cells have also been identified in the lungs of influenza virus- and RSV-infected mice. However, their significance in antiviral immunity is far from clear. In both of these acute infections the suggestion is that γ/δ T cells do not contribute to virus clearance[47,48]. However, their role in chronic/persistent viral infections or other mucosal infections, e.g. of the gut, have still to be determined. They may serve an immunoregulatory role, inhibiting or down-regulating an α/β T cell response.

References

1. Yokoyama WM, Seaman WE. Ly-49 and NKR-P1 gene families encoding lectin like receptors on NK cells. Annu Rev Immunol. 1993; 11: 613–636.
2. Bukowski JF, Warner JF, Dennert G, Welsh RM. Adoptive transfer studies demonstrating the antiviral effects of NK cells *in vivo*. J Exp Med. 1985; 161: 40–52.
3. Biron CA, Byron KS, Sullivan JS. Severe herpes virus infections in an adolescent without natural killer cells. N Engl J Med. 1989; 320: 1731–1735.
4. Janeway CA. A primitive immune system. Nature. 1989; 351: 108.
5. Joklik WK. Interferons. In: Fields BN, Knipe DM, eds. Virology. New York: Raven Press, 1990; 384–410.
6. Farrar AR, Schreiber R. The molecular cell biology of IFNγ and its receptor. Annu Rev Immunol. 1993; 11: 571.
7. Scalzo AA, Fitzgerald NA, Wallace CR, Gibbons AE, Smart YC, Burton RC, Shellam GR. The effect of the Cmv-1 gene, which is linked to the natural killer cell gene complex, is mediated by NK cells. J Immunol. 1992; 149: 581–589.
8. Porterfield JS. Antibody dependent enhancement of viral infectivity. Adv Virus Res. 1986; 31: 335–355.
9. Greve JM, David G, Meyer AM, Forte CP, Yost SC, Morlan CW, Karnack ME, McClelland A. The major human rhinovirus receptor is ICAM-1. Cell. 1989; 56: 839–847.
10. Staunton DE, Merluzzi VJ, Rothlein R, Barton R, Martin SD, Springer TA. A cell adhesion molecule, ICAM-1, is the major surface receptor for rhinoviruses. Cell. 1989; 56: 849–853.
11. Mendelsohn CL, Wimmer E, Racaniello VR. Cellular receptor for poliovirus: molecular cloning, nucleotide sequence and expression of a new member of the immunoglobulin super family. Cell. 1989; 56: 855–865.
12. Dalgleish AG, Beverley PCL, Clapham PR et al. The CD4 (T4) antigen is an essential component of the receptor for the AIDS retrovirus. Nature. 1984; 312: 763–767.
13. Weiss W, Brown JH, Cusacks S, Paulson JC, Skelhel JJ, Wiley DC. Structure of the influenza virus haemagglutinin complexed with its receptor, sialic acid. Nature. 1988; 333: 426–431.
14. Clements JE, Dederson FS, Narayan O et al. Genomic changes associated with antigenic variations of visna virus during persistent infection. Proc Nat Acad Sci USA. 1980; 77: 4454–4458.
15. Payne S, Parekh B, Montelaro RC, Issel CJ. Genomic alterations associated with persistent infection by equine infectious anaemia virus, a retrovirus. J Gen Virol. 1984; 65: 1395–1399.
16. Rossman MJ, Palmenberg AC. Conservation of the putative receptor attachment site on picornaviruses. Virology. 1988; 164: 373–382.
17. Gollins SW, Porterfield JS. A new mechanism for the neutralization of enveloped viruses by antiviral antibody. Nature. 1986; 321: 244–246.
18. Dimmock NJ. Neutralization of animal viruses. Curr Top Microbiol Imunol. 1993; 183.
19. Mandel B. Mechanisms of virus neutralization. In: Oldstone MBA, Notkins AL, eds. Concepts in Viral Pathogenesis. New York: Springer-Verlag, 1984; 32.
20. Cooper NR. Humoral immunity to viruses. In: Fraenkel-Conrat H, Wagner RR, eds. Comprehensive Virology. New York: Plenum Press, 1979: 123.
21. Bartholomew RM, Esser AF, Müller-Eberhard HJ. Lysis of oncornaviruses by human serum: Isolation of the viral complement (CI) and identification as p15E. J Exp Med. 1978;

147: 844–853.

22. Hirsch RL, Winkelstein JA, Griffin DE. The role of complement in viral infection. J Immunol. 1980; 124: 2507–2510.

23. Lachmann PJ, Rosen FS. Genetic defects of complement in man. Semin Immunopathol. 1979; 1: 339–353.

24. Sissons JGP. Antibody and complement-dependent lysis of virus-infected cells. In: Oldstone MBA, Notkins AL, eds. Concepts in Viral Pathogenesis. New York: Springer Verlag, 1984: 39.

25. Trinchieri G. Biology of natural killer cells. Adv Immunol. 1989; 47: 187–376.

26. Crowe JE, Murphy BR, Channock RM, Williamson RA, Barbas CF, Burton DR. Recombinant human respiratory syncitial virus (RSV) monoclonal antibody Fab is effective therapeutically when introduced directly into the lungs of RSV infected mice. Proc Natl Acad Sci USA. 1994; 91: 1386–1390.

27. Kohl S. Role of antibody-dependent cellular cytotoxicity in defense against herpes simplex virus infection. Rev Infect Dis. 1991; 13: 108–114.

28. Levine B, Hardwick JM, Trapp BD, Crawford TO, Bollinger RC, Griffin DE. Antibody-mediated clearance of alphavirus infection from neurons. Science. 1991; 254: 856–860.

29. Fujinami RS, Oldstone MBA. Alterations in expression of measles virus polypeptides by antibody: molecular events in antibody-induced antigenic modulation. J Immunol. 1980; 125: 78–85.

30. Halstead SB. Pathogenesis of Dengue: challenges to molecular biology. Science. 1988; 239: 476–481.

31. Kapoor AK, Nash AA, Wildy P, Phelan J, McLean CS, Field HJ. Pathogenesis of herpes simplex virus in congenitally athymic mice: the relative roles of cell-mediated and humoral immunity. J Gen Virol. 1982; 60: 225–233.

32. Jacobson S, Richart JR, Biddison WE, Satinsky A, Hartzman RJ, McFarland HF. Measles virus-specific T4+ human cytotoxic T cell clones are restricted by class II HLA antigens. J Immunol. 1984; 133; 754–757.

33. Yasukawa M, Zarling JM. Human cytotoxic T cell clones directed against herpes simplex virus-infected cells. Lysis restricted by HLA class II MB and DR antigens. J Immunol. 1984; 133: 422–427.

34. Lukacher AE, Morrison LA, Brachiale VL, Malissen B, Brachiale TJ. Expression of specific cytolytic activity by H-21 region-restricted, influenza-specific T lymphocyte clones. J Exp Med. 1985; 162: 171–187.

35. Scherle PA, Gerhard W. Functional analysis of influenza-specific helper T cell clones *in vivo*. T cells specific for internal viral proteins provide cognate help for B cell responses to the haemagglutinin. J Exp Med. 1986; 164: 1114–1128.

36. Jacobson S, Sekaly RP, Jacobson CL, McFarland HF, Long EO. HLA class II-restricted presentation of cytoplasmic measles virus antigens to cytotoxic T cells. J Virol. 1989; 63: 1756–1762.

37. Long EO, Jacobson S. Pathways of viral antigen processing and presentation to CTL. Immunol Today. 1989; 10: 45–48.

38. Koszinowski UH, Keil GM, Schwarz H, Schickendanz J, Reddehase MJ. A nonstructural polypeptide encoded by immediate-early transcription unit 1 of murine cytomegalovirus is recognised by cytolytic T lymphocytes. J Exp Med. 1987; 166: 289–294.

39. Borysiewicz LK, Hickling JK, Graham S, Sinclair J, Cranage MP, Smith GL, Sissons JGP. Human cytomegalovirus-specific cytotoxic T cells. Relative frequency of stage specific CTL recognizing the 72 kD immediate early protein and glycoprotein B expressed by recombinant vaccinia virus. J Exp Med. 1988; 168: 919–932.

40. Reddehase MJ, Rothbard JB, Koszinowski UH. A pentapeptide as minimal antigenic determinant for MHC class I-restricted T lymphocytes. Nature. 1989; 337: 651–653.

41. Welsh PRJ, Tonks P, Nash AA, Blakemore WF. The effect of L3T4 T cell depletion on the pathogenesis of Theiler's murine encephalomyelitis virus infection in CBA mice. J Gen Virol. 1987; 68: 1659–1667.

42. Borrow P, Tonks P, Welsh CJR, Nash AA. The role of CD8+ T cells in the acute and chronic phases of Theiler's murine encephalomyelitis virus-induced disease in mice. J Gen Virol. 1992; 73: 1861–1865.

43. Nash AA, Cambouropoulos P. The immune response to herpes simplex virus. Semin Virol.

1993; 4: 181–186.

44. Wu L, Morahan PS. Macrophages and other nonspecific defenses: role in modulating resistance against herpes simplex virus. In: Rouse BT, ed. Herpes simplex virus pathogenesis, immunobiology and control. New York: Springer-Verlag, 1992: 89.

45. Doherty PC. Virus infections in mice with targeted gene disruptions. Curr Opinion Immunol. 1993; 5: 479–483.

46. Ceredig R, Allan J, Tabi Z, Lynch F, Doherty PC. Phenotypic analysis of the cerebrospinal fluid inflammatory exudate in murine lymphocytic choromeningitis. J Exp Med. 1987; 165: 1539–1551.

47. Openshaw PJM. Pulmonary epithelial T cells induced by viral infection express T cell receptors α/β. Eur J Immunol. 1991; 21: 803–806.

48. Doherty PC, Allan W, Eichelberger M. Roles of $\alpha\beta$ and $\gamma\delta$ T cell subsets in viral immunity. Annu Rev Immunol. 1992; 10: 123–151.

5
The Immunology and Pathogenesis of Persistent Virus Infections

N. ALP and L. K. BORYSIEWICZ

INTRODUCTION

Infection by a virus usually initiates an immune response to the virus, as a result of which the infection is cleared. Viruses have, therefore, evolved ways of evading immune recognition which allow them to persist in individuals or, if clearance with lifelong protection is the outcome of initial contact with the host, to maintain themselves within the population. Examples of such mechanisms include infection in early childhood, as new susceptible hosts appear every 2–3 years (e.g. measles virus); the availability of a secondary host (often an animal reservoir, e.g. influenza virus)[1,2]; and modification of viral coat proteins by antigenic shift and drift (e.g. influenza virus haemagglutinin)[1]. It is also possible for a virus to persist in cells or animals of a species other than the natural host[2]. Although this may be an artificial phenomenon it provides important clues as to the nature of persistence in the intact host. Lastly, viruses may become persistent in a single host. The maintenance of such persistence requires a complex series of interactions between host and virus to be established and maintained to provide an asymptomatic virus–host equilibrium. This latter mechanism is the subject of this chapter.

The classical separation of virus infections into acute, chronic (persistent) and latent has become increasingly blurred. In a chronic or persistent infection there is a continued low level of turnover and shedding of the virus; a latent infection is characterized by restricted viral gene expression and no viral replication (Figure 1). Epstein–Barr virus (EBV) was previously considered to be an example of a virus that used the latter mechanism, with limited expression of virus proteins in transformed B cells. However, the existence of productive virus replication has recently been recognized, both in these cells and in the pharyngeal mucosa of most seropositive individuals[3].

99

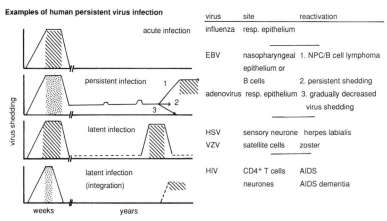

Figure 1 Example of human persistent virus infection

The range of viruses known to be capable of establishing a persistent infection has been extended to include archetypal viruses such as the enteroviruses (e.g. coxsackie B). Thus despite primary infection or control of acute childhood infections by vaccination, such agents can still be implicated in a number of chronic diseases of unknown aetiology.

The failure of the immune response to clear an infection is an implicit requirement for the establishment of persistence. This failure is influenced by both viral factors, such as cellular tropism, replication strategy and virus-induced immunosuppression, and host factors, including the balance between responses generated against the virus and the induction of immunopathology or autoimmunity. These factors will be considered separately for convenience, but it is their interaction in the intact host that will determine the nature and outcome of an individual virus infection.

VIRAL FACTORS IN THE ESTABLISHMENT AND MAINTENANCE OF PERSISTENT INFECTION

Viruses are obligate intracellular parasites, and therefore use the transcriptional and translational mechanisms of the host cell for their replication. In the case of an acute infection, this results in cell lysis and release of infectious virus: a classical example of this is infection of a cell by poliovirus. This non-enveloped, single-strand, 'positive sense' RNA virus enters the cell after interaction with a receptor – a member of the Ig superfamily of cell surface proteins. This receptor has restricted distribution in the host[4], and this in part determines viral tissue tropism, although this virus also has an enhanced ability to replicate in the nervous system, possibly related to structural differences in the 5′ non-coding region of the genome[5]. Following uptake into the cell, the virus is uncoated and the RNA serves as a direct template for translation of viral proteins. These can be divided into two types: structural proteins, which provide coat proteins for progeny virus, and non-structural proteins, which serve to modify or shut off host cell macromolecular synthetic pathways and are enzymes required for efficient replication of the viral genome. The viral RNA is then duplicated into a template (or negative sense strand) intermediate from which new virus 'genomic' RNA is produced. This is packaged and released by cell lysis (Figure 2).

Even with this simple lytic replication strategy a number of mechanisms may operate to allow the virus to persist. Hepatitis A virus, for example, is a picornavirus that infects human fibroblasts *in vitro*, but establishes a persistent infection, possibly by failing to shut off host cell protein synthesis which competes with, and ultimately balances, viral protein synthesis[6]. Similarly, coxsackieviruses establish persistent infection in cardiac tissue, as has been demonstrated by *in situ* hybridization studies. This is probably mediated by an accumulation of template negative strand RNA, which may form an excess of double-stranded RNA intermediates that block efficient RNA replication[7,8].

The above examples illustrate first, that molecular mechanisms of persistence vary for different viruses and at different tissue sites and second, and more contentiously, that as the genome and replicative cycle of a virus becomes more complex – often with increasing size – the number of possible mechanisms by which persistence can be achieved may increase.

The human herpesviruses, divided into α-herpesviruses (herpes simplex virus (HSV) type I and varicella-zoster virus (VZV)), β-herpesviruses (human cytomegalovirus; CMV) and γ-herpesviruses (EBV), all establish persistent infections. A common feature of these viruses is that replication occurs in three temporally regulated phases of gene expression, termed the immediate early (IE), early and late phases[9]. Following infection by HSV-I latency is established in sensory ganglion neurones. The nature of this latent infection is unknown, but the double-stranded DNA genome is probably maintained as episomes and in the form of long concamers[9]. Recently, attention has focused on a transcript (latency-associated transcript) of viral DNA which is found in latently infected ganglia and may be complementary to an important protein expressed during the IE phase of viral gene transcription. However, this mechanism has been questioned, as deletion of the LAT gene does not prevent the establishment of latent infection[10]. The factors initiating reactivation of latent virus, leading to virus shedding, are poorly understood at the molecular level, although physical trauma (UV light or direct damage to the ganglion or nerve fibre) and fever are well established clinical initiators. The induction of host cell proteins and factors which transregulate the IE genes may be an important element in allowing the induction of the replicative virus cycle from the quiescent state.

EBV establishes persistent infection in man, and transforms two different cell types. *In vivo*, EBV enters via the respiratory epithelium and then infects B cells. The virus may transform epithelial cells, resulting in nasopharyngeal carcinoma, or B cells, producing Burkitt's lymphoma. The cellular tropism is determined by the interaction between a viral envelope protein (gp340) and the C3D receptor. In the majority of B cells the virus is present in a latent form: the entire genome is maintained as a supercoiled episome with limited expression of seven viral proteins (EBNA 1–6 and latent membrane protein, LMP) within these cells. These proteins are responsible for maintaining genome replication during the cell cycle and, *in vitro*, for immortalizing the host cell. *In vitro*, the virus switches to a replicative cycle in 1 in every 10^3–10^6 cells: this change is mediated by the *BZLF-1* gene, which induces lytic replication in B cells[11]. The *BZLF-1* gene product is a series of nuclear polypeptides with molecular weights of 30–38 kD; these transactivate genes encoding three IE proteins: BLMF1, BMRF1 and BRLF1. These proteins are themselves transactivators of EBV genes and appear to be important for the initiation of a cascade leading to lytic replication[12].

There has been much debate over the true site of EBV persistence. Initially it was proposed that continuous low level productive infection in the oropharyngeal epithelium would result in repeated infection of B cells, and the low level of B cell infection (1 in 10^6–10^7 cells) was maintained by immune surveillance. This has been challenged by the observation that irradiation of the bone marrow can clear resident infection in bone marrow cells of a bone marrow transplant recipient, and that infection can then be established by an EBV serotype derived from donor bone marrow cells. The haematopoietic compartment itself may harbour a persistent reservoir of the virus. B cells in this compartment are immature and the EBV genome in these cells is in a highly methylated, and therefore inhibited, state. Occasional escape from this molecular restriction, perhaps concomitant with B cell maturation, might be sufficient to maintain the low level of B cell infection, and B cell traffic might infect oral epithelial cells, promoting virus shedding, not vice versa.

The site of human CMV persistence is unknown, although polymerase chain reaction (PCR) analysis has identified monocyte and polymorphonuclear cells in peripheral blood[13] and epithelial cells as potential sites. Expression of CMV genes occurs in a similar temporally regulated sequence to that seen in EBV. The control of IE gene expression is probably a key event which determines whether infectious progeny is produced following infection. This gene cluster is regulated by a strong promoter region which may be activated or inhibited by a number of viral and cellular factors that have only been partially identified. Human teratocarcinoma (T2) cells provide some insight into these mechanisms. T2 cells can be induced to differentiate by retinoic acid. Undifferentiated cells show little or no IE gene expression after CMV infection, but retinoic acid-induced differentiation is associated with the expression of IE gene products in most cells[14]. Transfection of undifferentiated cells with truncated IE constructs demonstrated the presence of a negative transcriptional factor that binds to a region of CMV DNA 300 base pairs upstream from the promoter[15]. IE gene products are capable of regulating not only the expression of early and late CMV genes, but can also enhance and inhibit the expression of their own genes[16]. The interplay of viral and host cell factors is thus essential to the switch between latency and persistent infection.

Another mechanism by which latency can be established is integration of virus genome into the host cell DNA. This strategy is employed by retroviruses, which encode a reverse transcriptase enzyme that converts the genomic viral RNA into complementary DNA, which can then recombine with the genome of the host cell. This mechanism provides a selective advantage to the virus by enabling the viral genome to persist and bypass a host generation by vertical transmission (transmission via the germ line of the host). However, integration may result in tumour development. Retroviruses such as human T lymphotropic virus (HTLV), murine leukaemia viruses and feline leukaemia virus can induce tumours either through the expression of a virus-encoded oncogene (e.g. Rous sarcoma virus), or through insertion of strong viral promoters adjacent to host oncogenes.

Horizontal transmission can be achieved by reactivation of the integrated virus. The control of this aspect of retroviral shedding is best exemplified by human immunodeficiency virus (HIV). The switch of productive infection by this virus is regulated by three genes – *tat*, *rev* and *nef* – which serve to maintain persistent infection. Again, there is interplay between the products of these genes and host cell factors, such as the enhanced expression of NFKB in activated T cells, which may upregulate viral as well as host genes, leading to increased shedding of virus.

Hepatitis B virus (HBV) also integrates into the host genome. The importance of such integration in relation to HBV persistence and the development of hepatocellular carcinoma has been established by epidemiological studies[17]. A number of HBV integration sites has been reported, including one in the cyclin gene of an early hepatocellular carcinoma cell line[18,19]. This gene is important in the control of cell division, and its disruption by viral insertion might contribute to tumourigenesis.

Persistent viruses are capable of remaining in a population of susceptible cells for extended periods; dual infection by another acute or persistent virus is therefore more likely. For example, HIV may be able to infect lymphoid and myeloid cells already persistently infected with CMV, and vice versa. These viruses may interact: CMV IE gene products can transactivate the HIV LTR, and hence initiate transcription and HIV gene expression[20]. Such interactions may offer an explanation for the more rapid progression of HIV infection in CMV-seropositive subjects.

Host cell machinery is required for the replication of persistent viruses, which utilize cellular as well as viral regulatory elements. These vary with the tissue that is infected and may in themselves dictate viral tropism. Viruses may also interfere with host cell replication, resulting in transformation and consequent neoplasia. However, these are relatively rare events in the context of the large number of possible persistent viral infections, suggesting that an efficiently regulated equilibrium is established not only at the level of the host cell, as discussed above, but also by direct interaction with the immune response.

THE IMMUNE RESPONSE TO PERSISTENT VIRUS INFECTION

The antigens expressed by the virion or by an infected cell act as powerful inducers of immune responses. During acute infection this results in clearance of the virus, coupled with prolonged, often lifelong, protection from reinfection. In persistent infections the virus is not cleared, but extension of the infection is controlled, probably with the establishment of an equilibrium between the virus and the specific response.

Primary infection produces immune responses similar to those described in Chapter 4 in the context of an acute virus infection. However, the role of these responses once persistence is established may be very different from that in acute infection. The requirements for control of the infection at the level of the infected cell, rather than the control of free virus, focuses attention on specific cellular rather than humoral mechanisms.

Innate immunity is mediated by physiological barriers such as the skin, the mucociliary escalator of the respiratory tract, the complement system, interferons, polymorphonuclear phagocytes, macrophages and natural killer (NK) cells. The innate immune response forms the first line of defence against parasitism: it is immediate, non-specific and non-adaptive, and its role in virus persistence is unknown.

Initial infection of a cell by a virus stimulates the release of interferon (IFN)-α and -β, which induces an 'antiviral state' in neighbouring cells. IFN-γ is a specific lymphokine that modulates the immune response to the infection. The complement system can be activated directly by virus infection, and the classical pathway can also be activated following antigen–antibody interactions. Complement can act by blocking receptors on the surface of the virus, reducing infectivity, by directly lysing enveloped viruses and virus-infected cells and by acting as an opsonin. These effects may be important in restricting the spread of virus once a focus of reactivation and virus shedding has been established, but overall they are probably more important in acute than persistent infections.

NK cells are predominantly CD16$^+$ in man, although they have not been completely characterized, and their receptors and ligands on infected cells have not been fully identified. They kill a variety of virus-infected cells and tumour cells without classical antigen specificity or MHC restriction. The best evidence for their role in protecting against persistent virus infection comes from experimental murine CMV infection: mice genetically deficient in NK activity, or whose NK cells have been depleted by administration of antibodies directed against asialoprotein-GM1 are susceptible to CMV infection. Protection against the infection can be restored by adoptive transfer of a clone of NK cells[21]. The nature of the susceptibility of CMV-infected fibroblasts to lysis by human NK cells has been shown to be dependent on the expression of non-structural genes, although it is a host cell protein, rather than a viral protein, that is probably recognized by the NK cells[22]. Such NK activity can be detected in CMV-seropositive and -seronegative individuals, suggesting that this is neither a sufficient nor an induced immune mechanism in persistent CMV infection. Furthermore, murine studies suggest that these cells may protect against primary infection rather than against reactivation. This is underlined by the genetic linkage between susceptibility to primary intraperitoneal CMV infection and the ability to produce IFN and generate NK responses in strains of mice bearing the *CMV-1* gene[23]. A single patient with NK cell deficiency and recurrent or severe HSV infections has been described, suggesting that infection by this herpes virus may be controlled by an effective NK cell response[24]. Thus although NK cells may be a hypothetical surveillance system which could restrict foci of reactivated virus without the commitment to maintaining an antigen-specific response, their role in persistent infection remains unclear.

An antibody response is elicited by most persistent viruses, and a variety of functionally distinct responses can be detected throughout the course of an infection. Evidence for the protective nature of these responses is limited. In man, passive immunization affords protection against primary challenge with VZV. However, the role of passive antibody following reactivation is questionable. High titres may restrict the spread of liberated infectious virus, but little convincing evidence of this has been published. In order to establish and maintain a persistent infection, a virus must evade this immune response. Generation of antibody responses was thought to facilitate the establishment of persistence by stripping viral antigens from the surface of the infected cell. This was proposed to be the mechanism in subacute sclerosing panencephalitis, a progressive neurological disorder occurring in $0.4–1.4/10^6$ children following measles virus infection. In this condition, very high levels of measles virus-specific antibody are maintained in the blood and are produced in the cerebrospinal fluid. *In vitro*, these antibodies, which are directed against the viral haemagglutinin, strip measles antigen from the surface of infected cells by capping. However, it is probable that persistence is in fact maintained by viral mutants escaping the control exerted by the presence of antibody[25].

Once a virus has established a persistent infection, neutralizing antibody must be evaded in order to permit spread of progeny virus. Equine infectious anaemia (EIA) virus is a lentivirus that causes a persistent infection. The primary virus infection is transmitted by contaminated blood, transferred by biting flies (*Stomoxys* spp.). Within 7–21 days the animal becomes weak, pyrexial and anaemic. About 80% of animals succumb to this initial illness; the remainder suffer from recurrent episodes of anaemia, and some develop glomerulonephritis. During the initial infection, the virus infects macrophages and lymphocytes, replicates and is released into the blood. The major virus glycoprotein (gp90) binds the virus to erythrocytes. Antibodies directed against gp90 mediate complement-dependent lysis of the erythrocytes. Virus–antibody complexes are also found in the basement membrane and mesangium of animals with glonerulonephritis. The antibody directed against gp90 is often poorly neutralizing, which may explain the persistence of the infection within macrophages[26]. Serum from horses suffering from repeated episodes of anaemia binds the virus isolated from the current or previous episodes of illness, but not that isolated from later episodes[26]. This implies that the viral gp90 undergoes considerable variation within the infected animal – new variants can be detected as little as 15 days after the preceding change. The variation in amino acids in this region is 0.5–3.2% within a single animal, and these changes are random: sera from different animals do not cross-react with new isolates. This mechanism of antigenic variation in a single host allows the virus to evade the antibody response, allowing periodic release of progeny virus and creating the possibility of horizontal transmission.

Antigenic variation of HIV via random point mutations has also been observed in infected patients. The antibody response to this virus is predominantly directed against the envelope glycoprotein gp120, but this molecule varies widely between HIV isolates, even those obtained sequentially from a single individual. The region of gp120 that interacts with the CD4 molecule is highly conserved: it is located in a cleft and shielded from immunoglobulin, preventing direct competitive inhibition by antibody, although a loop (V3 loop) nearby shows frequent variation and often binds neutralizing antibody[27]. In addition, soluble gp120 is shed from HIV-infected cells and may absorb anti-gp120 antibody. Free virus is neutralized by antibody, but only a small proportion of the antibody produced is neutralizing. Infectious virus may, therefore, remain in immune complexes, the entry of which into macrophages may be facilitated by Fc receptor-mediated endocytosis. The precise protective role of this antibody response remains unknown as a number of other immune responses, such as cytotoxic T lymphocytes, are detectable in these individuals. However, it is interesting that if the mechanisms of neutralizing antibody production and viral antigenic variation are entered into computer models as the most important determinants for progression of HIV infection to AIDS, the predicted reduction in $CD4^+$ cells and virus shedding follows a similar course to that seen clinically[28].

Antibody also contributes to the clearance of virus-infected cells by antibody-dependent cellular cytotoxicity (ADCC), which is mediated by binding of IgG to viral proteins on infected cells. Receptor-mediated binding of NK cells and lymphokine activated killer (LAK) cells to the Fc domain of the bound immunoglobulin triggers cytolysis of the virus-infected cell and destruction of intracellular virus. Although this effector mechanism is efficient *in vitro*, the protective nature of this process remains to be demonstrated *in vivo*.

VIRUS-SPECIFIC CELL-MEDIATED IMMUNITY

Clinical observations suggest that the development of humoral responses may be insufficient to control reactivation of persistent viral infection. Patients with primary immunoglobulin deficiency may develop acute picornaviral infection, but otherwise have few clinical problems related to persistent viruses. This is in contrast to patients with Di George syndrome, who have thymic aplasia and consequent deficiency of cellular immunity. Such patients with secondary immunodeficiency develop a range of functional antibodies in response to reactivation of viruses such as CMV, yet this response frequently fails to control the infection. Such observations have focused attention on the role of virus-specific immune responses.

A number of functionally distinct responses have been described. First, activated T cells secrete a variety of cytokines, such as IFN-γ, which may control virus spread, tumour necrosis factor, which may lyse cells directly, and BCGF and interleukins 2, 4 and 6, which augment other cellular and humoral effector mechanisms. The deletion of antigen-specific T cells may influence the development of protective immunity, even if such cells do not have a direct effector function. However, such studies also reveal that specific subsets of T cells may impair protection at defined sites of infection: for example, infection of the central nervous system by HSV is dependent on an effective CD8[+] response.

Delayed type hypersensitivity (DTH) responses have been studied in a number of experimental murine viral infections[29]. During primary HSV infection in mice, DTH, mediated by MHC Class II-restricted CD4[+] T cells, is the most important effector mechanism for clearance of virus from the site of inoculation[30]. This protective response can be adoptively transferred between animals. However, following influenza virus infection, the generation of a similar MHC Class II-restricted DTH response results in more rapid progression of disease. This again underlies the differences seen with different viruses and different sites of infection. Little is known about the relative importance or nature of this response in man, largely because no good *in vitro* assay system is available.

Cytotoxic T lymphocytes (CTL) appear to play a major role in limiting reactivation and spread of many persistent viruses. Koszinowski *et al.*[31] have shown CTL to be important in the immune control of murine CMV: selective deletion of the CD8[+] T lymphocyte subset leads to severe disease[32], while reconstitution with CMV-specific CTL lines or clones affords protection from lethal challenge[33]. In further experiments, these authors showed that CTL from persistently infected mice recognized fragments of the major IE protein (a non-structural phosphoprotein of 89 kD molecular weight) in an MHC Class I-restricted fashion. In addition, mice vaccinated with a recombinant vaccinia virus expressing the major IE gene were protected from lethal challenge, apparently by induction of CTL. These observations have been reinforced by the detection of relatively high numbers of human CMV-specific CTL precursors in the peripheral blood of seropositive individuals[34,35]. Part of this response was shown to be directed against determinants within the CMV 72 kD major IE protein. Subsequent studies have shown that input virion protein pp65 is an additional major CTL target[36]. This predominance of CTL directed against input and non-structural proteins might protect the host by killing cells nurturing reactivating virus at an early stage, before virus replication begins.

CTL are also important mediators of protective immunity during persistent EBV infection. Patients with a rare familial syndrome known as X-linked lymphoproliferative disease, or Duncan syndrome, are well until they are infected with EBV. They then develop a fulminant disease characterized by agammaglobulinaemia and B cell lymphoma. The immune defects identified in these patients include abnormal NK and EBV-specific CTL responses[37]. In normal individuals, EBV induces a CTL response. These cells recognize a number of latency-associated EBNA proteins[38]. During persistent infection, however, this precursor CTL population is maintained. Regression analyses[39] and limiting dilution assays have shown the frequency of EBV-specific CTLK precursors in normal individuals to be about 1:500–1:10000 peripheral blood mononuclear cells[40]. This proportion remains remarkably constant over periods of up to 5 years, in contrast to the declining immunity to acutely infective viruses such as influenza[41]. This suggests that restimulation of

EBV-specific CTL may be occurring: whether this is at the level of the oropharyngeal epithelium, circulating B cells or the haematopoietic compartment is still a matter for debate, although recent studies suggest that in lymphocytic choriomeningitis infection CTL numbers may be retained in the absence of continued restimulation[42].

The specific CTL response may not be the major protective mechanism following primary infection. During acute infectious mononucleosis there is polyclonal T cell activation[43], and cytotoxic activity can be demonstrated *in vitro* against allogeneic as well as EBV-infected target cells. This response is mediated by MHC Class I-restricted CTL which are clonally distinct from EBV-specific populations[44]. Others have described suppressor cells in patients with acute infectious mononucleosis, and clones derived from such patients prevent the outgrowth of immortalized B cells *in vitro* without direct cytotoxicity.

The extension of these studies to human lentiviruses and retroviruses such as HIV and HTLV-1 has identified a subpopulation of patients in whom direct virus-specific CTL activity can be detected[45]. Such activity is difficult to detect in other acute virus infections, and in most situations *in vitro* restimulation of a precursor CTL is used. During asymptomatic HIV infection CTL are present in PBM and at other tissue sites, and it has been suggested that their numbers decline as disease progresses. It is tempting to speculate that failure of this response may be a causal factor in disease progression, although it may also be indicative of advancing immunodeficiency. Similarly recent studies suggest that HIV may invade CTL-mediated immunity at least at the level of a single epitope[46].

VIRUS EVASION OF THE IMMUNE RESPONSE

Virus-specific cell-mediated immunity may play an important role in restricting persistent virus infections in the host. However, horizontal transmission requires localized shedding of virus and at least temporary escape from immunological control. Viruses have evolved a number of strategies to accomplish these ends.

Anatomical localization

The virus may persist at sites that are relatively inaccessible to the cellular immune response. Papillomaviruses, for example, are shed from differentiating epithelial surfaces, and clinical infection is present in the face of antibodies and T cell responses. However, cutaneous papillomavirus lesions ultimately undergo spontaneous resolution, with infiltration of $CD4^+/CD8^+$ T cells into the dermis and $CD8^+$ cells into the epithelium. Such temporary persistence in the epithelium may also be a feature of infection with adenoviruses and herpesviruses (EBV, HSV and VZV during reactivation, and CMV).

Direct interference with virus-specific immune responses

Infection of immunocompetent cells

Many persistent viruses infect immune cells which may abrogate responses generated against the virus. HIV is an obvious example, as is EIA virus, which infects macrophages. This may block the generation of activated T cells. Measles virus infects T cells, but replication within these cells only occurs once the T cell has been activated. *In vitro*, this infection abrogates the development of both primary and anamnestic immune responses: the *in vivo* counterpart to this effect may be manifest as the development of cutaneous anergy to antigens such as PPD. This defect may account for the high mortality associated with secondary infections that occur 2–3 weeks after primary measles.

Induction of tolerance

Tolerance may be induced following neonatal infection: lymphocytic chorio-meningitic virus (LCMV) infection in neonatal mice provides the clearest example of a virus persisting in a tolerant immune environment. A non-neutralizing antibody response is generated during this infection, implying that the helper T cell and B cell responses are not activated, but neither DTH nor a CTL response is present. This tolerance is virus-specific, and although it has been suggested that LCMV-specific CTL are clonally deleted[47], others have detected such cells in persistently infected mice[48]. The mechanism by which tolerance is sustained in this instance is, therefore, unknown. Although the virus itself is non-cytopathic, infection is not asymptomatic: the function of some host cells, such as those in the anterior pituitary, is disturbed, and the presence of the virus is thus potentially detrimental to the host.

Failure to develop specific immunity

The specific failure to develop an immune response to a virus is best exemplified by the 'slow' virus infections of the central nervous system. This situation may be partly a consequence of the 'host-derived' nature of the infectious particles, which leads to minor immunological differences remaining undetected.

PERSISTENT VIRUS-INDUCED IMMUNOPATHOLOGY AND AUTOIMMUNITY

Immune responses generated against persistent viruses can mediate tissue injury. The general question of the role of infectious organisms in the induction of immunopathology is discussed in Chapter 7 this section focuses only on examples related to persistent viruses.

Interactions between viruses and antibodies generate immune complexes which may themselves initiate a circulating immune complex disease, as occurs in Aleutian mink disease and LCMV infection. In the former disease, the generation of non-neutralizing but antigen-binding antibodies results in the generation of large quantitites of immune complexes which are ultimately deposited in the kidney. This condition may be a model for a number of diseases in man. The prodromal arthritis or arthralgias and urticarial skin rash seen in 10–20% of patients with acute HBV infection are accompanied by evidence of complement activation and immune complex production[49]. An association between persistent HBV infection and polyarteritis nodosa, a systemic necrotizing vasculitis, has also been described: complement, immunoglobulin and hepatitis B virus surface antigen (HBsAg) have all been demonstrated in arterial lesions.

Virus-specific T cells may also mediate immunopathology. Intracerebral inoculation of LCMV results in the death of normal adult mice. Mice immunosuppressed with cyclophosphamide survive, but adoptive transfer of LCMV-specific CTL again leads to death. Death is thought to result from cerebral oedema following damage to the blood–brain barrier mediated by virus-specific CTL.

In man, chronic active hepatitis B is associated with the production of virus-specific CTL. Persistent HBV infection can sometimes occur in the presence of minimal liver injury, suggesting that the virus itself is not necessarily cytopathic. However, other cases are associated with infiltration of CD8[+] T cells into the liver[50]. Cloning of these cells has shown them to be heterogeneous with respect to their specificity. The target for HBV-CTL has subsequently been identified as the core antigen of the virus (HBcAg), which is expressed on infected cells during active virus replication. Chu et al.[51] demonstrated increased expression of MHC Class I molecules on hepatocytes of patients with chronic active hepatitis, and showed that the antiviral activity in these patients is MHC Class I restricted. They suggested that upregulation of MHC Class I antigen expression in virus-infected cells potentiates the activity of infiltrating virus-specific CTL, leading to liver cell damage and hepatitis.

DTH reactions are generally mediated by CD4[+] T cells, but CD8[+] clones are also capable of recruiting macrophages to sites of viral replication. The mediation of immunopathology by such reactions has been suggested in experimental murine HSV infection, influenza and respiratory syncytial virus infection. Inoculation of HSV into the anterior chamber of the eye produces infection in the contralateral eye by intracerebral spread of virus. Delayed hypersensitivity reactions in the contralateral eye result in retinal damage, although this ocular pathology does not correlate with systemic immunity to the virus[52].

In man, the difficulty involved in unequivocally identifying a DTH response and separating it from other effector cells has made identification of similar phenomena difficult. However, DTH type responses may be involved in a number of diseases, such as CMV pneumonia.

The development of true virus-induced autoimmunity, as opposed to immunopathology, is difficult to detect[53]. Potentially pathogenic antibodies have been described in a number of experimental infections, and T cell responses directed against normal host cell antigens have been identified (e.g. murine coxsackie B3 infection and myocarditis)[54].

CONCLUSION

Many factors are involved in the initiation and facilitation of virus persistence. The virus must have the potential to persist: some have evolved methods for acute infection, others invariably establish a persistent infection in the host, while some may establish either acute or persistent infection, depending on the host environment. The specific environment of the host cell must also be able to support a persistent infection, and the virus must be able to maintain infection, whether chronic or latent, in the face of an immune response.

The ability to establish a persistent state has several advantages for the virus over acute infection. For example, the virus can maintain itself in a smaller 'community'. Mimms[55] has pointed out that an acute infection such as measles requires the virus to replicate in a susceptible host in order to maintain itself in the population. Its survival is dependent on large communities (500 000 or greater): the virus was absent from small closed communities, such as those of the Faroe Islands, and the population was non-immune. Introduction from external sources had catastrophic results. In contrast, persistent viruses are able to bypass a generation even without integrating into germline DNA: a community of 1200 is sufficient to maintain VZW. If vertical transmission from mother to offspring occurs, the size of the host community required is likely to be even smaller.

Even when persistence is established, the virus remains a parasite, and to date the establishment of true symbiosis has not been documented. However, the stability of the persistent state means that detrimental effects to the host may be very subtle. Litter size and frequency is reduced in colonies of wild mice infected with LCMV, indicating that long-term persistence in a community of animals is detrimental.

By definition, a persistent virus infection is not cleared by the host immune response. Does this mean that the immune response has failed? The immune response may still be judged a success if it maintains the autonomy of the host and prevents direct virus-induced tissue damage without itself causing pathology. In acute virus infections this is often not the case: immune responses can destroy normal as well as infected cells in an attempt to clear the pathogen. A persistent virus infection may make the induction of immunopathology or autoimmunity even more likely, since viral antigen is present for an extended period. Persistent viruses may have exerted an evolutionary pressure on the immune system to moderate the full force of the response, so that the virus can remain in the host while damage to healthy tissue is minimized.

In approaching the question of preventing or minimizing damage caused by persistent virus infection, the balance between virus factors and the host immune response is of paramount importance. Unlike the primary response to an acute virus, in which the sustained presence of antibody will ensure that parasitism is not established, the generation of such a response against a persistent virus may induce an immunopathological response. In order to develop effective prophylactic and therapeutic approaches to these viruses a detailed understanding of the nature of the virus–host equilibrium in each specific case is required.

References

1. Wiley DC, Skehel JJ. The structure and function of the haemagglutinin membrane glycoprotein of influenza virus. Annu Rev Biochem. 1987; 56: 365–394.
2. Krug RM. The influenza viruses. New York, London: Plenum Press, 1989.
3. Yao QY, Rickinson AB, Gaston JSH, Epstein MA. *In vitro* analysis of the Epstein Barr virus host balance in long term renal allograft recipients. Int J Cancer. 1985; 35: 43–54.
4. Koike S, Taya C, Kurata T, Abe S, Ise I, Yonekawa H, Nomoto A. Transgenic mice susceptible to poliovirus. Proc Natl Acad Sci USA. 1991; 88: 951–955.
5. Evans DMA, Dunn G, Minor PD, Schild GC, Cann AJ, Stanaway G, Almond JW, Currey K, Maizel JW. Increased neurovirulence associated with a single nucleotide change in a non-coding region of the Sabin type 3 poliovaccine genome. Nature. 1985; 314: 548–550.
6. Vallbracht A, Maier K, Stierhof YD, Wiedmann KH, Fiehmig B, Fleischer B. Liver derived cytotoxic T cells in hepatitis A virus infection. J Infect Dis. 1989; 160: 209–217.
7. Cunningham L, Bowles NE, Lane RJM, Dubowitz V, Archard LC. Persistence of enterovirus RNA in chronic fatigue syndrome is associated with the abnormal production of equal amounts of positive and negative strands of enteroviral RNA. J Gen Virol. 1990; 71: 1399–1402.
8. Archard L, Bowles NE, Cunningham L, Frecke CA, Olsen EGJ, Rose ML, Mearly B, Why HJF, Richardson PJ. Molecular probe for the detection of persisting enterovirus infection of human heart and their prognostic value. Eur Heart J. 1991; 12D: 56–59.
9. Roizman B, Sears AE. Herpes simplex viruses and their replication. In: Fields BN, Knipe DM, eds. Virology. New York: Raven Press, 1990: 1795–1841.
10. Ho DY, Mocarski ES. HSV latent RNA (LAT) is not required for latent infection in the mouse. Proc Natl Acad Sci USA. 1989; 86: 7596–7600.
11. Sample C, Kieff E. Molecular basis for Epstein-Barr virus induced pathogenesis and disease. Semin Immunopathol. 1991; 13: 133–146.
12. Alfieri C, Birkenbach M, Kieff E. Early events in Epstein-Barr virus infection of human B lymphocytes. Virology. 1991; 181: 595–610.
13. Taylor-Weidemann J, Sissons JGP, Borysiewicz LK, Sinclair JH. Monocytes as a major site of persistence of human cytomegalovirus in peripheral blood mononuclear cells. J Gen Virol. 1991; 72: 2059–2064.
14. Shelbourn SL, Sissons JGP, Sinclair JH. Expression of oncogenic ras in human teratocarcinoma cells induces partial differentiation and permissiveness for human cytomegalovirus infection. J Gen Virol. 1989; 70: 367–374.
15. Shelbourn SL, Kothari SK, Sissons JGP, Sinclair JH. Repression of human cytomegalovirus gene expression associated with a novel immediate-early regulatory region binding factor. Nucleic Acids Res. 1989; 17: 9165–9171.
16. Stamminger T, Felkenstein B. Curr Topics Microbiol Immunol. 1990; 154: 3–19.
17. Chisari FV. Hepatitis B virus biology and pathogenesis. Mol Genet Med. 1991; 2: 67–104.
18. Robinson WS. The role of hepatitis B virus in the development of primary hepatocellular carcinoma. Part I. J Gastroenterol Hepatol. 1993; 7: 622–638.
19. Robinson WS. The role of hepatitis B virus in the development of primary hepatocellular carcinoma. Part II. J Gastroenterol Hepatol. 1993; 8: 95–106.
20. Walker SM, Hagemeier C, Sissons JGP, Sinclair JH. Transregulation of the HIV long terminal repeat by HCMV involves the HIV TATA box region. J Virol. 1991.
21. Bukowski JF, Warner JF, Dennert G, Welsh RM. Adoptive transfer studies demonstrating the antiviral effect of natural killer cells *in vivo*. J Exp Med. 1985; 161: 40–52.
22. Borysiewicz LK, Graham S, Sissons JGP. Human NK lysis of virus infected cells – relationship to expression of the transferrin receptor. Eur J Immunol. 1986; 16: 405–411.

23. Scalzo AA, Fitzgerald NA, Simmons A, La Vista AB, Shellam GR. CMV-1, a genetic locus that controls murine cytomegalovirus replication in the spleen. J Exp Med. 1990; 171: 1469–1483.
24. Biron CA, Byron KS, Sullivan JL. Severe herpesvirus infections in an adolescent without natural killer cells. N Engl J Med. 1989; 320: 1731–1735.
25. Swoveland PT. Molecular events in measles virus infection of the central nervous system. Int Res Exp Pathol. 1991; 32: 255–275.
26. McGuire TC, O'Rourke KI, Parrymen LE. Immunopathogenesis of equine infectious anaemia lentivirus disease. Dev Biol Stand. 1990; 72: 31–37.
27. Nara PL, Garrity RR, Goldsmit J. Neutralization of HIV-1: a paradox of humoral proportions. FASEB J. 1991; 5: 2437–2458.
28. Nowak M. HIV mutation rate. Nature. 1990; 347: 552.
29. Nash AA. Different roles for the L3T4$^+$ and Lyt2$^+$ T cell subsets in the control of an acute herpes simplex virus infection of the skin and central nervous system. J Gen Virol. 1987; 68: 825–833.
30. Mester JC, Rouse BT. The mouse model and understanding immunity to herpes simplex virus. Rev Infect Dis. 1991; 13(Suppl. 11): S935–945.
31. Koszinowski UH, Del Val M, Reddehase MJ. Cellular and molecular basis of the protective immune response to cytomegalovirus infection. Curr Topics Microbiol Immunol. 1990; 154: 189–220.
32. Reddehase MJ, Weiland F, Muench K, Jonjic S, Lueske A, Koszinowski UH. Interstitial murine cytomegalovirus pneumonia after irradiation: characterization of cells that limit viral replication during established infection of the lungs. J Virol. 1985; 55: 264–273.
33. Reddehase MJ, Mutter W, Muench K, Buhring HJ, Koszinowski UH. CD8-positive T lymphocytes specific for murine cytomegalovirus immediate-early antigens mediate protective immunity. J Virol. 1987; 61: 3102–3108.
34. Borysiewicz LK, Graham S, Hickling JK, Mason PD, Sissons JGP. Human cytomegalovirus-specific cytotoxic T cells: their precursor frequency and stage specificity. Eur J Immunol. 1988; 18: 269–275.
35. Borysiewicz LK, Hickling JK, Graham S, Sinclair J, Cranage MP, Smith GL, Sissons JGP. Human cytomegalovirus-specific cytotoxic T cells. Relative frequency of stage-specific CTL recognizing the 72-kD immediate-early protein and glycoprotein B expressed by recombinant vaccinia viruses. J Exp Med. 1988; 168: 919–931.
36. Riddell SR. Restoration of viral immunity in immunodeficient humans by the adoptive transfer of T cell clones. Science. 1992; 257: 238–241.
37. Purtillo DT. X-linked immunoproliferative disease (XLP) as a model of Epstein-Barr virus-induced immunopathology. Semin Immunopathol. 1991; 13: 181–197.
38. Moss DJ, Misko IS, Scully TB, Apolloni A, Khanna R, Burrows SR. Immune regulation of Epstein-Barr virus: EBV nuclear antigen as a target for EBV-specific T cell lysis. Semin Immunopathol. 1991; 13: 147–156.
39. Rickinson AB, Moss DJ, Allen DJ, Wallace LE, Rowe M, Epstein MA. Reactivation of Epstein-Barr virus-specific cytotoxic cells by in vitro stimulation with the autologous lymphoblastoid cell line. Int J Cancer. 1981; 27: 593–601.
40. Alp NJ, Borysiewicz LK, Sissons JGP. Automation of limiting dilution cytotoxicity assays. J Immunol Methods. 1990; 129: 269–276.
41. McMichael AJ, Gotch FM, Noble GR, Beare PA. Cytotoxic T-cell immunity to influenza. N Engl J Med. 1983; 309: 13–17.
42. Lau LI, Jamieson BD, Somasundaram T, Ahmed R. Cytotoxic T-cell memory without antigen. Nature. 1994; 369:648–652.
43. Strang G, Rickinson AB. Multiple HLA class I-dependent cytotoxicities constitute the "non-HLA-restricted" response in infectious mononucleosis. Eur J Immunol. 1987; 17: 1007–1112.
44. Tomkinson BE, Maziarz R, Sullivan JL. Characterization of the T cell-mediated cellular cytotoxicity during acute infectious mononucleosis. J Immunol. 1989; 143: 660–670.
45. Gotch FM, Nixon DF, Alp NJ, McMichael AJ, Borysiewicz LK. High frequency of memory and effector gag specific cytotoxic T lymphocytes in HIV seropositive individuals. Int Immunol. 1990; 2: 707–712.
46. Phillips RE, Rowland-Jones S, Nixon DF et al. HIV genetic variation that can escape

cytotoxic T cell recognition. Nature. 1991; 354: 453–459.

47. Lehamnn-Grube F, Tijerina R, Zeller W, Chaturvedi UC, Lohler J. Age-dependent susceptibility of murine T lymphocytes to lymphocytic choriomeningitis virus. J Gen Virol. 1983; 64: 1157–1166.

48. Buchmeier MJ, Welsh RM, Dutko FJ, Oldstone MB. The virology and immunobiology of lymphocytic choriomeningitis virus infection. Adv Immunol. 1980; 30: 275–331.

49. Dienstag JL. Hepatitis B as an immune complex disease. Semin Liver Dis. 1981; 1: 45–57.

50. Meuer SC, Moebius U, Manns MM, Dienes HP, Ramadori G, Hess G, Hercend T, Meyer zum Buschenfelde K-H. Clonal analysis of human T lymphocytes infiltrating the liver in chronic active hepatitis B and primary biliary cirrhosis. Eur J Immunol. 1988; 18: 1447–1452.

51. Chu CM, Shyu WC, Kuo RW, Liaw UF. HLA class I antigen display on hepatocyte membrane in chronic active hepatitis B virus infection: its role in the pathogenesis of chronic type B hepatitis. Hepatology. 1988; 8: 712–717.

52. Metzger EE, Whittum-Hudson JA. The dichotomy between herpes simplex virus type 1-induced ocular pathology and systemic immunity. Invest Ophthalmol Vis Sci. 1987; 28: 1533–1540.

53. Borysiewicz LK. Virus infection and autoimmunity. In: Ballardie FW, ed. Autoimmunity in nephritis. UK: Harwood Academic Publ. 1993; 15–25.

54. Borysiewicz LK. Viral mycoarditis. Horizons Med. 1994; 5: 267–282.

55. Mimms CA. The pathogenesis of infectious disease, 4th edn. Oxford: Blackwell, 1992.

6
Immunopathology of HIV Infection

SUNIL SHAUNAK

INTRODUCTION

The acquired immune deficiency syndrome (AIDS), as defined by the Centre for Disease Control (CDC) surveillance criteria, is characterized by the development of opportunistic infections and/or malignancy in patients infected with the human immunodeficiency virus (HIV)[1-3]. The main indicator diseases are listed in Table 1. The laboratory hallmark of HIV infection is a progressive and irreversible decline in the number and function of CD4$^+$ lymphocytes (T-helper subset), with the eventual development of a clinical immunodeficiency state. Death ensues 5–15 years after infection with the virus, by which time opportunistic infections and malignancy have supervened to cause additional immunosuppression. Since the description of the original syndrome, HIV-1 and HIV-2 have been identified and successfully cultured, and several strains have been sequenced. Epidemiological studies have defined the modes of transmission. Therapeutic interventions have reduced both morbidity and mortality from HIV and from opportunist infections. Nevertheless the pandemic continues: over half a million people have developed AIDS and millions more carry the virus[4].

The AIDS pandemic is best viewed as a series of separate epidemics that now overlap in both time and place. There are three broad epidemiological patterns. In regions with pattern 1 (USA, Canada, Western Europe, Australasia, North America and parts of South America) HIV has spread mainly amongst homosexual and bisexual men and injecting drug users. Those with heterosexually acquired infection form a small proportion of cases. In areas showing pattern 2 epidemiology (the remainder of Africa and South America), most people have acquired HIV heterosexually, and the ratio of infected males to females is approximately one. AIDS has so far had the most profound effects in these regions: for example, 8 million of an estimated 13 million people infected with HIV world-wide reside in sub-Saharan Africa. A third pattern is found in Asia and the Pacific, Eastern Europe, and the

Table 1 CDC surveillance case definition for AIDS

Diseases diagnosed definitively without confirmation of HIV infection in patients without other causes of immunodeficiency

Candidiasis of the oesophagus, trachea, bronchi, or lungs

Cryptococcosis, extrapulmonary

Chronic intestinal cryptosporidiosis >1 month duration

Cytomegalovirus (CMV) infection of any organ except the liver, spleen, or lymph nodes in patients >1 month old

Herpes simplex infection, mucocutaneous (>1 month duration) or of the bronchi, lungs, or oesophagus in patients >1 month duration

Kaposi's sarcoma in patients <60 years old

Primary central nervous system lymphoma in patients <60 years old

Lymphoid interstitial pneumonitis (LIP) and/or pulmonary lymphoid hyperplasia (PLH) in patients <13 years old

Mycobacterium avium complex or *M. kansaii*; disseminated

Pneumocystis carinii pneumonia

Progressive multifocal leukoencephalopathy

Toxoplasmosis of the brain in patients >1 month old

Invasive cervical carcinoma

Diseases diagnosed definitively with confirmation of HIV infection

Multiple or recurrent pyogenic bacterial infections in patients <13 years old

Coccidioidomycosis, disseminated or extrapulmonary

Histoplasmosis, disseminated

Chronic intestinal isosporiasis >1 month

Kaposi's sarcoma, any age

Primary CNS lymphoma, any age

Non-Hodgkin's lymphoma – small, noncleaved lymphoma; Burkitt or non-Burkitt type; or immunoblastic sarcoma

Mycobacterium avium complex or *M. kansasii*; disseminated or extrapulmonary

Mycobacterium, other species or unidentified species; disseminated or extrapulmonary

M. tuberculosis, any site

Salmonella septicaemia, recurrent

Diseases diagnosed presumptively with confirmation of HIV infection

Candidiasis of the oesophagus

CMV retinitis

Kaposi's sarcoma

Lipoid interstitial pneumonitis in patients <13 years old

Disseminated mycobacterial disease (not cultured)

Pneumocystis carinii pneumonia

Toxoplasmosis of the brain in patients >1 month old

HIV encephalopathy

HIV wasting syndrome

Recurrent pneumonia

Pulmonary tuberculosis

Middle East, where HIV was probably introduced rather later than elsewhere. Recent studies, however, indicate that there is a high incidence of new seroconversions taking place in these areas. WHO is concerned that the epidemic in Asia may ultimately dwarf all others in scope and in impact.

THE HUMAN IMMUNODEFICIENCY VIRUSES

HIV-1 is an RNA virus which belongs to the lentivirus group of the retroviridae family. In common with other members of this group (visna/

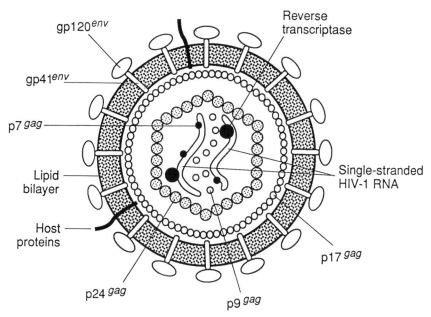

Figure 1 Schematic diagram of the HIV-1 virion. Each of the virion proteins making up the envelope (gp120^{env} and gp41^{env}) and nucleocapsid (p24^{gag}, p17^{gag}, p9^{gag} and p7^{gag}) is identified. In addition, the diploid RNA genome is shown associated with reverse transcriptase, an RNA-dependent DNA polymerase

maedi virus, equine infectious anaemia virus, caprine arthritis/encephalitis virus), it is a non-transforming virus which generates a cytopathic or lytic effect on cells *in vitro* and causes a persistent infection following integration of HIV proviral DNA into the host genome. The group now contains the human viruses HIV-1 and HIV-2, the related simian immunodeficiency viruses SIV, and the more distantly related feline leukaemia virus (FIV) and bovine leukaemia virus (BIV). HIV-1 is pandemic, whereas HIV-2 has been isolated almost entirely from patients who live in or have visited West Africa. HIV-2 shares close antigenic cross-reactivity and nucleotide sequence homology with SIV, and is more distantly related to HIV-1[5,6]. Infection with HIV-2 produces a clinical syndrome of AIDS which is similar to that seen with HIV-1[7,8], except that the rate of progression to AIDS may be slower than is seen with HIV-1. SIV also causes an immunodeficiency syndrome (Simian AIDS, SAIDS) in Asian Old World monkeys, but not in African Old World monkeys or in New World monkeys.

Structure and protein products

The structure of HIV-1 (Figure 1) is representative of the group. Two single-stranded copies of RNA are non-covalently linked to the gag protein p15; p24 is the most abundant core protein and together with p18 they comprise

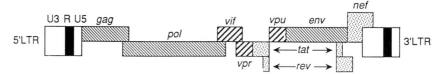

Figure 2 Genomic structure of HIV-1. Each of the nine known genes of HIV-1 are shown, and their recognized primary functions summarized. The 5' and 3' long terminal repeats (LTRs) containing regulatory sequences recognized by various host transcription factors are also depicted, and the positions of the tat and rev response elements (TAR [transactivation response] element and rev RNA response element) are indicated

the major gag structural proteins. RNA-dependent DNA polymerase (reverse transcriptase), encoded by the *pol* gene, is closely associated with the RNA genome. The outer envelope of HIV consists of a lipid and protein membrane which is derived from the host cell membrane and in which a transmembrane glycoprotein (gp41) anchors the extracellular glycosylated protein gp120.

The proviral genome of HIV-1 and HIV-2 is 9–10 kb long. Sequencing data from several different HIV-1 strains have shown that the structural genes *gag* (group antigen) and *pol* (polymerase) are more conserved than *env* (envelope). Several other genes have been identified which encode for proteins whose function is to regulate viral replication. Tat (transactivator) proteins accelerate the production of viral proteins (including itself) by as much as 1000 times. The *cis*-acting sequence required for tat activity is the transactivation response region (*TAR*) which is located immediately downstream of the cap site residues $+1$ to $+79$ and forms part of the 5' untranslated (U5) region of all the mRNAs encoded by HIV[9]. Interaction of *TAR* and tat facilitates transcriptional elongation, increases mRNA stability and enhances translation.

nef (negative regulatory factor) was so called because nef proteins were believed to have a negative regulatory effect on viral transcription and replication. However, there are now numerous conflicting reports on whether nef has a negative effect, no effect, or a positive effect on viral transcription and replication. Such discrepancies have occurred with researchers using the same virus and the same cell lines. It is likely that any effect of nef on the growth of lentiviruses *in vitro* is probably small, at least under standard cell culture conditions.

The viral protein rev (regulator of virion protein) serves as a switch which determines whether only non-structural regulatory proteins will be made or whether viral particles can also be made. The role of vif (virion infectivity factor) has not been clearly established, but it seems to have a dramatic effect on virus replication and is thought to play a role in virion infectivity. VpU (viral protein U) allows proper virion assembly, packaging, budding and release of infectious virus. Regulatory proteins therefore affect the production not only of structural gene proteins but also that of regulatory gene proteins including themselves.

Cells arrested in the G_0 phase have few if any viral transcripts. Following cellular activation, nuclear factors which activate interleukins and their receptors also lead to the transcription of HIV. Initially, low levels of short viral transcripts are synthesized, with accumulation of tat. On reaching a threshold, tat greatly increases the expression of TAR-containing RNA transcripts. Controlled viral replication depends upon a balance being maintained between positive and negative regulatory factors such that when an infected cell dies enough virions are released to infect other cells.

The CD4 receptor for HIV

The CD4 antigen was identified as an essential component of the receptor for infection by HIV following the observation that the development of AIDS was associated with a decline in the CD4$^+$ lymphocyte count. The *in vitro* tropism of HIV for CD4$^+$ lymphocytes was demonstrated using monoclonal antibodies specific for CD4 which blocked HIV infection and syncytium formation, as well as by VSV(HIV) pseudotype plating experiments[10,11]. Transfer of the cDNA for the human CD4 receptor to cells lacking it (HeLa cells) made them susceptible to infection by HIV[12]. In contrast, cDNA inserts of the human CD4 receptor into murine T cells resulted in binding of HIV to the cell surface receptor, but no entry of the virus into cells. These findings suggest that a second cell surface receptor is required for entry of the virus once binding to the CD4 receptor has occurred.

The CD4 antigen acts as the receptor not only for HIV-1, but also for HIV-2 and SIV. It is also present on monocytes and macrophages and is presumed to play a central role in the entry of virus into these cells[13,14]. HIV binds to the CD4 receptor through the gp120 envelope glycoprotein with an affinity constant of 10^{-9} M. The receptor site has been mapped using monoclonal antibodies to a conserved region of gp120 and C3, within amino acid residues 413–456[15]. It is believed that for viral entry to occur gp120 must first bind to CD4. A secondary conformational change in the HIV transmembrane protein gp41 then leads to fusion (in a pH-independent manner) of the virus membrane with that of the host[16,17]. On brain and bowel cells (which are negative for CD4) galactosyl ceramide is thought to be the receptor for HIV-1[18,19].

Strain variations

There is increasing evidence to suggest that the biological properties of molecularly cloned viruses vary considerably from clone to clone[20,21]. Active retroviral replication results in changes in the structural genes such that defective virus particles are produced which, although replication incompetent, have been implicated in the pathogenesis of the immunodeficiency syndrome[22–24]. It is now clear that HIV is constantly evolving *in vivo*. Isolates obtained from patients with asymptomatic HIV infection grow slowly, and usually do so only in primary cell cultures. They produce low titres of reverse transcriptase activity and have been termed slow/low viruses. Isolates established from patients with AIDS are capable of continuous viral replication in CD4$^+$ lymphocyte and monocyte cell lines[24,26]. Even isolates

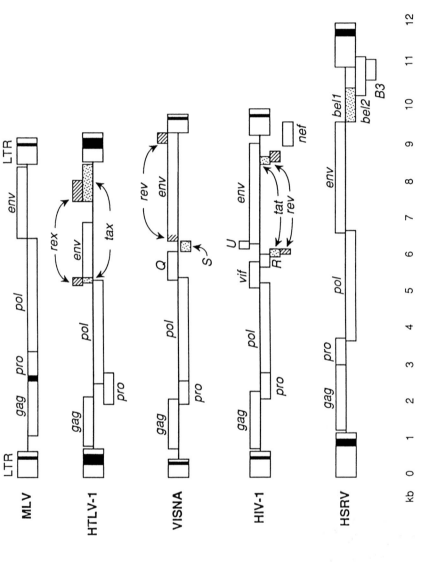

Figure 3 Representative retroviral proviruses. Shown are the genomic organization of MLV, a typical simple retrovirus, and of four representative complex retroviruses. Although all known viral genes are named and drawn approximately to scale, this listing is not exhaustive. Known transcriptional activators are marked by stippling, while known post-transcriptional regulators are indicated by hatching. LTRs are indicated by large terminal boxes, with the R

obtained sequentially from the same patient show differences in their replicating ability and cytopathic effect[20,26]; those taken from patients with AIDS having an expanded host cell tropism *in vitro*, faster replication rates and a greater cytopathic effect[27,28]. A large number of related but genotypically distinguishable variants evolve in parallel *in vivo*, with rapid/high variants becoming more common during the course of the infection. The immune mechanisms underlying the emergence of such variants and their relationship to the progression of clinical disease remain to be determined.

Mechanisms of cytopathic effect

A given individual is infected with several different isolates of HIV-1 throughout the course of the disease. Some of these isolates produce high titres of reverse transcriptase and grow rapidly in peripheral blood mononuclear cells (fast/high viruses) while others produce low titres of reverse transcriptase activity and grow slowly (slow/low viruses)[25,26]. Isolates obtained sequentially from the same patient show differences in their ability to replicate in PBMN cells and in their cytopathic effect[20,26]. Furthermore, isolates taken from patients with AIDS have an expanded host cell tropism *in vitro*, compared with isolates from patients with asymptomatic HIV infection[27,28]. This difference in the biological properties of viral isolates has been confirmed using molecularly cloned viruses[20,21].

Although a progressive loss of CD4[+] T lymphocytes is central to the immune defect in AIDS, the precise mechanisms underlying the quantitative as well as the functional defects still remain to be defined. Infection *in vitro* of any cell expressing CD4 can lead to one of several possible outcomes.

Syncytia formation

Single cell killing and syncytia formation is through a direct HIV-mediated cytopathic effect[29,30]. Single cell killing may result from the accumulation of unintegrated proviral DNA and/or from defects in post-translational processes which interfere with the processing of heteronuclear cellular RNA and which lead to the arrest of normal cellular processes[31,32]. Syncytium formation involves fusion of the cell membrane of an infected cell with the cell membranes of uninfected CD4[+] cells and the formation of multinucleated giant cells. As many as 500 uninfected cells can combine to form a multinucleated giant cell with the subsequent death of both the original infected cell and that of uninfected T cells.

Antibody-dependent cellular cytotoxicity

Although the major effect of antibodies against HIV-1 is attributed to their neutralizing properties, some antibodies which are directed against regions of the envelope of HIV-1 may have an additional protective function which is related to their ability to mediate antibody-dependent cellular cytotoxicity. This leads to the death of HIV-infected cells which express viral envelope proteins on their surface[33].

Autoimmune mechanisms

Non-polymorphic determinants of MHC Class II molecules, particularly HLA-DR and HLA-DQ, share some degree of structural homology with the gp120 and gp41 proteins of HIV-1[40], and antibodies to these HIV-1 proteins can therefore cross-react with MHC Class II molecules. Antibodies which react with MHC Class II molecules have been found in the serum of patients with HIV-1 infection. These antibodies could therefore prevent the interaction between CD4 and MHC Class II molecules on antigen-presenting cells, thereby impairing the cellular interaction which is required for efficient antigen presentation and inhibiting the antigen-specific functions which are mediated by helper $CD4^+$ T cells[34,35].

Anergy

Complexes of gp120–anti-gp120 bind to CD4, and the $CD4^+$ cells then become refractory to further *in vitro* stimulation via their CD3 molecules[36]. Similarly, *in vitro*, peripheral blood mononuclear cells inoculated with HIV-1 do not respond to stimulation with anti-CD3 antibodies[35]. These observations have led to the hypothesis that a negative signal is delivered to $CD4^+$ cells after CD4 has bound to gp120 or to gp120–anti-gp120 complexes. In this regard, anti-gp120 antibodies have recently been detected on $CD4^+$ T lymphocytes in patients with AIDS[38].

Superantigens

Several authors have reported that endogenous or exogenous retroviral-encoded superantigens stimulate murine $CD4^+$ T cells *in vivo* and that this leads to anergy or deletion of a substantial percentage of $CD4^+$ T cells with specific V_β regions[39,41]. This has led to the hypothesis that a superantigen (either retrovirally encoded or unrelated to HIV-1) may play an important part in the immunopathogenesis of HIV-1 infection[42]. Consistent with this hypothesis have been reports that patients with HIV-1 infection have disturbances of T cell subgroups bearing certain specific V_β regions[43].

Programmed cell death

This is a mechanism whereby the body eliminates autoreactive clones of T cells. Since apoptosis can be induced in mature murine $CD4^+$ T cells after cross-linking CD4 molecules to one another and triggering of the T cell antigen receptor[44], there has been speculation that cross-linking of the CD4 molecule by gp120 or gp120–anti-gp120 immune complexes prepares the cell for programmed cell death which then occurs when an MHC Class II molecule complexed to an antigen binds to the T cell antigen receptor[45]. Thus the mere activation of a prepared cell by a specific antigen or superantigen could lead to the death of the cell without direct infection by HIV-1.

PRIMARY HIV-1 INFECTION

Patients with primary HIV infection can present clinically with an abrupt onset of a febrile illness resembling acute mononucleosis. Symptoms can include lymphadenopathy, pharyngitis, rash, myalgia, arthralgia, diarrhoea, headache, nausea and vomiting[46]. Shallow ulcers can occur in the mouth, oesophagus or in the genital area[47]. Neurological involvement (meningoence-phalitis) also occurs but is uncommon. These symptoms and signs can be associated with a transient leucopenia, atypical lymphocytosis, increased numbers of banded neutrophils and thrombocytopenia[48]. Symptomatic primary HIV-1 infection that comes to medical attention typically occurs 2–6 weeks after exposure to HIV-1 and usually resolves within 1–2 weeks. The symptoms coincide with a high-grade viraemia, as indicated by the presence of p24 antigenaemia, plasma viraemia and a high titre of HIV-1 in peripheral blood mononuclear cells. The HIV strains associated with acute infection are uniformly macrophage tropic[49]. Resolution is coincident with the emergence of detectable HIV-specific antibody and an increase in cytotoxic T lymphocytes[50,51]. A host IgM (variable) and IgG response develop within 7–14 days and almost always within 3 months[52].

The general activation of the immune system during this time is reflected by increases in serum neopterin, a breakdown product secreted from activated macrophages indicating increased cellular activation, β_2-microglobulin, a component of major histocompatibility complex Class I indicating increased cellular turnover, and α-interferon[53,54]. The activation of the immune response is characterized by the appearance of activated T cells in the circulation.

Responses to antigen and mitogen are impaired during primary HIV-1 infection. Patients have a reduced response to both pokeweed mitogen and to phytohaemagglutinin (PHA). Antigen-specific responses can remain impaired for up to 6–12 months after the primary infection[55].

The immunological profile typically shows an initial reduction in total lymphocyte count followed by transient increases in CD8[+] lymphocytes and inversion of the CD4:CD8 cell ratio[51]. Although in some subjects the number of CD4[+] lymphocytes may recover to the level prior to infection, the overall trend in HIV-infected persons is a progressive decrease in these cells. In vitro, autologous CD8[+] lymphocytes are capable of suppressing HIV replication in peripheral blood mononuclear cells[56]. Transient increases in the numbers of CD8[+] cells and activated CD8[+] cells can also be found in acute infections with other viruses such as cytomegalovirus and Epstein-Barr virus and therefore may represent a non-specific immune response against viral infections. However, HIV-1 is the first chronic viral disease associated with prominent cytotoxic T lymphocyte activity[33].

Although HIV-1 is believed to disseminate widely during the early stages of infection, the immunological response results in a rapid decline in the level of the viraemia within weeks and the acute syndrome subsides. It is likely, however, that viral replication is never completely curtailed, since it is detectable in lymph nodes during apparently quiescent stages of infection[57]. The events described above probably occur even in those patients who do not have a clinically recognizable acute seroconversion syndrome.

Following acute infection of T cells by HIV *in vitro*, there is a transient reduction in the expression of HLA DR on the cell surface[58]. Cells which survive the cytopathic effect of the virus have a decreased level of expression of CD4 molecules on their cell surface. Expression of interleukin-2 (IL-2) is also decreased, despite normal expression of the IL-2 receptor gene[59]. This functional defect in the expression of IL-2 may contribute to the antigen-specific defect which requires IL-2 for amplification.

During the early course of asymptomatic HIV infection, the proliferative responses of peripheral blood lymphocytes and purified populations of CD4$^+$ lymphocytes to PHA, tetanus toxoid and/or calcium ionophore do not demonstrate a functional defect in T cell function[60].

Other as yet undetermined factors are clearly important at this early stage of infection in patients whose acute illness lasts for more than 14 days. The rate of progression to CDC IV within 3 years is eight times higher in this group of patients than in patients who have mild symptoms. CD4$^+$ lymphocyte counts are similar in these two groups at the time of seroconversion and for a period of 6 months thereafter[52]. It is possible that the severity of symptoms at the time of seroconversion reflects the degree of active viral replication. Similarly, parameters of humoral immunity to HIV at seroconversion affect outcome in terms of disease progression. No immune response to HIV at the time of infection or in the subsequent course of the illness unequivocally clears virus from the host.

ASYMPTOMATIC HIV INFECTION

After recovering from their seroconversion illness, most patients have a period of clinical latency during which they are clinically asymptomatic. During this period, which can last for several years, almost all patients have a gradual depletion of their CD4$^+$ T cells. Although it can be difficult to detect virus in the peripheral blood at this time, viral replication continues in lymphoid organs and the spectrum of immunological events which are triggered by the virus is evident within lymph nodes.

SYMPTOMATIC HIV INFECTION

The inevitable outcome of the progressive deterioration of the immune system is the development of clinically apparent disease. A re-examination of lymphoid tissue from patients during the early stages of the disease has shown a high burden of HIV-1 in lymphoid tissues, both as extracellular virus trapped in the follicular dendritic cell network of the germinal centres and as intracellular virus[61,62]. HIV replicates, albeit at low levels, during the early, asymptomatic phase of the disease. As the disease progresses, the level of replication in lymphoid tissue increases.

The development of the AIDS-related complex (ARC) is usually associated with a fall in the CD4$^+$ lymphocyte count to $<200/\mu l$. This decrease is due to a fall in the CD4$^+$ TQ1$^+$ subset (inducer function) with normal CD4$^+$ TQ1$^-$ subset (helper function) cells. The total number of CD8$^+$ cells remains normal or increases. Within the CD8$^+$ group of cells, CD8$^+$ 9.3$^+$ cells (suppressor T cell) increase and CD8$^+$ 9.3$^-$ (cytotoxic T cell) cells decrease.

AIDS

Progression to AIDS is associated with an inversion of both the cytotoxic/suppressor cell ratio and the CD4/CD8 ratio to less than 1.0. Concomitant infections, especially with cytomegalovirus, cause wide fluctuations in the number of suppressor/cytotoxic cells which is reflected in the CD4/CD8 ratio. Consequently the most consistent indicator of the severity of immune dysfunction is the CD4$^+$ lymphocyte count. The percentage CD4$^+$ lymphocyte count is a more reliable indicator for the longitudinal follow-up of patients than the absolute CD4 count because it is not affected by day-to-day fluctuations in either the total white cell count or the percentage of total lymphocytes[63]. In late-stage AIDS, all lymphoid cells, including those which are CD8$^+$, are depleted due to both HIV itself as well as to opportunistic infections which may independently cause bone marrow suppression[64].

In patients with AIDS, the CD4$^+$ lymphocyte is unable to mount a proliferative response to soluble antigens such as tetanus toxoid. This abnormality is seen with both unfractionated cells and with purified CD4$^+$ cells[65]. It is not due to a defect in antigen-presenting cells and implies a selective depletion or a selective functional impairment of a specific subset of T helper/inducer cells. It is also reflected in the defective autologous mixed lymphocyte reaction of peripheral blood mononuclear cells from patients infected with HIV in which CD4$^+$ lymphocytes fail to proliferate[66]. These defects are thought to reflect abnormalities at the level of the cell surface rather than at a subcellular level. gp120 bound to CD4 was thought to interfere with MHC Class II function, but this now seems unlikely. Using homologue-scanning mutagenesis, Lamarre found that gp120 binding could be abolished without affecting MHC Class II binding and vice-versa[67], indicating that the gp120 and MHC Class II binding sites of CD4 are distinct and can be separated.

In assays used to assess the ability of CD4$^+$ cells to help and CD8$^+$ cells to suppress immunoglobulin production by pokeweek mitogen-stimulated B cells *in vitro*, the CD4$^+$ cells from patients with AIDS demonstrate little or no helper function, in contrast to CD8$^+$ cells from the same patients which exhibit normal suppressor function[68,69]. These results confirm that the overall defect in patients with AIDS remains a failure of helper and inducer cell function rather than increased suppressor cell function.

LYMPHOID ORGANS IN HIV-1 INFECTION

It has recently become clear that the lymphoid organs are a major anatomical site in which HIV-1 becomes established and in which it is propagated in both the short and long term. Most studies, of necessity, focus on HIV infection of peripheral blood mononuclear cells, but it is important to remember that the lymphocytes in the peripheral blood at any given time represent only 2% of the total lymphocyte pool[70]. Therefore, in certain pathogenic processes involving lymphoid cells, the peripheral blood may not accurately reflect the status of the disease. Furthermore, specific immune responses are generated predominantly in the lymphoid organs rather than in the peripheral blood[71].

Studies using the standard polymerase chain reaction (PCR) to detect HIV DNA and reverse transcriptase PCR to detect HIV RNA have found 5–10 times more HIV-infected cells and higher concentrations of both regulatory and structural messenger RNA in the lymphoid organs (lymph nodes, adenoids and tonsils) of patients than in their peripheral blood. This viral burden in lymphoid organs is greater than that in the peripheral blood throughout the period of clinical latency[72].

In early and intermediate disease HIV particles, complexed with antibodies and complement, accumulate in lymph nodes, where they are trapped within the network of follicular dendritic cells within germinal centres[73]. Follicular dendritic cells function during the normal immune response to trap antigens in the environment of the germinal centre and to allow the presentation of antigen to competent immune cells[74]. This is an efficient means of initiating and propagating an appropriate immune response to antigenic challenge, be it microbial or environmental. The progression to clinical HIV-related disease is associated with the degeneration of the network of follicular dendritic cells and the loss of the ability of lymphoid organs to trap HIV particles, thereby contributing to an increase in viraemia.

In the late stages of HIV disease, the architecture of the lymph nodes is disrupted and the network of follicular dendritic cells dissolves, removing the mechanisms for trapping virions. HIV is thus free to recirculate, a finding that has been interpreted to be a reflection of a massive increase in the total viral burden in late-stage disease. However, rather than representing a true increase in viral burden, these high levels of viraemia in AIDS may reflect, at least in part, the recirculation of HIV particles removed from the constraints of lymph node entrapment.

The increased viral load in lymph nodes has recently been confirmed by culturing mononuclear cells obtained from lymph nodes. The mean titre of virus was 60 times higher in lymph nodes from CDC Stage III patients than in blood[75]. Co-cultures of mononuclear cells from the lymph nodes also became positive before those from blood.

The gut is another major lymphoid organ in the body, and as many as

5–50% of all lymphocytes are contained within it, distributed as Peyer's patches, lamina propria, lymphoid cells and aggregates of intra-epithelial lymphocytes. Infection in gut-associated lymphoid tissue is similar to that in peripheral lymph nodes, with trapping of virus on follicular dendritic cells which then act as reservoirs of latent and replicating virus[76]. It is likely that other reservoirs of HIV exist in other locations within the body and that they also contribute to the total body load of infectious, replicating HIV-1.

EFFECTS OF CYTOKINES

Although infection with HIV-1 is associated with increased production of a number of cytokines, both *in vitro* and *in vivo*, the relative roles of each of these cytokines during HIV infection is not clear. It remains to be established whether these cellular products act as cofactors to influence CD4$^+$ cell destruction or compromise their function[77]. For example, B cells isolated from HIV-infected individuals spontaneously secrete high levels of tumour necrosis factor α and IL-6 *in vitro*[78]. Since activated B cells within the germinal centres of lymph nodes of HIV-infected individuals are in close proximity to latently infected CD4$^+$ T cells in the paracortical area of the nodes, as well as to HIV-infected CD4$^+$ T cells that have infiltrated the germinal centres, cytokine secretion may play an important role in the microenvironment of the lymph node. Recent reports suggest that there may be a progressive imbalance in the T cell limbs of the immune system of HIV-infected individuals, with a selective defect in T_{H1} responses mediated by IL-2 and γ-interferon (IFN-γ) and a predominance of T_{H2} responses mediated by IL-4, IL-5, IL-6 and IL-10[79].

MONOCYTES AND MACROPHAGES

Early studies on macrophages were hampered by a lack of growth factors for *in vitro* cultivation, and by the use of a strain of HIV (IIIb) which was subsequently shown to be incapable of infecting human macrophages[27]. Gendelman subsequently showed that human monocytes cultivated with colony stimulating factor-1 can be easily infected with HIV and that the virus replicates in these cells to very high levels[80]. After intracellular maturation, HIV buds into intracytoplasmic vacuoles, with only rare budding of the virus onto the cell surface. Despite continuous viral production there is little or no cytopathic change, with the formation of only a few giant cells and a moderate decrease in CD4 expression[81].

Strains derived from brain or lung tissue exhibit a particular monocyte tropism with high reverse transcriptase activity, in contrast to infection of CD4$^+$ T lymphocytes in which infection is often poorly productive[27,82]. Reverse transcriptase activity in monocytes (as in T cells) seems to depend upon the degree of cell activation rather than on cell proliferation, presumably because replication can involve unintegrated DNA[27]. As a result, the number of HIV antigen-positive cells and reverse transcriptase activity increases considerably in monocytes and U937 cells which have been stimulated with IFN-γ, granulocyte-macrophage colony stimulating factor and IL-2[83,84].

The number of circulating monocytes is decreased in patients with ARC or AIDS[85]. Functional abnormalities, such as a reduced production and secretion of IL-1 and reduced ability to respond to chemotactic stimuli, are not evident until the development of AIDS[86]. Defects in the intracellular killing of *Toxoplasma gondii* and *Chlamydia psittacii* are also likely to reflect defective production of lymphokines because they can be corrected by prior exposure to IFN-γ[87]. Receptor-specific phagocytosis (Fc and C3 receptor-mediated clearance) is impaired in patients with AIDS in contrast to non-immune (non-specific) mechanisms, which remain intact[88].

Interest in the role of the macrophage *in vivo* in HIV-1 infection increased following reports that antibody-mediated enhancement may be an important alternative mechanism for the infection of monocyte-macrophage derived cells which bear Fc receptors[89,90]. In contrast to neutralizing antibodies, enhancing antibodies do not prevent fusion of the virus with the cell but rather facilitate uptake of the virus–antibody complex through binding of the Fc portion of the antibody molecule to Fc receptors on the cell surface. The particular Fc receptor subtype involved has not yet been determined. *In vitro*, the enhancing effect of such antibodies can be as much as 10^4 fold, providing neutralizing antibodies are absent or diluted out; *in vivo*, such antibodies could alter the course of the disease[91]. The phenomenon is, however, far less significant than that seen in dengue virus infection and reflects a temporary increase in the rate of infection rather than an increase in the overall level of infection.

It remains unclear whether enhancement is separable from the conventional CD4-dependent mechanism of entry. Two groups have reported that monoclonal antibodies (OKT4 and Leu 3a) directed against the CD4 receptor block enhancement, while another has reached the opposite conclusion[92–94]. It may be that enhancing antibodies serve to concentrate the virus on the macrophage surface prior to its transfer to CD4 molecules and entry by normal mechanisms. An alternative or additional mechanism may involve components of human complement. Cells bearing receptors for human complement would attract complement-fixing antibodies attached to HIV, similar to the way in which Fc receptors bind antibody–HIV complexes. There also seems to be a requirement for CD4 in this situation. Enhancement has not been documented in animal studies of HIV or SIV vaccine testing, and more specifically it has not been found in humans immunized with HIV antigens. The issue needs to be resolved in order to ensure that any potentially harmful epitopes are eliminated from a potential vaccine.

Primary monocytes derived from peripheral blood do not seem to be highly susceptible to HIV infection, despite the fact that more than 90% of them express the activation marker HLA-DR[95,96]. In contrast, non-dividing differentiated macrophages can be infected with HIV-1 with relative ease[97]. In the latter case, differentiation has taken place at the time of productive infection and cell division has stopped. The window of susceptibility to infection by HIV-1 seems to be relatively narrow, because terminally differentiated macrophages are difficult to infect with HIV-1[98].

These observations place further emphasis on the role of tissue macrophages as an important site of virus replication; this is particularly well demonstrated by HIV-1 infection of the brain[99]. It still remains to be established whether monocytes are infected by HIV-1 in the blood stream and then carry the virus into extravascular compartments, or whether they become infected after leaving the vascular system and migrating into tissues where they then become the major source of virus replication.

References

1. Classification system for HTLV III virus infections. MMWR. 1986; 35: 334–339.
2. Revision of the CDC surveillance case definition for AIDS. MMWR. 1987; 36 (Suppl 1): 1–15.
3. CDC surveillance case definition for AIDS. MMWR. 1992: 41 (RR-17).
4. Perriens J, Piot P. World wide epidemiology of HIV infection. In: Neu HC, Levy JA, Weiss JA, eds. Frontiers of Infectious Diseases, Focus on HIV. New York: Churchill Livingstone, 1993: 3–19.
5. Chakrabarti L, Guyader M, Alizon M et al. Sequence of SIV from macaque and its relationship to other human and simian retroviruses. Nature. 1987; 328: 543–547.
6. Franchini G, Gurgo C, Guo HG et al. Sequence of SIV and its relationship to HIV. Nature. 1987; 328: 539–543.
7. Clavel F, Mansinho K, Chamaret S et al. HIV Type 2 infection associated with AIDS in West Africa. New Engl J Med. 1987; 316: 1180–1185.
8. Le Guenno BM, Barabe P, Griffet PA et al. HIV-2 and HIV-1 AIDS cases in Senegal: clinical patterns in immunological perturbations. J AIDS. 1991; 4: 421–427.
9. Muesing MA, Smith DA, Capon DJ. Regulation of mRNA accumulation by a HIV trans-activator protein. Cell. 1987; 48: 691–701.
10. Dalgleish AG, Beverley PCL, Clapham PR et al. The CD4 antigen is an essential component of the receptor for the AIDS retrovirus. Nature. 1984; 312: 763–767.
11. Klatzmann D, Champagne E, Chamaret S et al. T-lymphocyte T4 molecule behaves as the receptor for human retrovirus LAV. Nature. 1984; 767–768.
12. Maddon PJ, Dalgeish AG, McDougal JS et al. The T4 gene encodes the AIDS virus receptor and is expressed in the immune system and the brain. Cell. 1986; 47: 333–348.
13. Ho DD, Rota TR, Hirsh MS. Infection of monocyte/macrophages by HTLV III. J Clin Invest. 1986; 77: 1712–1715.
14. Crowe S, Mills J, McGrath MS. Quantitative immunocytofluorographic analysis of CD4 antigen expression and HIV infection of human peripheral blood monocyte/macrophages. AIDS Res Hum Retroviruses. 1987; 3: 135–138.
15. Lasky LA, Nakamura G, Smith DH et al. Delineation of a region of the HIV type I gp 120 glycoprotein critical for interaction with the CD4 receptor. Cell. 1987; 50: 975–985.
16. Stein BS, Gowda SD, Lifson JD et al. pH-independent HIV entry into CD4+ T cells via virus envelope fusion to the plasma membrane. Cell. 1987; 49: 659–668.
17. McClure MO, Marsh M, Weiss RA. HIV-1 virus infection of CD4 bearing cells occurs by a pH independent mechanism. EMBO J. 1988; 7: 513–518.
18. Harouse JM, Bhat S, Spitalnik SL et al. Inhibition of entry of HIV-1 into neural cell lines by antibodies against galactosyl ceramide. Science. 1991; 253: 320–323.
19. Yahi N, Baghdiguian S, Moreau H et al. Galactosyl ceramide (or a closely related molecule) is the receptor for HIV-1 on human colon epithelial HT29 cells. J Virol. 1992; 66: 4848–4854.
20. Fisher AG, Ensoli B, Looney D et al. Biologically diverse molecular variants within a single HIV-1 isolate. Nature. 1988; 334: 444–447.
21. Sakai K, Dewhurst S, Ma X et al. Differences in cytopathogenicity and host cell range among infectious molecular clones of HIV-1 simultaneously isolated from an individual. J Virol. 1988; 4078–4085.
22. Aziz DC, Hanna Z, Jolicoeur P. Severe immunodeficiency disease induced by a defective murine leukaemia virus. Nature. 1989; 338: 505–508.

23. Hartley JW, Frederickson TN, Yetter RA *et al.* Retrovirus-induced murine acquired immunodeficiency syndrome; natural history of infection and differing susceptibility of inbred mass strains. J Virol. 1989; 63: 1223–1231.

24. Overbaugh J, Donahue PR, Quackenbush SL *et al.* Molecular cloning of a FeLV that induces fatal immunodeficiency disease in cats. Science. 1988; 239: 906–910.

25. Asjo B, Morfeldt-Manson L, Albert J *et al.* Replicative capacity of HIV from patients with varying severity of HIV infection. Lancet. 1986; ii: 660–662.

26. Cheng-Mayer C, Seto D, Tateno M, Levy JA. Biologic features of HIV-1 that correlate with virulence in the host. Science. 1988; 240: 80–82.

27. Gatner S, Markovits P, Markovitz DM *et al.* The role of mononuclear phagocytes in HTLV III infection. Science. 1986; 233: 215–219.

28. Koyanagi Y, Miles S, Mitsuyasu RT *et al.* Dual infection of the central nervous system by AIDS viruses with distinct cellular tropisms. Science. 1987; 236: 819–822.

29. Lifson JD, Reyes GR, McGrath MS *et al.* AIDS retrovirus induced cytopathology: giant cell formation and involvement of the CD4 antigen. Science. 1986; 232: 1123–1127.

30. Sodroski J, Goh WC, Rosen C, Campbell K, Haseltine WA. Role of the HTLV-3/LAV envelope in syncytium formation and cytopathicity. Nature. 1986; 322: 470–474.

31. Levy JA, Kaminsky LS, Morrow WJW *et al.* Infection by the retrovirus associated with AIDS. Ann Intern Med. 1985; 103: 694–599.

32. Koya Y, Linstrom E, Fenyo EM *et al.* HIV infection may interfere with hnRNA processing in cells. V International Conference on AIDS. Stockholm, June 1988; 2573.

33. Fauci AS (Moderator). Immunopathogenic mechanisms in HIV-1 infection. Ann Intern Med. 1991; 114: 678–693.

34. Golding H, Robey FA, Gates FT III *et al.* Identification of homologous regions in HIV-1 gp41 and human MHC Class 2 B1 domain. J Exp Med. 1988; 167: 913–923.

35. Golding H, Shearer JM, Hillman K *et al.* Common epitope in HIV-1 gp41 and HLA Class II elicits immunosuppressive autoantibodies capable of contributing to immune dysfunction in HIV-1 infected individuals. J Clin Invest. 1989; 83: 1430–1435.

36. Mittler RS, Holfmann MK. Synergism between HIV-gp 120 and gp120-specific antibody blocking human T cell activation. Science. 1989; 245: 1380–1382.

37. Linette GP, Hartzmann RJ, Ledbetter JA, June CH. HIV-1 infected T cells show a selective signalling defect after perturbation of the CD3/antigen receptor. Science. 1988; 241: 573–576.

38. Amadori A, de Silvestro G, Zamarchi R *et al.* CD4 epitope masking by gp120-antibody complexes: potential mechanism for CD cell function downregulation in AIDS patients. J Immunol. 1992; 148: 2709–2716.

39. Frankel WN, Rudy C, Coffin JM, Huber BT. Linkage of MLS genes to endogenous mammary tumour viruses of inbred mice. Nature. 1991; 349: 526–528.

40. Marrack P, Kushnir E, Kappler J. Maternally inherited superantigen coded by a mammary tumour virus. Nature. 1991; 349: 524–526.

41. Woodland DL, Happ MP, Gollob AJ, Palmer E. An endogenous retrovirus mediating deletion of T cells? Nature. 1991; 349: 529–530.

42. Janeway C. MLS: makes a little sense. Nature. 1991; 349: 459–461.

43. Imberti L, Sottini A, Bettinardi A *et al.* Selective depletion in HIV infection of T cells that bear specific T cell receptor V_β sequences. Science. 1991; 254: 860–862.

44. Newell MK, Haughn LJ, Maroun CR, Julius MH. Death of mature T cells by separate ligation of CD4 and the T cell receptor for antigen. Nature. 1990; 347: 286–289.

45. Groux A, Torpier G, Monte D *et al.* Activation-induced death by apoptosis in CD4-positive T cells from HIV-1 infected asymptomatic individuals. J Exp Med. 1992; 175: 331–340.

46. Pedersen C, Lindhardt BO, Jensen BL *et al.* Clinical course of primary HIV infection: consequences for subsequent course of infection. Br Med J. 1989; 299: 154–156.

47. Gaines H, Sydow M, Pehrson PO *et al.* Clinical picture of primary HIV infection presenting as a glandular fever like illness. Br Med J. 1988; 297: 1363–1368.

48. Tindall B, Barker S, Donovan B *et al.* Characterisation of the acute clinical illness associated with HIV infection. Arch Intern Med. 1988; 148: 945–949.

49. Zhu T, Mo H, Wang N *et al.* Genotypic and phenotypic characterisation of HIV-1 in patients with primary infection. Science. 1993; 261: 1179–1181.

50. Clark SJ, Saag MS, Decker WD *et al.* High titres of cytopathic virus in plasma of patients

with symptomatic HIV infections. New Engl J Med. 1991; 324: 954–960.

51. Daar ES, Moudgil T, Meyer RD et al. Transient high levels of viraemia in patients with primary HIV-1 infection. New Engl J Med. 1991; 324: 961–964.

52. Von Sydow M, Gaines H, Sonnerborg A. Antigen detection in primary HIV infection. Br Med J. 1988; 296: 238–240.

53. Gaines H, von Sydow MAE, von Stedingk LV et al. Immunological changes in primary HIV infection. AIDS. 1990; 4: 995–999.

54. Sonnerborg AB, von Stedingk LV, Hansson LO et al. Elevated neopterin and β-2 microglobulin levels in blood and cerebrospinal fluid occur early in HIV infection. AIDS. 1989; 3: 277–283.

55. Pedersen C, Dickmeiss E, Gaub J et al. T cell subset alterations and lymphocyte responsiveness to mitogens and antigen during severe primary infection with HIV: a case series of seven consecutive HIV seroconverters. AIDS. 1990; 4: 523–526.

56. Walker CM, Moody DJ, Stites DP et al. CD8 + lymphocytes can control HIV infection in vitro by suppressing virus replication. Science. 1986; 234: 1563–1566.

57. Fauci AS. Multifactorial nature of human immunodeficiency virus disease: implication for therapy. Science. 1993; 262: 1011–1018.

58. Mann DL, Lesane F, Blattner WA et al. HLA DR is involved in the HIV receptor. III International Conference on AIDS, Washington DC, 1987; 209.

59. Fauci AS. The HIV virus: infectivity and mechanisms of pathogenesis. Science. 1988; 239: 617–622.

60. Gurley RJ, Ikeuchi K, Byrn RA et al. CD4 + lymphocyte function with early HIV infection. Proc Natl Acad Sci USA. 1989; 86: 1993–1997.

61. Pantaleo G, Graziosi C, Demarest JF et al. HIV infection is active and progressive in lymphoid tissue during the clinically latent stage of disease. Nature. 1993; 362: 355–358.

62. Embretson J, Zupancic M, Ribas JL et al. Massive covert infection of helper T lymphocytes and macrophages by HIV during the incubation period of AIDS. Nature. 1993; 362: 359–362.

63. Kessler HA, Landay A, Pottage JC Jr et al. Absolute number versus percentage of T-helper lymphocytes in HIV infection. J Infect Dis. 1990; 161: 356–357.

64. Lane HC, Masur H, Gelmann EP et al. Correlation between immunologic function and clinical subpopulations of patients with AIDS. Am J Med. 1985; 78: 417–422.

65. Lane HC, Depper JM, Greene WC et al. Qualitative analysis of immune function in patients with AIDS: Evidence for a selective defect in soluble antigen recognition. New Engl J Med. 1985; 313: 79–84.

66. Gupta S, Safai B. Deficient autologous mixed lymphocyte reaction in Kaposi's sarcoma associated with a deficiency of Leu 3 + responder T cells. J Clin Invest. 1983; 71: 296–300.

67. Lamarre D, Ashkenazi A, Fleury S et al. The MHC binding and gp120 binding functions of CD4 are separable. Science. 1989; 245: 743–746.

68. Benveniste E, Schroff R, Stevens RH et al. Immunoregulatory T cells in men with AIDS. J Clin Immunol. 1983; 3: 359–367.

69. Lane HC, Masur H, Edgar LC et al. Abnormalities of B cell activation and immunoregulation in patients with AIDS. New Engl J Med. 1983; 309: 453–458.

70. Westerman J, Pabst R. Lymphocyte subsets in the blood: a diagnostic window on the lymphoid system? Immunol Today. 1990; 11: 406–410.

71. Parrott DM, Wilkinson PC. Lymphocyte locomotion and migration. In: de Weck AL, ed. Differentiated lymphocyte functions. Progress in Allergy, Vol. 28. Basel: Karger, 1981: 193–284.

72. Wood GS. The immunohistology of lymph nodes in HIV infection: a review. In: Rotterdam H, Racz P, Greco MA, Cockerell CJ, eds. Progress in AIDS Pathology Vol. 2. New York: Field and Wood, 1991; 25–32.

73. Speigel H, Herbst H, Niedobitek G et al. Follicular dendritic cells are a major reservoir for HIV-1 in lymphoid tissues facilitating infection of CD4 + T helper cells. Pathology. 1992; 140: 15–22.

74. Steinman RM. The dendritic cell system and its role in immunogenicity. Annu Rev Immunol. 1991; 9: 271–296.

75. Lafeuillade A, Tamalet C, Pellegrino P et al. High viral burden in lymph nodes during early stages of HIV infection. AIDS. 1993; 11: 1527–1541.

76. Fox CH, Kotler D, Tierney A, Wilson CS, Fauci AS. Detection of HIV-1 RNA in the lamina propria of patients with AIDS and gastrointestinal disease. J Infect Dis. 1989; 159: 467–471.

77. Poli G, Fauci AS. Cytokine modulation in HIV expression. Semin Immunol. 1993; 5: 165–173.

78. Rieckmann P, Poli G, Fox CH, Kehrl JH, Fauci AS. Recombinant gp120 specifically enhances tumour necrosis factor-alpha production and immunoglobulin secretion in B lymphocytes from HIV infected individuals but not from seronegative donors. J Immunol. 1991; 147: 2922–2927.

79. Clerici M, Shearer GM. TH 1–TH 2 switch as a critical step in the etiology of HIV infection. Immunol Today. 1993; 14: 107–111.

80. Gendelman HE, Orenstein JM, Martin MA et al. Efficient isolation and propagation of HIV on recombinant CSF-1 treated monocytes. J Exp Med. 1988; 167: 1428–1441.

81. Folks TM, Justement J, Kinter A et al. Cytokine-induced expression of HIV-1 in a chronically infected promonocyte cell line. Science. 1987; 238: 800–802.

82. Koenig S, Gendelman HE, Orenstein JM et al. Detection of AIDS virus in macrophages in brain tissue from AIDS patients with encephalopathy. Science. 1986; 233: 1089–1093.

83. Ruscetti FW, Mikovits JA, Kalyanaraman VS et al. Analysis of effector mechanisms against HTLV I and HTLV III infected lymphoid cells. J Immunol. 1986; 136: 3619–3624.

84. McCartney-Francis N. III International Conference on AIDS. Washington 1987; 84.

85. Sei Y, Petrella RJ, Tsang P et al. Monocytes in AIDS. New Engl J Med. 1986; 315: 1611–1612.

86. Smith PD, Ohura K, Masur H et al. Monocyte function in AIDS: defective chemotaxis. J Clin Invest. 1984; 74: 2121–2128.

87. Murray HW, Rubin BY, Masur H et al. Impaired production of lymphokines and gamma interferon in AIDS. New Engl J Med. 1984; 310: 883–889.

88. Bender BS, Davidson BL, Kline R et al. Role of the mononuclear phagocyte system in the immunopathogenesis of HIV infection and AIDS. Rev Infect Dis. 1988; 10: 1142–1154.

89. Zagury D, Bernard J, Cheynier R et al. A group specific anamnestic immune reaction against HIV-1 induced by a candidate vaccine against AIDS. Nature. 1988; 332: 728–731.

90. Suthipto S et al. V International Conference on AIDS. Montreal 1989 (Abst C Th Co 45).

91. Murphey-Corb M, Martin LN, Davison-Fairburn B et al. A formalin-inactivated whole SIV vaccine confers protection in macaques. Science. 1989; 246: 1293–1297.

92. Takeda A, Tuazon CU, Ennis FA. Antibody-enhanced infection by HIV-1 via Fc receptor-mediated entry. Science. 1988; 242: 580–583.

93. Robinson WE Jr, Montefiori DC, Mitchell WM. Antibody-dependent enhancement of HIV-1 infection. Lancet. 1988; i: 790–794.

94. Homsy J, Meyer M, Tateno M et al. The Fc and not CD4 receptor mediates antibody enhancement of HIV infection in human cells. Science. 1989; 244: 1357–1360.

95. Rich EA, Chen ISY, Zack JA et al. Increased susceptibility of differentiated mononuclear phagocytes to productive infection with HIV-1. J Clin Invest. 1992; 89: 176–183.

96. Schuitemaker H, Kootsra NA, Kopelman MHGM et al. Proliferation-dependent HIV infection of monocytes occurs during differentiation into macrophages. J Clin Invest. 1992; 89: 1154–1160.

97. Weinberg JB, Matthews TJ, Cullen BR, Malim MH. Productive HIV infection of non-proliferating human monocytes. J Exp Med. 1991; 174: 1477–1482.

98. Valentin A, von Gegerfelt A, Matsuda S et al. In vitro maturation of mononuclear phagocytes and susceptibility to HIV-1 infection. J AIDS. 1991; 4: 751–759.

99. Rudge P (ed.). Neurological aspects of human retroviruses in international practice and research. London, Baillière Tindall, 1992; vol. 1.

7
The Immunopathology of Viral and Bacterial Infections

J. G. P. SISSONS

INTRODUCTION

The immune system has evolved largely to enable the host to resist and overcome infection. However it is now clearly established that the immune response against infectious agents can, in some circumstances, be more responsible for the pathogenesis of the ensuing disease than any effects directly attributable to the agent itself. This ability of the immune response to produce damage to the organism is referred to as immunopathology. It is inevitably easier to demonstrate immunopathology in experimental models than in human disease, and this is where it has been shown most unequivocally. This chapter discusses examples of immunologically mediated disease associated with microbial infection in humans, with reference to experimental models where necessary to illustrate the mechanisms involved. Normal aspects of the immune response to viruses and bacteria are discussed elsewhere in this volume: however many micro-organisms have evolved mechanisms to subvert these immune responses and examples which show how such mechanisms are involved in pathogenesis are also covered here.

Rather more emphasis is given to evidence from viral systems as most studies have been undertaken in this area[1].

MOLECULAR ASPECTS OF PATHOGENESIS

Although this chapter focuses in particular on the involvement of the immune response in pathogenesis – immunopathogenesis – pathogenesis is a much wider area than this. Pathogenesis is the mechanism by which micro-organisms produce disease in the host, although it must be realised that most infections do not produce disease in the host. Virulence is the term used to describe the ability of an individual micro-organism to produce disease in a particular host, compared with other related members of its family.

Pathogenesis is the outcome of interactions between micro-organism and host, so both viral and host factors need to be considered. As microbial agents on the one hand, and cell biology and the host immune response on the other, become understood at a molecular level it becomes possible to explain pathogenesis in molecular terms, although the number of variables involved makes this a wide subject. An increasing number of genes that determine virulence and pathogenesis are being described for individual microbial agents. Viral genomes were the first complete genomes to be sequenced, and until very recently the large viral DNA genomes (such as cytomegalovirus, or vaccinia virus) remained the largest contiguous pieces of DNA of any sort to have been sequenced. A great deal of information can be derived from the microbial genomic sequence: genetic homology to other micro-organisms can be reecognized and facilitates classification; identification of homologues of other microbial genes and of cellular genes enables function of the products to be predicted; genetic variation or mutation can be identified and related to pathogenesis; and analysis of the genome by deletion and mutation becomes possible. The use of deletion and mutation analysis to identify genes involved in pathogenesis is particularly fruitful when a good animal model of disease exists, allowing the disease phenotype of the altered micro-organism to be studied *in vivo*.

IMMUNOPATHOLOGY OF VIRUS INFECTION

It is now well appreciated that the immune response against viruses can cause tissue damage and may have a pathogenic effect as well as a protective one[2]. Virus immunopathology has been particularly well studied in certain experimental models, such as lymphocytic choriomeningitis virus (LCMV) infection of mice[3]; human examples also exist but are rather harder to prove. In addition to pathology produced directly or indirectly by the antiviral immune response, viruses may infect immunocompetent cells and induce ineffective or abberant immune responses. These two broad areas of pathogenic interaction between viruses and the immune system are considered below (and see Table 1 and recent reviews[2,4]).

Pathology induced by the antiviral response

Antibody

Antibody can be responsible for immunopathology in several ways. In some circumstances antibody can facilitate virus infection of cells which express Fc receptors. This phenomenon, named antibody-dependent enhancement, was first described for dengue virus. When non-neutralizing antibody against dengue virus is added to the virus in the presence of macrophages *in vitro*, the virus replicates to much higher titres. This results from antibody–virus

Table 1 Examples of *in vivo* immunopathology resulting from the immune response to viruses

Mechanism	Virus	Host	Comment
Inappropriate antibody production	Measles	Man	Killed vaccine enhanced disease following natural or live vaccine exposure
	RSV	Man	Killed vaccine enhanced bronchiolitis following natural infection
	Dengue	Man	Non-neutralizing antibody enhances virus replication in macrophages
Immune complex disease	Hepatitis B	Man	Associated with arthralgia, rash, glomerulonephritis and periarteritis nodosa
	Aleutian disease	Mink	Immune complex disease with glomerulonephritis
	LCMV	Mouse	Immune complex disease with glomerulonephritis; severity strain-dependent
	LDH	Mouse	Less severe than LCMV; low incidence of nephritis
	Infectious anaemia	Horse	Immune complex disease related to antigen. Antigenic variation in viral glycoproteins within the individual host
	Infectious peritonitis virus	Cat	Circulating immune complexes and disseminated intravascular coagulation (DIC)
T-cell mediated	Measles	Man	Rash of measles dependent on T cell response
	Mumps	Man	Possible meningoencephalitis
	LCMV	Mouse	Fatal meningoencephalitis following intracerebral injection
	Influenza	Mouse	Td cells may enhance pneumonia
	Coxsackie	Mouse	Late phase of myocarditis
Enhanced mediator release	Dengue	Man	Haemorrhagic syndrome due to procoagulant release by infected macrophages

complexes binding to Fc receptors and entering the macrophages by receptor-mediated endocytosis, in addition to the normal route of entry. This *in vitro* phenomenon has been adduced as a possible factor in the pathogenesis of the dengue shock syndrome (DSS). Subjects at risk of DSS are those who have experienced dengue virus infection, and acquire a second infection with a different serotype of the virus: this may be associated with shock and intravascular coagulation, particularly in children. It is hypothesized that non-neutralizing antibody from the first infection may mediate enhancement allowing more widespread infection of macrophages, consequent mediator release and shock[5]. A similar mechanism has been described *in vitro* for other flaviviruses. The complement fragment C3b has also been reported to produce a similar enhancement effect in the presence of antibody, acting on the CR3 receptor on the macrophage, which binds complexes of antibody and flavivirus with C3b on them[6]. There has been considerable interest in whether antibody to the envelope protein of human immunodeficiency virus (HIV) can produce enhancement by facilitating virus entry into monocyte/macrophages. Although certain antibodies to the env protein have been shown to produce this effect *in vitro*, its significance *in vivo* is unknown[7,8].

Antibody can also be involved in the development of virus-induced immune complex disease. Animal models of chronic immune complex disease induced by persistent virus infections include the glomerulonephritis associated with LCMV or lactic dehydrogenase virus infection in mice, and with Aleutian disease in mink, which is caused by persistent parvovirus infection[9-11]. In these models, soluble complexes of viral antigen and antibody are deposited in tissues with filtering basement membranes, such as the renal glomerulus, joint synovium and choroid plexus. The glomerulonephritis may ultimately be fatal, particularly in infections with relatively non-cytopathic viruses such as LCMV.

These models have stimulated investigations into whether human diseases with an immune complex aetiology may be associated with persistent virus infections. The arthralgias and rash associated with many acute human virus infections such as hepatitis B may have an immune complex basis. Clear evidence for an association between persistent human virus infections and chronic immune complex disease is harder to find. However there is an association between persistent hepatitis B virus (HBV) infection and membranous glomerulonephritis, although this type of nephritis is not common in persistent HBV infection. HBV e antigen has recently been detected in the glomeruli, suggesting an immune complex aetiology[12]. The mechanism underlying the association between rubella and parvoviruses and arthritis has again not been clearly proven, although an immune complex aetiology is plausible.

Effector T lymphocytes

A large body of work has delineated the beneficial role of T cells in the resolution of experimental virus infections – cytotoxic T lymphocytes (CTL) which kill virus-infected cells, and T cells mediating delayed hypersensitivity (DTH) have been particularly well studied. Given that viruses are intracellular parasites, it is perhaps not especially surprising that host defence mechanisms designed to eliminate virus-infected cells should sometimes produce tissue damage in the process. The best known experimental example in which virus-specific CTL produce tissue damage is again that of LCMV: intracerebral inoculation of virus into adult mice results in their death. They survive if immunosuppressed with cyclophosphamide, despite persistent LCMV infection in the brain; however adoptive transfer of LCMV-specific CTL to these survivors then causes death[9]. The LCMV-specific CTL attack virus-infected cells and produce cerebral oedema, and it is this rather than the virus infection of the brain which leads to death. In mice infected with influenza virus a pathogenic role for DTH T cells, restricted in expression of their effector function by Class II MHC products, has been shown: transfer of influenza-specific DTH cells to naive virus-infected mice accelerates their death. Further work suggested that this mechanism is normally held in check by suppressor T cells[13].

As yet there are no clearly defined human counterparts to these experimental models, but there are candidates. It has been suggested, for instance, that liver injury during chronic HBV infection may be produced by HBV-specific

CTL lysing virus-infected hepatocytes. Formal proof of this hypothesis is made difficult by the absence of any tissue culture system for HBV, which limits *in vitro* experiments. However, CTL that apparently recognize determinants in HBcAg and HBeAg have been described in the peripheral blood of patients with chronic liver disease. Infiltrating CD8$^+$ cells can be shown in the liver, and there is evidence that these are HBV-specific CTL[14,15]. Immunosuppression ameliorates HBV-associated chronic active hepatitis. Administration of interferon-α (IFN-α) results in the disappearance of markers of HBV replication in about one-third of chronic HBV carriers: at least part of the mechanism for this effect may be the induction of Class I MHC expression on hepatocytes (which normally express only a low amount) by IFN-α, rendering them susceptible to lysis by CTL. In fact IFN-α administration is often accompanied by transient evidence of worsening liver function, which could be consistent with hepatocyte damage due to cytotoxic effector cells. In support of this concept, it has been shown in transgenic mice that express HBV envelope protein in the liver that HBV envelope-specific CD8$^+$ CTL can produce liver injury *in vivo*[16]. It has also been proposed that the virus-specific CTL detectable in the CSF during mumps meningitis may be tissue damaging, but this is speculative[17].

The more recent recognition of two types of T cells, T_{H1} and T_{H2}, with distinct patterns of cytokine release (see below), raises the question of whether these may account for any of the pathogenic effects of virus infections. Respiratory syncitial virus (RSV) may be associated with the development of wheezy bronchiolitis in children, and there is some evidence from a mouse model that this could be mediated by RSV-specific T_{H2} cells promoting eosinophilia and bronchoconstriction[18].

Virus infection of immunocompetent cells

Some viruses produce direct pathogenic effects both via and on the immune system by infecting immunocompetent cells, often with effects on their function. As a generalization, those viruses which establish persistent infection seem frequently to infect, and persist in, cells of the immune system. Lymphocytes and monocytes undergo activation and differentiation from a resting state in response to external signals, and for viruses within them the induction of virus gene transcription (which depends in part on cellular transcriptional factors) is frequently linked to the associated changes in transcription of cellular genes. Each of the major classes of immunocompetent cells may be infected by particular viruses.

Virus receptors may be the major determinants of tropism of the virus and hence of pathogenicity, and for several viruses which infect immunocompetent cells these are molecules involved in immune responses. Prime examples are Epstein-Barr virus (EBV) and the CR2 complement receptor, which defines its tropism for B cells[19] and human immunodeficiency virus (HIV) and the CD4 molecule[20]. Although MHC molecules have been suggested as receptors for certain viruses there is no definitive proof of their being so for any virus.

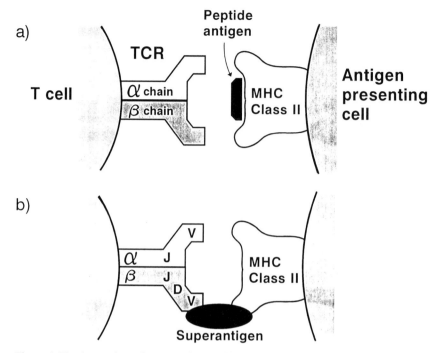

Figure 1 The interaction of superantigens with the T cell receptor. (a) Normal antigen presentation; (b) the binding of superantigens

T cells

A number of retroviruses infect T cells in animals and man. HIV and its interaction with T cells is covered in more detail in Chapter 6. The first human retrovirus to be described, HTLV 1, also infects $CD4^+$ T cells, and is causally associated with adult T cell leukaemia and tropical spastic paraparesis. HTLV 1 is transforming rather than lytic, and this may be related to the ability of the virus to induce interleukin-2 (IL-2) receptor expression as a consequence of transactivation of the cellular IL-2 receptor gene by the tax transactivator protein of the virus[21]. Retrovirus integration and replication require activation and division of T cells, and it has recently been shown that at least some T cell tropic retroviruses have the ability to stimulate T cell division by encoding proteins which act as superantigens. Superantigens, described in more detail below, are proteins with the ability to induce a potent T cell proliferative response by combining with MHC Class II molecules to form ligands which stimulate T cells via the V_β element of the T cell receptor. This has been convincingly shown for mouse mammary tumour virus, and the ability to stimulate T cell division by a superantigen effect would be a clear advantage to T cell-tropic retroviruses. No human equivalent of the endogenous mouse retroviral superantigens has yet been described. However it has been suggested that acquired human retroviruses (such as HIV) might act as superantigens, and that this could contribute to the T cell pathology they produce. Reports of selective depletion of a common set of V_β elements in individuals with HIV infection[22], and that HIV selectively stimulates and replicates in CD4 cells with particular V_β elements *in vitro*[23] are compatible with (but not proof of) HIV encoding a superantigen.

The most recently described herpesvirus, human herpesvirus 6 (HHV 6), also infects human T cell lines *in vitro*, although it probably persists in monocytes. Apart from producing the clinical syndrome of roseola infantum as a primary infection in children, HHV 6 has not been conclusively causally associated with illness, nor has any definite functional effect on T cells been attributed to the virus[24].

Measles virus has been demonstrated in peripheral blood T cells during acute infection, and impairment of T cell responses has been shown; this may cause clinically significant immunosuppression[25].

B cells

EBV is the principal human virus whose biology is intimately linked with the B cell. EBV is a polyclonal B cell activator *in vitro*. The virus persists in B cells as circular episomes of DNA, viral gene expression being limited to a small set of genes needed for episomal maintenance as the B cell divides. EBV also persists in oropharyngeal epithelial cells. The frequency of EBV-carrying B cells in peripheral blood is about 1 in 10 000: *in vitro* culture of peripheral blood mononuclear cells with cyclosporin A (which inhibits EBV-specific cytotoxic T lymphocytes) results in the outgrowth of EBV-transformed B cells, suggesting that CTL are important in controlling EBV transformation of B cells *in vivo*. The factors determining the different forms of EBV replication and gene expression are unclear. EBV plays a role in the aetiology of B cell lymphomas in immunosuppressed individuals and in nasopharyngeal carcinoma[26].

Monocytes/macrophages

Human monocytes can be infected with a number of different viruses. Their capacity to migrate to tissues and acquire a different activated phenotype (as tissue macrophages) makes them an important route by which viruses can disseminate and reactivate at local tissue sites, including the nervous system. They appear to play an important role in the pathogenesis of lentiretrovirus infections for these reasons, as shown experimentally for visna virus in sheep[27], which is carried in a transcriptionally inactive form until the monocyte differentiates into a macrophage. It is now clear that monocytes also play an important role in the pathogenesis of HIV infection – there are monocyte-tropic strains of HIV and replication of the virus in monocytes is enhanced by monocyte activation (see Chapter 6 for further details).

Amongst the human herpesviruses, human cytomegalovirus (CMV) is carried in monocytes. The virus can be detected by the polymerase chain reaction (PCR) in the monocytes of all carriers, where it appears to be latent: there is no CMV gene expression or production of infectious virus. Although *in vitro* infection of monocyte lines does not result in virus gene expression, phorbol-ester-induced differentiation of cells results in transcriptional activation of CMV immediate-early (IE) genes. Similarly, exposure of infected monocytes from normal seropositive donors to differentiating agent results in induction of IE gene expression in endogenous CMV[28]. Current available evidence, again using PCR, suggests that HHV6 also persists in monocytes. Reactivation of these viruses is thus linked closely to the state of activation/differentiation of the cells and, as for visna, the monocyte/macrophage can potentially carry the virus into the nervous system and other organs.

Virus evasion of the immune response

Viruses have evolved a number of mechanisms for evading the immune response.

Latency

A number of viruses persist in the host in a transcriptionally silent state, and as no proteins are produced they are invisible to the immune response. The clearest example is the alpha herpesviruses (e.g. herpes simplex virus, HSV) which establish classical latency in neuronal cells in sensory ganglia, whence they periodically reactivate and are transported down the axon to infect cells at the nerve ending. Little or no viral transcription occurs for most of the time, the only consistent transcript detected in HSV latency in neurones being the LAT (latency-associated) transcript which is not expressed as protein and whose function is uncertain. The molecular events involved in latency are complex and not completely elucidated: it is likely that latency depends in large part on control of virus transcription, exerted by the presence or absence of specific cellular nucleic acid binding proteins. In the case of HSV, a factor called Oct 1 that is required for transcription of viral immediate early genes is only present at low levels in neurones[29]. It is worth noting that the cellular sites of persistent virus infection frequently include cells which may be less accessible to the immune system, such as epithelial or neuronal cells, in addition to cells of the immune system itself (as in the case of HIV).

Antigenic variation

Some viruses have the ability to exhibit variation in their antigenic structure. This is, to a large extent, a reflection of the replicative strategy of those particular viruses which show this phenomenon, and which leads to their genomic variation. For instance the intrinsic mutation rate of some viruses may be high. Positive-strand RNA viruses are dependent on viral RNA polymerase, which has a high error rate for transcription (1 in 10^4 base pairs read)[30]. In the absence of a proof-reading or repair system, such as applies to DNA, these errors are rapidly compounded and transmitted to progeny particles, thereby maintaining high resolution rates and a high level of antigenic variation.

Another example is influenza virus which has a segmented (negative-strand) RNA genome which can undergo genetic mixing with other strains of the virus, including avian and animal strains, to produce 'reassortants'. This process leads to antigenic shift, an abrupt change in the haemagglutinin (HA) gene due to incorporation of the HA from a different strain. The more gradually operating phenomenon of antigenic drift is produced by variation in the amino acids situated on projecting loops around the receptor-binding pocket on the HA molecule which are the target for neutralizing antibody – the amino acids in the floor of the pocket are highly conserved[31].

The lentiretroviruses also exhibit great genomic diversity, and multiple variants with different sequences may be found in a single persistently infected host[32]. This diversity results from multiple single point nucleotide substitutions as a result of copying errors by the viral reverse transcriptase. Such substitutions in the *env* gene of HIV result in antigenic variation in the envelope protein, which is an important target for neutralizing antibody. Such antigenic variants may then be subjected to a degree of *in vivo* selection because of their failure to be neutralized by pre-existing antibody[33]. The question also arises of whether HIV 'escape mutants' may emerge which are not recognized by CTL[34]. The resultant continual emergence of new antigenic variants is probably a contributory factory in the pathogenesis of the lentiretroviruses and has been best documented in equine infectious anaemia and visna virus infection in sheep[35].

Altered expression of immunoregulatory molecules

Recent evidence from several *in vitro* systems suggests that viruses can modulate the expression of cell surface molecules involved in the induction and effector components of the immune response. This can have clear functional consequences *in vitro*, although it remains to be seen whether the same applies *in vivo*.

Adenovirus can down-regulate the amount of Class I MHC molecules on the cell surface, to the point where the infected cell can no longer be recognized by adenovirus-specific CTL. This effect is mediated by a specific adenovirus gene product (encoded in the E3 region), which is responsible for the retention of Class I MHC molecules in the endoplasmic reticulum[36]. Human CMV infection is also associated with a 10-fold reduction in Class I MHC expression on the surface of infected cells, accompanied by an apparent abrogation of the ability of the cell to present other exogenous antigens (such as other viruses) in the context of Class I MHC. This appears more likely to be a post-transcriptionally mediated effect[37].

It is now appreciated that a range of adhesion molecules, in addition to the T cell receptor interaction with antigen plus MHC, are important in target/effector cell binding and recognition. These include the interactions between ICAM 1 and LFA 1, and between LFA 3 and CD2. Further recent work indicates that expression of these adhesion molecules can be modulated by viruses: EBV transformation may be associated with reduced expression of LFA 1. Burkitt lymphoma lines which show this are resistant to lysis by EBV-specific CTL[38], although this may also relate to their expression of a limited number of EBV encoded proteins, mainly EBNA-1 which is not recognized by CTL. CMV can induce an increase in surface expression of ICAM 1 which, together with the down-regulation of MHC Class I, could relate to the increased susceptibility to NK cell lysis shown by CMV-related cells[39].

Virus-encoded homologues

The sequencing of complete viral genomes has led to the recognition that some viruses encode for proteins with homologies to human proteins involved in the immune response. Having identified such homologous genes it is possible to make deletion mutants lacking the homologue and observe the effect on pathogenicity, although this is only possible where there is an animal model. Poxviruses are particularly striking: vaccinia virus has genes homologous to those for the IL-2 receptor, serpins (serine proteinase inhibitors) and the complement control proteins (C4 binding protein and factor H). The vaccinia virus protein with homology to the C4 binding protein can inhibit the classical pathway of complement activation, and deletion of the serpin homologues decreases pathogenicity[40]. Vaccinia virus also has a homologue of the IL-1β receptor, and Shope fibroma virus has a homologue of tumour necrosis factor receptor: both are secreted in soluble form from infected cells and may act as 'decoys' for the cytokines – their deletion diminishes pathogenicity[41,42]. Herpes simplex virus encodes a glycoprotein (gC) which acts as a C3b receptor. CMV encodes a glycoprotein which is homologous to the Class I MHC heavy chain and a homologue of a G-protein coupled receptor whose ligand is a C–C chemokine, MIP 1α: whether these have any pathogenic function, and the underlying mechanism, remain to be determined[43]. EBV possesses a gene (*BCRF1*) with homology to a cytokine synthesis inhibitory factor (IL-10) produced by murine T_{H2} cells, and with similar functional activity[42]. The full pathogenetic significance of most of these homologues remains to be assessed, but the degree of homology and their retention by the viruses concerned suggests that they may be 'captured' cellular genes that confer some selective advantage on the virus (reviewed in ref. 45).

Viruses and autoimmunity

There are several potential mechanisms by which viruses could induce autoimmune responses. These include polyclonal activation of B cells, production of anti-idiotypic antibodies against antiviral antibodies which might then simulate a viral protein and bind to cell surface receptors and 'molecular mimicry' where viral epitopes shared with host antigens result in the production of cross-reactive antibody or T cells[46] (see below). Animal models for all these mechanisms exist, but none of them have been unequivocally shown to operate in humans. Other possible mechanisms can also be envisaged, such as viral interference with normal suppressor cell regulation, but are still more speculative.

Cross-reactivity between viral and host epitopes

The ever-increasing amount of protein sequence information, and the ability to perform rapid homology searches, has revealed various homologies between viral proteins and epitopes on normal host proteins. In some cases these homologous sequences have been shown to induce immunological cross-reactivity. For example, a number of viral polypeptides contain sequences showing homology with the encephalitogenic peptide of myelin basic protein, suggesting a possible basis for 'post-viral demyelination', in which peptide-specific T cells induced by a virus infection might cross-react with myelin and produce injury[46]. Although speculative, this sort of mechanism offers one possible explanation of the way in which autoimmunity may be induced. The ability to respond to particular peptides might be linked to specific MHC gene products and thus vary between individuals, which could be one potential explanation for the known MHC associations of these diseases. However it should be emphasized that there are other possible explanations for autoimmunity besides this phenomenon of molecular mimicry.

Expression of viral proteins in transgenic mice

In several recent experiments isolated viral genes have been expressed in a tissue-specific manner as transgenes. Expression of influenza HA in the pancreas of mice induced insulin-dependent diabetes and lymphocytic infiltration of the islets. Similar experiments have been reported for the LCMV glycoprotein expressed as a transgene in the pancreas: when the mice were later infected with LCMV they developed diabetes as a consequence of an immune response to the glycoprotein[47]. It seems likely that peripheral T cells do not become tolerant to the viral transgene in the pancreas which has not been presented to them on antigen-presenting cells: however subsequent viral infection allows expression on presenting cells, inducing a response to the transgene. Such experiments probably tell us more about the mechanisms by which immunological tolerance is produced than they do about virus pathogenesis. However they do show that viral antigens can induce tissue-specific immunologically mediated disease with very similar pathology to the human autoimmune counterpart.

IMMUNOPATHOLOGY OF BACTERIAL INFECTION

Bacterial infections may also induce immunopathology, in some cases by analogous mechanisms to those described above for viruses but in others by mechanisms specific for bacteria. Examples are discussed below, and some immunopathological aspects of mycobacterial infection are dealt with in Chapter 2.

Pathology induced by the antibacterial response

Normal host resistance to bacteria is dependent mainly on antibody, complement and neutrophils. Bacterial infections can also provoke immuno-pathological tissue damage by mechanisms similar to those described above.

Antibody

Bacterial infections may also result in immune complex disease, but this is only of significance where the infection is chronic and bacterial antigens are released into the circulation over a period of time. The two classic human diseases in which this occurs are bacterial endocarditis and infected ventriculo-atrial shunts, where sustained release of bacterial antigen leads to formation of circulating complexes and consequent glomerulonephritis and other manifestations of immune complex disease[48]. The direct role of the bacterial infection in causing the immune complex disease is clearly shown by the response to antibacterial chemotherapy which can lead to resolution of the nephritis and other manifestations of the immunopathology.

T cells

As most bacteria are extracellular pathogens, effector T cells play a less central role in their elimination than does antibody; however they are particularly important for those bacteria which are intracellular. Delayed-type hypersensitivity reactions are a characteristic feature of mycobacterial infections and play an important role in their resolution. However they may also account for tissue damage, as occurs in the tuberculoid form of leprosy, in which few bacilli are in evidence and skin and nerves are infiltrated with lymphocytes and macrophages[49]. Two distinct classes of $CD4^+$ T cells distinguished by their differential production of cytokines have recently been recognized: in the mouse T_{H1} cells produce IL-2, IFN-γ and TNFβ, whereas T_{H2} cells produce IL-4, IL-5, IL-6, IL-10 and IL-13. The T_{H1} cytokines predominantly favour enhancement of cellular immunity, particularly activ-ation of microbicidal activity in macrophages. The T_{H2} cytokines particularly favour the development of B cells into antibody producing cells, but may also down-regulate the activity of T_{H1} cells through the action of IL-4 and IL-10. T_{H2} cells may thus limit the potentially tissue damaging consequences of T_{H1} cytokines[50]. There is increasing evidence that the balance between these two phenotypically distinct types of T cell is important in the pathogenesis of infectious diseases, particularly those caused by intracellular parasites and bacteria. The clearest example is that of the intracellular protozoan *Leishmania major*: strains of mice which recover from leishmaniasis show a T_{H1} response[51,52]. While there is as yet less clear-cut evidence for the importance of the T_{H1}/T_{H2} balance in human microbial disease, leprosy is a possible example where this balance is important in pathogenesis. Lepromatous leprosy is characterized by the presence of many intracellular organisms and T cells isolated from lesions have been shown predominantly to secrete IL-4: conversely in tuberculoid leprosy there are very few organisms but considerable immunopathological tissue damage, and a predominance of IFN-γ producing T cells[53]. This would be consistent with the idea that one of the functions of T_{H2} cells may be to hold in check the potentially tissue damaging effects of T_{H1} cells.

Bacterial infection of immunocompetent cells

Intracellular bacteria

A number of bacteria, including mycobacteria, *Legionella*, *Listeria*, and salmonellae are facultative intracellular parasites. Rickettsiae and chlamydiae are obligate intracellular bacteria. These intracellular bacteria particularly invade macrophages (as a general rule lymphocytes and neutrophils are not targets for intracellular bacteria). *Legionella*, *Salmonella* and mycobacteria share the interesting property of being able to exist and replicate within the phagolysosome. The mechanisms by which they resist inactivation (in a location specifically designed to kill bacteria) are not completely known, but they involve the bacteria somehow 'remodelling' the phagosome[54]. Thus *Legionella* inhibits fusion of the phagosome with the lysosome, and mycobacteria-containing phagosomes do not acidify and show a selective lack of the lysosomal proton-ATPase responsible for normal acidification of the lysosome[55]. *Listeria* and some rickettsiae avoid inactivation by escaping from the phagolysosome into the cytoplasm. *Listeria* achieves this using listeriolysin – deletion of this gene makes the organism avirulent[56]. These bacteria may have other mechanisms of resistance to being killed in macrophages: salmonellae carry a specific gene (*phoP*) which enables them to resist the microbicidal peptides (called 'defensins') present in the lysosomes of neutrophils and macrophages[57]. Infected macrophages may nevertheless become capable of killing intracellular bacteria in phagosomes when the macrophage itself is activated, principally by IFN-γ.

Bacterial evasion of the immune response

The mechanisms by which bacteria resist intracellular killing described above are one example of evasion of host defence but bacteria show many others.

Antigenic variation

Variation in bacterial antigens may occur between different strains of the same species, but not usually within a given strain (e.g. the M types of streptococci do not elicit cross-protective antibody). However, some species of bacteria can show antigen variation within a strain. One of the best studied examples is the variation which occurs in the pilin genes of gonococci whose products make up the bacterial pili: this variation occurs by the transfer of silent promoterless pilin (*pil*S) genes into the locus for expressed pilin (*pil*E) genes, by homologous recombination[58]. Other examples of bacterial antigenic variation are seen in *Borrelia hermsii*, the spirochaete which causes relapsing fever, whose surface variable major protein changes with each episode of fever by a mechanism involving non-reciprocal gene exchange. Some bacteria may also undergo antigenic variation by transfer of genes between strains by transformation (e.g. the antigenic mosaicism in the IgA proteases of gonococci)[59].

Properties of the bacterial capsule

Most bacteria possess the ability to synthesize a capsule external to their cell wall: these nearly always consist of high molecular weight polysaccharides. The structure of these capsules is frequently not conducive to complement activation: their surface may promote the degradation of C3 or inhibit assembly of the alternative pathway C3 convertase: the capsule of type b *Haemophilus influenzae*, for example, is relatively resistant to complement activation, and this type is associated with 95% of invasive disease. The lipopolysaccharide of some salmonellae confers relative resistance to complement inactivation, associated with its having long O side-chains. Finally, the capsules may prevent access of antibody and complement components (such as the membrane attack complex) to the underlying cell wall.

Some carbohydrate determinants of capsules, such as the group B meningococcal capsule, are particularly difficult to raise antibodies against. In this case there is a homology between group B carbohydrate and neural cell adhesion molecule (N-CAM), which may contribute to its poor immunogenicity[59-61].

Immunopathogenic effects of bacterial toxins

The exo- and endotoxins of bacteria have diverse effects on many organs. This section deals only with their effects on the immune system.

Bacterial exotoxins as superantigens

A recently described property of certain bacterial exotoxins is their ability to act as superantigens – so called because of their ability to induce a potent T cell proliferative response by combining with MHC Class II molecules to form ligands which stimulate T cells via the V_β element of the T cell receptor. In normal antigen presentation, T cells recognize conventional antigens not as whole proteins but as short peptide fragments derived from the protein by intracellular processing, and bound in a groove on the heavy chain of the MHC Class I and Class II molecules. Particular amino acid residues at critical points in the peptide sequence anchor the peptide in the groove, and this interaction is relatively specific for each of the different allelic forms of MHC molecules. Hence a complex of peptide and MHC molecule (and the MHC molecule must be the same allelic form as that on the T cell) is recognized by the T cell receptor (TCR), with consequent activation of the T cell and expression of its effector functions. The TCR consists of α and β chains, each composed of variable (V) and joining (J) segments (with an additional diversity (D) segment for the β chain): these segments are encoded by separate genes which undergo DNA rearrangement to give very many different combinations. The association of peptides with MHC alleles on the one hand, and the diversity of the TCR on the other, allows T cells to recognize a huge number of antigens while conferring extreme specificity on this recognition. This means that only a small fraction of all T cells will respond to any given antigen.

Superantigens do not conform to this conventional pathway of antigen presentation, but simultaneously activate large numbers of T cells by bypassing the normal route of intracellular processing, and binding directly as intact proteins to Class II MHC molecules at a site distinct from the peptide binding groove[62]. They also bind to most allelic forms of Class II molecules rather than to restricted alleles as do conventional peptide antigens. The superantigen/MHC complex then reacts with the TCR through the V segment of the β chain (V_β), rather than with the normal antigen-binding site on the TCR composed of both α and β chains. Furthermore superantigens react with *all* T cells carrying a particular V_β gene: there are some 50 different V_β genes in humans, and so a superantigen reacts with more than 1 in 50 T cells whereas a conventional peptide antigen will react with 1 in 10^4–10^6 T cells.

Two groups of proteins have been shown to act as superantigens, one exogenous to the host and the other carried endogenously in the host genome[63]. The first group are nearly all bacterial exotoxins[63,64], including the exotoxins produced by staphylococci that cause food poisoning (entero-toxins A, B, C1–3, D and E), toxic shock syndrome (TSST-1), and the scalded skin syndrome (exfoliating toxins A and B), pyrogenic exotoxins A, B, C and D of group A streptococci, and enterotoxins of *Clostridium perfringens* and *Yersinia enterocolitica*. *Mycoplasma arthritidis* also produces a superantigen[65]. The bacterial exotoxin superantigens are relatively small proteins which bind to Class II molecules with high affinity and each stimulates T cells through a number of different V_β segments: they are particularly strong T cell mitogens and activate both CD4$^+$ and CD8$^+$ T cells (whereas conventional antigens presented by Class II MHC molecules only activate CD4$^+$ T cells).

The second class of superantigens has only been clearly defined in the mouse. A group of antigens capable of stimulating a strong mixed lymphocyte reaction between mice of the same MHC haplotype was recognized some time ago: these were termed minor lymphocyte stimulating (MLs) determi-nants. They again act by binding to Class II MHC molecules and stimulating large numbers of T cells through their V_β elements. It has now been established that MLs determinants are proteins encoded by genes of mouse mammary tumour viruses integrated and vertically transmitted in the mouse genome[66]. They are in effect self antigens and, as with any self antigen encountered by T cells during their maturation in the thymus, T cells which react with MLs determinants are clonally eliminated in their early development with consequent 'skewing' of the animal's V_β T cell repertoire. An interesting consequence of this is that the mice are then resistant to infection with exogenous mammary tumour viruses.

The way in which superantigens activate T cells may well be relevant to the pathogenesis of infectious disease[67]. The ability of bacterial exotoxins to activate large numbers of T cells with consequent release of cytokines could directly account for their pathogenic effects and the clinical syndromes they produce: for instance experimental staphylococcal enterotoxin shock depends on superantigen-induced release of TNF mediated via T cells[68]. Widespread activation of T cells, with selective representation of particular V_β elements, is also a feature of some inflammatory joint diseases linked with infective agents and of Kawasaki disease[69,70]: superantigen effects could account for this. It seems clear that superantigens are yet another example of microbial pathogens evolving mechanisms to use and subvert the immune response.

Bacterial endotoxin

Bacterial endotoxin or lipopolysaccharide (LPS) is a component of the outer cell wall of gram-negative bacteria, and is composed of outer polysaccharide and inner lipid A moieties. It is responsible for most features of the syndrome of gram-negative shock. LPS binds to LPS-binding protein, an acute phase protein, and this complex then binds to the CD14 molecule on macrophages, causing their activation. This in turn results in release of TNF-α and IL-1, which are probably the principal mediators of endotoxin shock[71]: both have effects on endothelium causing procoagulant release and hence the coagulopathy associated with the syndrome. Certainly antibodies to TNF block most of the effects of endotoxin in the whole animal[72]. The C3H/HeJ mouse strain is genetically resistant to the effects of endotoxin and this resistance appears to be due to failure of macrophage activation.

Endotoxin also causes antibody-independent complement activation by direct activation of C1 by lipid A, and by activation of the alternative pathway. Endotoxin is also a powerful polyclonal B cell activator. Further aspects of the biochemistry and immunology of endotoxin are discussed in recent reviews[73].

Bacteria and autoimmunity

Considerable circumstantial evidence suggests that bacteria may be involved in the pathogenesis of certain diseases which are believed to have an autoimmune component. Although the associations have been recognized for a considerable time definitive proof for any mechanism involved is harder to come by.

Streptococci

Particular types of streptococci have been implicated in the aetiology of rheumatic fever and nephritis. Acute post-streptococcal glomerulonephritis results from infection with a limited number of serotypes of group A streptococci. What exactly it is that renders these strains nephritogenic is still unclear[74,75]. Streptococcal antigens have been reported in glomeruli, but an immune complex mechanism does not really count as 'autoimmune' and whether streptococci induce antibodies which cross-react with glomerular antigens has not been definitively shown.

In the case of acute rheumatic fever, there is more evidence for streptococci inducing cross-reactive antibodies. Pharyngeal infection with β-haemolytic group A streptococci can cause rheumatic fever about 3 weeks later. Cross-reactivity between components of streptococcal M proteins and human cardiac antigens in the sarcolemmal membrane and in cardiac mysion and valvular glycoproteins has been described[75,76]. The small number of individuals who develop rheumatic fever may have an immunogenetic predisposition: an association with HLA-DR2 and DR4 has been reported.

Reactive arthritis and ankylosing spondylitis

There is a clear association between reactive arthritis and preceding infection with *Yersinia enterocolitica*, shigellae, salmonellae and *Campylobacter*. This and other seronegative spondyloarthropathies are very strongly associated with the Class I MHC allele HLA-B27. Ankylosing spondylitis itself has been more tentatively associated with *Klebsiella pneumoniae*, and a hexapeptide shared by the *Klebsiella* nitrogenase protein and HLA-B27 has been described. Antibodies to this sequence that cross-react with the two proteins have been reported in the sera of patients with ankylosing spondylitis[78]. This 'molecular mimicry' has generated much interest but there is no consensus on the role of this mechanism in the pathogenesis of these disorders. Furthermore, co-expression of HLA-B27 and β_2-microglobulin as transgenes in rats (but not mice) resulted in an inflammatory disease with similar features to human spondyloarthropathy in one of the transgenic lines, without any obvious requirement for an associated infective agent[79]. Thus the nature of the association between bacteria and these diseases still remains obscure.

THE PATHOPHYSIOLOGICAL EFFECTS OF CYTOKINES

A large number of mediators are released from monocytes and lymphocytes (but sometimes other cells as well), usually consequent upon their activation in the course of the immune response, and the basic biology of these monokines and lymphokines (or simply cytokines) is the subject of much current research. Most of these factors were originally described and named for their biological activities; however their molecular characterization, usually achieved by the cloning and expression of the genes, has revealed that multiple biological activities often reside in a single molecular species. This has frequently rendered previous nomenclature inapposite and/or redundant. The availability of these factors as pure proteins produced from the recombinant DNA, apart from facilitating their study *in vitro*, has also allowed them to be administered *in vivo* to experimental animals, and in some cases to human subjects. These factors may have a role in the pathogenesis of infectious disease – the examples quoted here have all been invoked as pathogenetic factors in addition to their role in the normal immune response. Table 2 summarizes the current nomenclature and characteristics of these factors: it should be emphasised that this is a rapidly evolving field and hence this can only be a provisional description.

Interferons

The interferons were all originally described for their antiviral effect, but are now recognized to have many other actions, particularly antiproliferative and immunomodulatory effects[80,81]. Three types of IFN are recognized: α, β and γ. There are about 20 IFN-α genes, one IFN-β gene (IFNβ_2 is now synonymous with IL6 – see below) and one IFN-γ gene[82].

The administration of pharmacological doses of recombinant IFN to patients causes fever and malaise, which may be dose limiting. This suggests that they may be responsible for these same symptoms during natural infection, although IL-1 and TNF can also produce fever. Production of IFN-γ by T_{H1} cells in response to intracellular mycobacteria may be responsible for tissue injury at the site of infection. T_{H2} cells have been proposed to play a role in suppressing the activity of T_{H1} cells, and hence limiting the potentially harmful effects of T_{H1} cytokines.

Interleukins

Full descriptions of the pro-inflammatory interleukins are available elsewhere[81]. Here we deal with those which currently appear likely to play a particularly significant role in the pathogenesis of infectious disease.

Interleukin 1 (IL-1)

This has a major immunoregulatory role in providing a signal for T cell activation. However it also causes fever, and the effects of the factor previously known as endogenous pyrogen are all reproduced by IL-1. The production of fever by IL-1 involves a direct action on the hypothalamus by which its thermoregulatory centre is reset – there is no firm evidence that IL-1 crosses the blood–brain barrier, but this resetting is associated with locally increased synthesis of prostaglandin E_2 (PGE$_2$), which may be a major mediator of the effect. IL-1 also causes tissue catabolism, and a specific peptide fragment of IL-1 has been shown to produce muscle proteolysis. IL-1 is a major mediator of the acute phase response, causing hepatocytes to increase

Table 2 The pro-inflammatory cytokines

	Protein (human)	Source	Receptors (human)	Principal actions
IL-1α	Mature 159 aa	Macrophages, keratinocytes, endothelial cells, some T and B cells	Type 1 binds IL-1α, IL-1β Type II binds IL-1β > IL-1α Both Ig superfamily	CNS effects – fever, sleep, anorexia Role in endotoxin shock Bone and cartilage resorption Induces acute phase response
IL-1β	Mature 153 aa			
TNFα	Mature 157 aa	Macrophages, many other cell types	55 kD mediates antiviral, gene induction effects. 75 kD mediates T cell proliferation	T cell – induces cytokines Macrophages – activation Endothelial cells and adipocytes Role in endotoxin shock
IL-6	Mature 190 aa	Macrophages, fibroblasts, T cells, endothelial cells	gp80, binds IL-6 gp130, transduces signal	Induces acute phase response Growth factor and mitogen for B and T cells
IFN-α and -β	165–172 aa 14 IFN-α proteins 1 IFN-β protein	IFN-α – many cells IFN-β – fibroblasts and others	Same receptor	Antiviral, antiproliferative Increase NK cell activity
IFN-γ	143 aa	T cells, NK cells	52 kD, most cells	Activates macrophages Up-regulates Class II MHC

synthesis of the acute phase proteins which include antiproteases, haptoglobin, complement components (C3, C4 and factor B), fibrinogen and ferritin. However it is the 100–1000 fold increase in C-reactive protein and amyloid A protein which is most dramatic and suggests that these two proteins play some special role in the response to infection. IL-1 also has significant effects on endothelial cells, including induction of expression of the adhesion molecule ICAM1, which probably explains the increased endothelial adherence of circulating mononuclear cells caused by IL1, increased synthesis of PGI_2 and PGE_2, and induction of a plasminogen activator inhibitor. The net effect of these actions would be decreased blood flow and local coagulation, as may occur in endotoxin shock: as a further complication, cultured endothelial cells can themselves release IL-1 in response to endotoxin[83].

Interleukin 2 (IL-2)

This is the major autocrine growth factor for activated T cells. Infusion of high doses of recombinant IL-2 into humans (as used for cancer therapy) results in fever. *In vitro*, high doses of IL-2 induce IL-1 and TNF release from large granular lymphocytes. However, on the basis of present evidence, it seems unlikely that IL-2 is itself an endogenous pyrogen under physiological circumstances[81].

Interleukin 6 (IL-6)

This was formerly known both as IFN-β_2 and B cell stimulating factor 2. In addition to its antiviral and B cell stimulating activities, IL-6 also has the ability to produce fever (in rabbits) with similar kinetics to IL-1, and to enhance the production of hepatic acute phase proteins. There are thus similarities between the actions of IL-1 and IL-6 and both are produced by a wide range of cells, including fibroblasts and endothelial cells. IL-1, IL-6 and TNF are coordinately released from activated monocytes and all are inducers of the acute phase response[81].

Tumour necrosis factor (TNF)

TNF has already been mentioned above in the context of endotoxin. TNFα is encoded on human chromosome 6, close to the complex encoding the major histocompatibility genes – another cytotoxic protein, lymphotoxin (TNFβ), is encoded close by, upstream of the TNFα gene, and these two proteins show about 45% nucleotide sequence homology. Purified or recombinant TNFα is a 17 kD protein which forms a trimer (allowing it to aggregate its receptor). TNF appears to be responsible for many, if not all, of the pathological effects of endotoxin, as discussed above. TNF can also produce fever directly by a hypothalamic action involving release of prostaglandin E_2, but TNF also induces release of IL-1, which itself produces fever. This ability of one cytokine to induce release of another is a recurring complication of attempts to dissect the primary actions of many of the cytokines discussed here. This also applies to the effects of TNF on endothelial cells: TNF has direct effects on endothelial cells similar to those of IL-1. There are two receptors for TNFα: both are expressed on most cells and to some extent they probably account for its differing actions. The 55 kD TNFα receptor is thought to mediate cytotoxicity, antiviral activity and NFKβ induction (through which TNF induces expression of other cellular genes), whilst the 75 kD receptor mediates T cell proliferation[84]. The factor originally named cachectin for its ability to induce cachexia in experimental animals is identical to TNF. Attempts to produce the cachectic syndrome in animals (rats or mice) by direct administration of recombinant human TNF have not been easy, and it appears that any cachectic effect of TNF in isolation may be produced by induction of anorexia[85].

Despite its adverse effects, TNF must have beneficial actions since it has been so highly conserved, at least in mammals. TNF has definite antiviral effects which are synergistic with those of IFN, and can augment the killing of C. albicans by neutrophils. There is also the activity for which it is named, and it may play some role in resistance to tumours in vivo. The mechanism of its antiviral effect is probably somewhat different from that of the interferons. TNF is reported to inhibit the replication of a number of DNA and RNA viruses but can also lyse cells infected with some viruses (vesicular stomatitis and adenoviruses)[86]. A protein encoded in the E3 transcription unit of adenovirus has been reported specifically to inhibit lysis of infected cells by TNF (deletion mutants for E3 are susceptible to lysis) suggesting that this virus has evolved a mechanism to counter the antiviral actions of TNF[87].

Thus, of the factors considered here, IFN, IL-1, IL-6 and TNF appear likely on present evidence to be of particular importance in the pathophysiology of infectious disease. All can act as endogenous pyrogens and inducers of acute phase proteins, and their other actions may explain aspects of the pathogenesis of infectious disease, such as, for instance, disseminated intravascular coagulation. IL-1, IL-6 and TNF are all released from activated monocytes and can induce production of each other: Il-1 and TNF can induce IL-6 and TNF can induce IL-1 production[81]. The other interleukins are of course also relevant to infection in the wider context of their role in regulating the immune response.

CONCLUSION

A better understanding of the immunopathology of bacterial and viral infections might be expected to have clinical consequences in several ways: by throwing light on the pathogenesis of microbial diseases and hence possibly their therapy, by suggesting microbial causes for diseases of unknown aetiology, and by contributing to vaccine design.

Vaccine-induced immunopathology

A thorough knowledge of their immunology and immunopathogenesis seems likely to eventually benefit vaccine design, particularly with respect to the more complex persistent viruses and to bacteria. There is clear precedent for the possibility that vaccines may cause adverse reactions by virtue of the immune responses they induce. The killed vaccine against respiratory syncitial virus (RSV) was associated with more severe illness in vaccinees than controls when they subsequently encountered the wild type virus, as was the killed measles vaccine. This was associated with failure of these vaccines to produce antibody to the F protein of the viruses. Possible explanations for this phenomenon include the development of an Arthus reaction, or the involvement of DTH[88]. Recent work on the LCMV model, using recombinant vaccinia viruses expressing LCMV genes as vaccines, has shown that some recombinant vaccines can also enhance the severity of disease[3].

Given the complexity of the immune response, and the strategies evolved by micro-organisms to evade it and produce infection, it is perhaps not surprising that the clash between the two should produce pathology. It seems certain that further examples of immunopathogenic disease caused by microbial infection will emerge.

References

1. Marrack P, Kappler J. Subversion of the immune system by pathogens. Cell. 1994; 76: 323–332.
2. Sissons JGP, Borysiewicz LK. Viral immunopathology. Br Med Bull. 1985; 41: 34–40.
3. Oehen S, Hengartner H, Zinkernagel RM. Vaccination for disease. Science. 1991; 251: 195–198.
4. Mims CA, White DO. Viral pathogenesis and immunology. Oxford: Blackwell Scientific, 1984.
5. Halstead SB. Pathogenesis of dengue: challenges to molecular biology. Science. 1988; 239: 476–481.
6. Cardosa MJ, Porterfield JS, Gordon S. Complement receptor mediates enhanced flavivirus replication in macrophages. J Exp Med. 1983; 158: 258–263.
7. Homsy J, Meyer M, Tateno M et al. The Fc and not the CD4 receptor mediates antibody enhancement of HIV infection in human cells. Science. 1989; 244: 1357–1360.
8. Robinson WE Jr, Kawamura T, Gorny MK et al. Human monoclonal antibodies to the human immunodeficiency virus type 1 (HIV-1) transmembrane glycoprotein gp41 enhance HIV-1 infection in vitro. Proc Natl Acad Sci USA. 1990; 87: 3185–3189.
9. Oldstone MBA, ed. Lymphocytic choriomeningitis virus. Curr Topics Microbiol. 1987; 133: 134.
10. Buchmeier et al. The virology and immunobiology of lymphocytic choriomeningitis virus infection. Adv Immunol. 1980; 30: 275–331.
11. Porter DD, Larsen AE, Porter HG. Aleutian disease of mink. Adv Immunol. 1980; 29: 261.
12. Lai KN, Li PKY, Lui SF, Au TC, Tam JSL, Tong KL, Lai FMM. Membranous nephropathy related to hepatitis B in adults. N Engl J Med. 1991; 324: 1457–1463.
13. Ada GL, Leung K-N, Ertl H. An analysis of effector T cell generation and function in mice exposed to influenza A or Sendai viruses. Immunol Rev. 1981; 58: 5–24.
14. Barnaba V, Franco A, Alberti A, et al. Recognition of hepatitis B virus envelope proteins by liver infiltrating T lymphocytes in chronic HBV infection. J Immunol. 1989; 143: 2650–2655.
15. Nayersina R, Fowler O, Guilhot S et al. HLA A2 restricted cytotoxic T lymphocyte responses to multiple hepatitis B surface antigen epitopes during hepatitis B virus infection.

J Immunol. 1993; 150: 4659–4671.

16. Moriyama T, Guilhot S, Klopchin K et al. Immunobiology and pathogenesis of hepatocellular injury in hepatitis B virus transgenic mice. Science. 1990; 248: 361–364.

17. Kreth HW, Kress HG, Ott HF, Eckert G. Demonstration of primary cytotoxic T cells in venous blood and cerebrospinal fluid of children with mumps meningitis. J Immunol. 1982; 128: 2411–2415.

18. Alwan WH, Kozlowska WJ, Openshaw PJM. Distinct types of lung disease caused by functional subsets of antiviral T cells. J Exp Med. 1994; 179: 81–89.

19. Nemerow GR, Houghton RA, Moore MD, Cooper NR. Identification of the epitope in the major envelope of Epstein Barr virus that mediates viral binding to the B lymphocyte EBV receptor (CR2). Cell. 1989; 56: 369–377.

20. Capon DJ, Ward RHR. The CD4-gp120 interaction and AIDS pathogenesis. Annu Rev Immunol. 1991; 9: 649–678.

21. Ruben S, Poteat H, Tan TH, Kawakami K, Roeder R, Haseltine W, Rosen CA. Cellular transcription factors and regulation of IL-2 receptor gene expression by HTLV-I tax gene product. Science. 1988; 241: 89–92.

22. Imberti L, Sottini A, Bettinardi A et al. Selective depletion in HIV infection of T cells that bear specific T cell receptor Vβ sequences. Science. 1991; 254: 860–862.

23. Laurence J, Hodtsev AS, Posnett DN. Superantigen implicated in dependence of HIV-1 replication in T cells on TCR Vβ expression. Nature. 1992; 358: 255–259.

24. Lopez C, Honess RW. Human herpesvirus 6. In: Fields BN, Knipe DM, eds. Virology. New York, Raven Press, 1990: 2055–2062.

25. Whittle HC, Dossetor J, Odinlojn S, Bryceson ADM, Greenwood BM. Cell mediated immunity during natural measles infection. J Clin Invest. 1978; 62: 678–684.

26. Rickinson AB, Murray RJ, Brooks J et al. T cell recognition of Epstein-Barr virus associated lymphomas. Cancer Surv. 1992; 13: 53–80.

27. Narayan O, Clements JE. Lentiviruses. In: Fields BN, Knipe DM, eds. Virology. New York, Raven Press, 1990: 1571–1589.

28. Taylor-Weidman J, Sissons JGP, Sinclair J. Induction of endogenous human cytomegalovirus gene expression after differentiation of monocytes from healthy carriers. J Virol. 1994; 68: 1597–1604.

29. Stevens JG. Overview of herpes virus latency. Semin Virol. 1994; 5: 191–196.

30. Holland J, Spindler K, Horodyski F, Grabam E, Nichol S, Van de Pol S. Rapid evolution of RNA genomes. Science. 1982; 215: 1577–1585.

31. Wiley DC, Skehel JJ. The structure and function of the haemagglutinin membrane glycoprotein of influenza virus. Annu Rev Biochem. 1987; 56: 365–394.

32. Meyerhans A, Cheynier R, Albert J, Seth M, Kwok S, Sninsky J, Morfeldt-Måonson L, Asjö B, Wain-Hobson S. Temporal fluctuations in HIV quasispecies in vivo are not reflected by sequential HIV isolations. Cell. 1989; 58: 901–910.

33. Albert J, Abrahamsson B, Nagy K, Aurelius E, Gaines H, Nystrom G, Fenyo EM. Rapid development of isolate-specific neutralising antibodies after primary HIV-1 infection and consequent emergence of virus variants which resist neutralisation by autologous sera. AIDS. 1990; 4: 107–112.

34. Philips RE, Rowland-Jones S, Nixon DF, et al. Human immunodeficiency virus genetic variation that can escape cytotoxic T cell recognition. Nature. 1991; 354: 453–459.

35. Clements JE, Godovin SL, Montelero RC, Narayan O. Antigenic variation in lentiviral diseases. Annu Rev Immunol. 1988; 6: 139–159.

36. Burgert H-G, Kvist S. An adenovirus type 2 glycoprotein blocks cell surface expression of human histocompatibility class 1 antigens. Cell. 1985; 41: 987–997.

37. Warren AP, Ducroq DH, Lehner PJ, Borysiewicz LK. Human cytomegalovirus infected cells have unstable assembly of MHC class I complexes and are resistant to lysis by cytotoxic T lymphocytes. J Virol. 1994; 68: 2822–2829.

38. Inghirami G, Grignani F, Sternas L et al. Down-regulation of LFA-1 adhesion receptors by C-myc oncogene in human lymphoblastoid cells. Science. 1990; 250: 682–686.

39. Borysiewicz LK, Rodgers B, Morris S et al. Lysis of human cytomegalovirus infected fibroblasts by natural killer cells – demonstration of an interferon independent component requiring expression of early viral proteins and characterisation of effector cells. J Immunol. 1985; 134: 2695–2710.

40. Traktman P. Poxviruses: an emerging portrait of biological strategy. Cell. 1990; 62: 621–626.

41 Alcami A, Smith GL. A soluble receptor for interleukin-1β encoded by vaccinia virus: a novel mechanism of virus modulation of the host response to infection. Cell. 1992; 71: 153–167.

42. Smith CA, Davis T, Anderson D *et al.* A receptor for tumor necrosis factor defines an unusual family of cellular and viral proteins. Science. 1990; 248: 1019–1023.

43. Beck S, Barrell BG. Human cytomegalovirus encodes a glycoprotein homologous to MHC class 1 antigens. Nature. 1988; 331: 269–272.

44. Moore KW, Vieira P, Fiorentino DF, Trounstine ML, Khan TA, Mosmann TR. Homology of cytokine synthesis inhibitor factor (IL-10) to the Epstein-Barr virus genome BCRF1. Science. 1990; 248: 1230–1234.

45. Gooding LR. Virus proteins that counteract host immune defenses. Cell. 1992; 71: 5–7.

46. Oldstone MBA. Molecular mimicry and autoimmune disease. Cell. 1987; 50: 819–820.

47. Ohashi PS, Oehen S, Buerki K *et al.* Ablation of 'tolerance' and induction of diabetes by virus infection in viral antigen transgenic mice. Cell. 1991; 65: 305–317.

48. Neugarten J, Gallo GR, Baldwin DS. Glomerulonephritis in bacterial endocarditis. Am J Kidney Dis. 1984; 3: 371–379.

49. Rees RWJ. Animal models in leprosy. Br Med Bull. 1988; 44: 650–664.

50. Paul WE, Seder RA. Lymphocyte responses and cytokines. Cell. 1994; 76: 241–251.

51. Liew FY. Functional heterogeneity of CD4+ T cells in leishmaniasis. Immunol Today. 1989; 10: 40–45.

52. Sher A, Coffman RL. Regulation of immunity to parasites by T cells and T cell-derived cytokines. Annu Rev Immunol. 1992; 10: 385–409.

53. Salgame P, Abrams JS, Clayberger C *et al.* Differing lymphokine profiles of functional subsets of human CD4 and CD8 T cell clones. Science. 1991; 254: 279–282.

54. Small PLC, Ramakrishnan L, Falkow S. Remodeling schemes of intracellular pathogens. Science. 1994; 263: 637–639.

55. Sturgill-Koszycki S, Schlesinger PH, Chakraborty P *et al.* Lack of acidification in *Mycobacterium* phagosomes produced by exclusion of the vesicular proton-ATPase. Science. 1994; 263: 678–681.

56. Kaufmann SHE. Immunity to intracellular bacteria. In: Paul WE, ed. Fundamental immunology. New York: Raven Press, 1993: 1251–1286.

57. Fields PI, Croisman EA, Heffron F. A *Salmonella* locus that controls resistance to microbicidal proteins from phagocytic cells. Science. 1989; 243: 1059–1062.

58. Meyer TF, Gibbs CP, Haas R. Variation and control of protein expression in *Neisseria*. Annu Rev Microbiol. 1990; 44: 451–457.

59. Gotschlich EC. Immunity to extracellular bacteria. In: Paul WE, ed. Fundamental immunology. New York: Raven Press, 1993: 1287–1308.

60. Cooper NR. Complement evasion strategies of microorganisms. Immunol Today. 1991; 12: 327–331.

61. Joiner KA, Brown EJ, Frank MM. Complement and bacteria: chemistry and biology in host defense. Annu Rev Immunol. 1984; 2: 461–471.

62. Moller G, ed. Superantigens. Immunol Rev. 1993; 131: 1–200.

63. Marrack P, Winslow GM, Choi Y *et al.* The bacterial and mouse mammary tumour virus superantigens: two different families of proteins with the same function. Immunol Rev. 1993; 131: 79–92.

64. Bowness P, Moss PAH, Tranter H *et al. Clostridium perfringens* enterotoxin is a superantigen reactive with human T cell receptors Vβ 6.9 and Vβ 22. J Exp Med. 1992; 176: 893–896.

65. Cole BC. The immunology of *Mycoplasma arthritidis* and its superantigen MAM. Curr Topics Microbiol Immunol. 1991; 174: 107–119.

66. Winslow GM, Scherer MT, Kappler JW *et al.* Detection and biochemical characterization of the mouse mammary tumour virus 7 superantigen (Mls-1ᵃ). Cell. 1992; 71: 719–730.

67. Johnson HM, Russell JK, Pontzer CH. Superantigens in human disease. Sci Am. 1992; 266: 92–101.

68. Miethke T, Wahl C, Heeg K *et al.* T cell mediated lethal shock triggered in mice by the superantigen staphylococcal enterotoxin B: critical role of tumour necrosis factor. J Exp Med. 1992; 175: 91–98.

69. Paliard X, West SG, Lafferty JA *et al.* Evidence for the effects of a superantigen in rheumatoid arthritis. Science. 1991; 253: 325–329.
70. Abe J, Klotzin BL, Jinjo K *et al.* Selective expansion of T cells expressing T cell receptor variable regions Vb2 and Vb8 in Kawasaki disease. Proc Natl Acad Sci USA. 1992; 89: 4066–4070.
71. Beutler B, Cerami AC. The biology of cachectin/TNF – a primary mediator of the host response. Annu Rev Immunol. 1989; 7: 625–656.
72. Beutler B, Milsark IW, Cerami AC. Passive immunisation against cachectin/tumour necrosis factor protects mice from lethal effect of endotoxin. Science. 1985; 229: 869–871.
73. Cohen J. Gram-negative shock. In: Lachman PJ *et al.*, eds. Clinical aspects of immunology. Oxford: Blackwell Scientific, 1993: 1469–1480.
74. Johnston KH, Zabriskie JB. Purification and partial characterisation of the nephritis strain-associated protein from *Streptococcus pyogenes* group A. J Exp Med. 1986; 163: 697–712.
75. Williams RC. Autoimmunity and infection. In: Lachman PJ *et al.* eds. Clinical aspects of immunology. Oxford: Blackwell Scientific, 1993: 1671–1686.
76. van de Rijn I, Zabriskie JB, McCarty M. Group A streptococcal antigens cross reactive with myocardium. J Exp Med. 1977; 146: 579–599.
77. Ayoub EM, Barrett DJ, MacLaren NK, Krischer JP. Association of human class II HLA antigens with rheumatic fever. J Clin Invest. 1986; 77: 2019–2026
78. Schwimmbeck PL, Yu DTY, Oldstone MBA. Autoantibodies to HLA-B27 in the sera of patients with ankylosing spondylitis and Reiter's syndrome: molecular mimicry with *Klebsiella pneumoniae*. J Exp Med. 1987; 166: 173–181.
79. Hammer RE *et al.* Spontaneous inflammatory disease in transgenic rats expressing HLA-B27 and B2m. Cell. 1990; 63: 1099–1112.
80. Joklik WK. Interferons. In: Fields BN, Knipe DM, eds. Virology. New York: Raven Press, 1990: 383–410.
81. Durum SK, Oppenheim JJ. Proinflammatory cytokines and immunity. In: Paul WE, ed. Fundamental immunology. New York: Raven Press, 1993; 801–835.
82. Farrar MA, Schreiber RD. The molecular biology of interferon gamma and its receptor. Ann Rev Immunol. 1993; 11: 571–612.
83. Dinarello CA, Cannon JG, Wolff SM. New concepts on the pathogenesis of fever. Rev Infect Dis. 1988; 10: 168–169.
84. Tartaglia LA, Goeddel DV. Two TNF receptors. Immunol Today. 1992; 13: 151–153.
85. Spiegelman BM, Hotamisligil GS. Through thick and thin: wasting, obesity and TNFo. Cell. 1993; 73: 625–627.
86. Wong GHW, Goeddel D. Tumour necrosis factors α and β inhibit virus replication and synergise with interferons. Nature. 1986; 323: 819–822.
87. Gooding LR, Elmore LW, Tollefson AE, Brady HA, Wold WSM. A 14700 MW protein from the E3 region of adenovirus inhibit cytolysis by tumour necrosis factor. Cell. 1988; 53: 341–346.
88. Kim HW, Leikin SL, Arrobio JO, Brandt CD, Channock RM, Parrott RH. Cell mediated immunity to respiratory syncytial virus infection induced by inactivated vaccine or by injection. Pediatr Res. 1976; 10: 75–78.

8
The Pattern of Infection in Immunodeficiency

A. D. B. WEBSTER

INTRODUCTION

Although experiments in animals can tell us something about the mechanisms of protection against infection, the relevance to human disease is usually uncertain. The study of rare immunodeficiency disorders has enabled us to make some clear statements on the critical role of individual host defence mechanisms against infection. It is likely that new genetically determined defects in relatively minor aspects of host defence or inflammation (e.g. lymphokines) will soon be discovered and enlighten us on the efficiency of the many 'back-up' mechanisms for dealing with infecting organisms. The problem with many of the known severe immunodeficiency disorders, such as severe combined immunodeficiency, is that more than one cell type is involved, making it difficult to link the clinical pattern of infection with any specific defect. Furthermore, it can be difficult to locate the immune defect in patients who are chronically infected with an organism, since the infection itself may cause secondary 'abnormalities' in the immune system, as is seen in mucocutaneous candidiasis. Nevertheless, studies in patients with immunodeficiencies involving antibody production and neutrophil function have enabled us to link defence mechanisms to specific infections. Most of these studies have been undertaken on patients in advanced countries, and the results may not apply to individuals in the Third World who are more frequently exposed to a wider range of organisms. In this situation a relatively minor defect in an amplifying or back-up mechanism may be potentially lethal.

The known defects in host defence will be discussed, beginning with the relatively non-specific and primitive mechanisms of phagocytosis originally described by Metchnikov, followed by complement, and finally the more sophisticated mechanisms involving cellular immunity and antibodies. I shall concentrate on the relatively well characterized inherited disorders and will only briefly discuss some of the more speculative primary and secondary deficiencies in phagocytes and cellular immunity.

DEFECTS IN PHAGOCYTES (Table 1)

The critical importance of neutrophils and macrophages is beyond question, as shown by the common occurrence of fatal bacterial and fungal septicaemia in patients with profound leucopenia (Figure 1). The most dramatic example of such a defect is reticular dysgenesis, in which an inherited defect causes a block in the differentiation of a primitive leucocyte stem cell, with absence of circulating neutrophils, macrophages and lymphocytes. Affected infants only survive a few days or weeks without a successful bone marrow transplant[1]. Selective absence of the monocyte/macrophage series has not been described, probably because this is incompatible with fetal survival, perhaps because these cells are involved in the formation of the brain[2]. If this is true, then some macrophage-like cells must be produced during the development of fetuses with reticular dysgenesis.

Neutropenia

Infants with severe forms of inherited neutropenia die early from septicaemia, usually due to staphylococci, but also due to gram-negative organisms such as *Pseudomonas* and *Klebsiella*[3]. These organisms are not efficiently phagocytosed by neutrophils in the absence of antibody and complement, and complete absence of the third complement component leads to a similar clinical outcome (see below). The MRC Leukaemia Trial showed a close relationship between mortality from infection and neutropenia induced by cytotoxic drugs[4]. In this case, antibody production may also have been impaired by the drugs.

There is evidence to suggest that the monocyte/macrophage series can compensate for an absence of neutrophils. First, rare individuals with very low neutrophil counts remain healthy[5]. Furthermore, the monocyte count may rise during the neutropenic troughs in cyclic neutropenia, and probably prevents life-threatening infection during this period[6]. Studies on these patients strongly suggest that adequate numbers of circulating neutrophils are important for the control of mucocutaneous infection with low-grade pathogens, particularly staphylococci and *Candida*. Staphylococcal skin boils characteristically occur in the neutropenic troughs, associated with malaise and fever indicating a bacteraemia. Mucosal ulceration of the mouth and vagina is common, although the organisms responsible are usually not clear. Chronic gingivitis is a common feature of neutrophil dysfunction, and shows that neutrophils in the crevicular fluid and gingival mucosa are important in the control of the growth of commensal organisms in the mouth. In general, circulating neutrophil counts below $500/\mu l$ are associated with infection.

Table 1 Clinically significant phagocyte defects

	Condition	Type/inheritance	Typical infection
Neutrophils	Neutropenia	Autosomal recessive Acquired { drugs autoimmune	*Staphylococcus/Pseudomonas/E. coli/Klebsiella* sp. septicaemia *Aspergillus* sp./*Candida*
	Chronic granulomatous disease (CGD)	Autosomal recessive X-linked	Chronic *Staphylococcus/Aspergillus/Salmonella* infections
	Leucocyte adhesion molecule deficiency (LAD)	Autosomal recessive	Chronic staphylococcal skin sepsis Gram-negative infections
	Chediak–Higashi	Autosomal recessive	Staphylococcal skin and *E. coli* urinary infections
	Hyper-IgE syndrome	Autosomal recessive	Staphylococcal and *Candida* infections
Macrophages/reticuloendothelial system	Absent spleen	Congenital Splenectomy	Pneumococcal/*H. influenzae* septicaemia
	Malakoplakia	Acquired	Chronic *Klebsiella/E. coli* urinary tract infections
	Whipple's disease	Acquired	Chronic 'bacillus' infection of gut
	Mucocutaneous candidiasis	Autosomal recessive Acquired	Candidiasis on mucous membranes, oseophagus and nail beds

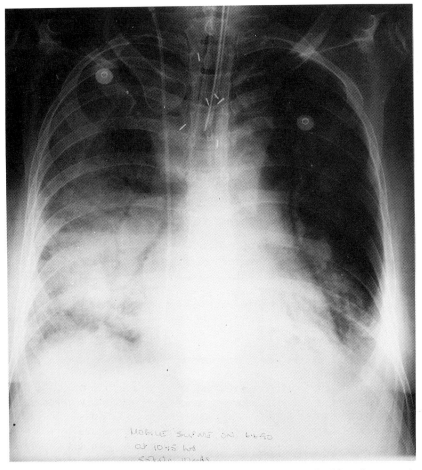

Figure 1 Lung radiograph showing extensive consolidation due to a mixed fungal pneumonia (Aspergillus and Mucor) in a patient with severe neutropenia. The patient died a few days later

FUNCTIONAL NEUTROPHIL DEFECTS

Chronic granulomatous disease (CGD)

Phagocytosis and the release of microbicidal proteins from cytoplasmic granules into the phagocytic vacuole is normal in this rare autosomal or X-linked recessive disorder. There is, however, a failure to kill some fungi and catalase-positive bacteria, including staphylococci, *Serratia marcescens* and *Aspergillus*[7]. At a molecular level, there is a failure to generate microbicidal reactive oxygen-derived products within the phagocytic vacuole due to inherited defects in the components of the NADPH oxidase system[8]. Patients characteristically present with cervical or inguinal suppurative lesions, originating from an infected lymph node. Abscesses in the gut, liver and

162

bone also occur, together with chronic inflammatory bowel disease due to granulomatous changes in the mucosa of the small and large bowel. Chronic *Salmonella* enteritis may also occur, associated with fatal septicaemia. Catalase-negative organisms such as pneumococci and streptococci are killed normally: they generate their own hydrogen peroxide within the phagocytic vacuole and 'self-destruct'. Meticulous clinical care and the administration of prophylactic antibiotics such as co-trimoxazole allows many of these patients to experience long periods free from infection. The disease demonstrates that containment of organisms within phagocytes, although it may prevent fulminant infection, is not an adequate defence mechanism in itself.

Myeloperoxidase deficiency

Myeloperoxidase is abundant in neutrophils and has the ability to oxidize halides to potentially bactericidal compounds. Partial myeloperoxidase deficiency is common, occurring in about 1% of the population, but this is not associated with increased susceptibility to infection[9]. Early reports suggested an association of complete deficiency with chronic infection, but a number of affected healthy individuals have now been described[10]. It may be an important back-up mechanism in the presence of other functional defects, and one could speculate on the outcome in a patient with both CGD and myeloperoxidase deficiency.

Chediak-Higashi disease

This inherited autosomal recessive disorder is characterized by oculocutaneous albinism, peripheral neuropathy and the frequent development of a leukaemia-like terminal phase with pancytopenia[11]. The basic abnormality is unknown, but cytoplasmic granules form abnormal, large secondary lysosomes. These lysosomes prevent neutrophils from squeezing through narrow spaces, such as those between vascular endothelial cells, and this may lead to a relative neutropenia at extravascular sites of infection. There is also a partial defect in bactericidal killing which is probably due to failure of cytoplasmic granules to fuse with the phagocytic vacuole and discharge their contents. These defects lead to a susceptibility to staphylococcal skin sepsis and to upper and lower respiratory tract infections due to a variety of organisms. The terminal 'leukaemic' phase is thought to be caused by a lymphotropic viral infection secondary to a defect in cellular immunity (see below).

Hyper-IgE syndrome

Patients with this rare disorder have chronic eczematoid dermatitis, coarse facial features, allergic phenomena such as asthma and sinusitis and recurrent infections with a variety of organisms, particularly staphylococci and *Candida albicans*[12]. Chronic staphylococcal abscesses in the skin are characteristic:

the lack of surrounding erythema and inflammation led to the term 'cold abscesses' and to the eponym Job's syndrome. Deep-seated abscesses, including osteomyelitis, also occur and some patients present with muco-cutaneous candidiasis. A prerequisite for the diagnosis is a very high serum IgE, usually > 5000 iu/l and sometimes as high as 90 000 iu/l. Levels of specific IgE antibodies to a variety of organisms are raised, but this in itself is not thought to compromise host defence. There is good evidence of a defect in neutrophil chemotaxis caused by as yet unidentified factors in the plasma. It is likely that the defect is caused by an autosomally inherited defect in the regulation of IgE production which causes down-regulation of neutrophil chemotaxis; histamine may be one of the factors involved and treatment with an H_2 antagonist is useful in some patients. Others may benefit from plasmaphoresis in acute situations, or regular intravenous immunoglobulin therapy, which reduces the serum IgE level through an unknown mechanism.

Leucocyte adhesion molecule defects (LAD)

Neutrophils express heterodimeric molecules belonging to the integrin superfamily; these enable cells to adhere to and migrate through vascular endothelium. These heterodimers (Leu-CAM) consist of a distinct α subunit (CD11a, b or c) non-covalently linked to a common β subunit (CD18). Autosomal recessively inherited point mutations in the β subunit cause a failure of neutrophil adhesion and migration[13]. There is a spectrum of clinical severity: some patients survive into the fourth decade with chronic gingivitis and recurrent indolent deep-seated skin ulceration which leave unsightly paper-thin scars[14] (Figure 2). The more severely affected usually die in the first few years of life with overwhelming sepsis due to *Pseudomonas aeruginosa*, *Escherichia coli*, *Klebsiella* and staphylococci; characteristically there is marked neutrophilia with no pus formation. Delayed separation of the umbilical cord at birth with omphalitis is a feature, suggesting that the integrins are involved in contraction and sealing of the cord. They also seem to be involved in graft rejection, since LAD patients have an unexpectedly good prognosis following receipt of unrelated bone marrow grafts. Inherited defects in the selectins, another class of adhesion molecules which mediate the initial rolling of neutrophils along the vascular endothelium, has not been reported but theoretically could cause a similar but less severe clinical pattern.

MACROPHAGES AND THE RETICULO-ENDOTHELIAL SYSTEM

The spleen

This organ is clearly not essential for defence against infection since its absence is compatible with life-long normal health. However, there is a slight risk of fatal septicaemia, and this may be more marked in children and infants[15]. Apart from acting as a substantial reservoir of cells involved in

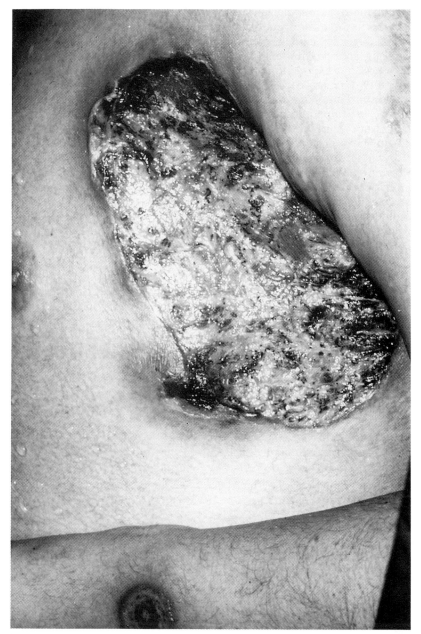

Figure 2 Large ulcerating skin lesion in the axilla, and an early lesion on the forearm, in a 20-year-old patient with leucocyte adhesion deficiency (LAD). This patient had < 10% expression of the CD11b/c integrin molecules on the surface of his neutrophils. Histology showed numerous neutrophils within capillaries, but a failure of these cells to move into the surrounding tissue

the immune response, the spleen is thought to act as an efficient 'filter' for blood-borne organisms and may prevent rapid multiplication of certain bacteria after they initially enter the blood stream, allowing the host time to mount an antibody response. This seems to be particularly important for pneumococci, which multiply rapidly in the blood stream in the absence of antibodies. Pneumococcal septicaemia and meningitis is a well recognized complication in infants with congenital asplenia, and after splenectomy for trauma or lymphoreticular malignancy. It is customary to administer prophylactic penicillin following splenectomy, although some would argue that ampicillin is more appropriate since there is also a risk of *Haemophilus influenzae* septicaemia. The risk of septicaemia seems to decrease with time following splenectomy, and there is still some debate as to whether life-long prophylactic antibiotics are required. This apparent decreasing risk may be due to the formation of a larger repertoire of antibodies to different pneumococcal strains, and it is common practice nowadays to increase this by immunizing patients with pneumococcal vaccines[16].

Macrophages

A number of metabolic storage diseases due to inherited defects in degradative enzymes are associated with the accumulation of metabolic substrates in macrophages and other cells. These include Gaucher's, Niemann–Pick, Crabbe and Fabry's diseases. None of these is associated with an obviously increased susceptibility to infection, probably because young cells which have not accumulated substrate function adequately. Chronic granulomatous disease (CGD) is the only inherited metabolic disease of macrophages (and neutrophils) which leads to chronic infection.

Absence of all macrophage Fc receptors has not been described. However, genetic deficiency of the high-affinity FcR1 receptor is compensated by FcR2 receptors, and affected individuals are healthy[17]. Furthermore, about one-third of normal healthy individuals have a genetic variant in the control of Fc receptors, but this seems to have no clinical significance in the Western world[18].

Defects in microbicidal activity

Malakoplakia

This rare sporadic disease is characterized by the presence of large macrophages containing lysosomal inclusions (Michaelis–Gutmann bodies). These macrophages contain viable bacteria, often *E. coli* or *Klebsiella* species[19]. The urinary tract is usually involved, with a chronic granulomatous cystitis. The circulating macrophages show subtle abnormalities *in vitro*, with depressed bactericidal killing and poor lysosomal enzyme release. The intracellular cGMP level is low, and there are claims that acetylcholine agonists, which raise cGMP levels *in vitro*, have been helpful in patients[20]. This may be a rare autosomal defect which is only significant when there are other reasons for bacterial cystitis.

Mucocutaneous candidiasis

This rare condition has a variety of underlying aetiologies. The severe type begins in childhood with chronic *Candida* infection of the mucous membranes and nails, causing the characteristic drumstick fingers, oro-genital thrush, and sometimes swollen, chronically inflamed lips. In some cases there is additional skin infection with low-grade pathogens such as staphylococci. About one-third of cases are associated with multiple endocrinopathies. Until recently, most investigations were undertaken on patients who were heavily infected, but effective antifungal drugs, such as ketoconazole are now available and can virtually eliminate the infection, making it easier to interpret any *in vitro* defects found.

There is a lack of consistency in the abnormalities found between patients. The critical mechanisms in the skin or mucous membranes for controlling *Candida* are not yet understood, but both monocyte/macrophages and T cells are likely to be involved because of the common association of mucocutaneous candidiasis with severe combined immunodeficiency and AIDS. Monocyte chemotaxis and *Candida* killing was reduced in a family where more than one member was affected, and there was a failure of the monocytes to produce interleukin-1 (IL-1) in response to stimulation with lipopolysaccharide (LPS)[21].

Whipple's disease

This is a rare chronic infection of the gut with an unknown organism, or a related group of still unclassified organisms, which usually occurs in middle-aged men. Electron microscopy shows infiltrating macrophages in the lamina propria filled with bacilli, and special staining shows an accumulation of PAS-like material which is thought to be derived from the bacteria[22]. There is controversy over whether an underlying broad defect in cellular immunity exists, since delayed hypersensitivity and *in vitro* T cell mitogenic responses are often depressed, even after the infection is eradicated with antibiotics[23]. Bjerknes *et al.*[24] showed that circulating monocytes, or macrophages derived from them *in vitro*, killed but failed to degrade bacteria. Such a defect would be expected to cause susceptibility to a variety of organisms, whereas these patients only have a problem with the Whipple's bacillus. The possibility of a specific T cell receptor defect for a critical epitope on these bacteria is possible, particularly since there is a markedly raised incidence of the HLA-B27 histocompatibility antigen in affected patients[25].

Other chronic infections

In general, there is a correlation between the ability of macrophages to kill large intracellular parasites such as *Trypanosoma cruzi* and *Toxoplasma gondii in vitro* and the formation of reactive oxygen species. However, this is not a spontaneous event, and lymphokines derived from T cells are required to activate the macrophages; one important lymphokine is interferon

(IFN)-γ[26]. A primary defect in IFN-γ has not yet been described, so it is not clear whether there are other compensatory mechanisms for activating macrophages. The killing of mycobacteria within macrophages also depends upon this mechanism, which has been demonstrated *in vivo* by the conversion of lepromatous leprosy into the tuberculoid form with IFN-γ treatment[27]. Other factors are probably involved, however, as indicated by the presence of a resistance gene for mycobacterial infection in mice, which is expressed in macrophages[28]. The current state of knowledge suggests that there may be genetically determined variations in the level of macrophage activation, and that these may determine the outcome of mycobacterial and some parasitic infections. The genes involved are likely to regulate lymphokine production, and not to be coding genes for molecules such as IFN-γ. Further knowledge of the interplay between T cells and macrophages, together with some technical advances for *in vitro* analysis, is required before different patterns of response between individuals can be identified.

Secondary defects in macrophage function probably account for the opportunistic parasitic infections, such as those with *Pneumocystis carinii* and *Toxoplasma gondii* which occur in patients with AIDS or after bone marrow transplantation[29,30]. Alveolar macrophages from such patients showed depressed intracellular killing and uptake of oxygen following phagocytosis of micro-organisms; this may be due to inadequate production of IFN-γ by T cells[31].

DEFECTS IN CELLULAR IMMUNITY

Selective T cell deficiencies (Table 2)

Two rare, selective defects of T cells demonstrate that a severe deficiency in the numbers and function of T cells is compatible with survival, and does not always lead to life-threatening infections. However, most, if not all, surviving patients with these defects have some residual T cell function, which is probably enough to respond to antigens and activate macrophages for the killing of micro-organisms.

Purine nucleoside phosphorylase (PNP) deficiency

This autosomal recessive disease is due to the inheritance of two abnormal alleles on chromosome 14. The most severely affected patients have very few circulating T lymphocytes, but normal numbers of NK cells and B cells, and normal monocyte/macrophage function[32]. In the absence of PNP, deoxyguanosine (dGuo) accumulates in the plasma: this has been shown *in vitro* to inhibit mitogen- and antigen-induced T cell proliferation, probably by altering the levels of intracellular guanine nucleotides. It is suggested that B lymphocytes escape inhibition because they lack the metabolic pathway to convert DGuo to these nucleotides[33]. Formal *in vitro* studies on the monocytes/macrophages from these patients, or from normal individuals in the presence of PNP inhibitors, have not been published; however, pilot

Table 2 Immunodeficiency predominantly affecting T cell function

	Condition	Type/inheritance	Characteristic infections
Selective T cell defects	Thymic aplasia	Fetal malformation	Cytomegalovirus/varicella/vaccinia (autoimmune phenomena)
	Purine nucleoside phosphorylase deficiency	Autosomal recessive	
Severe combined immunodeficiency (SCID)	IL-2 receptor γ-chain defect	X-linked	Opportunistic infections with
	Adenosine deaminase deficiency	Autosomal recessive	a) Fungi
	MHC Class II lymphocyte defect	Autosomal recessive	*Candida*
	Reticular dysgenesis	Autosomal recessive	*Cryptococcus neoformans*
			Pneumocystis carinii
			Histoplasma capsulatum
			b) Viruses
			Cytomegalovirus
			Varicella zoster
	AIDS	Acquired	*Polyoma*
			c) Protozoa
			Giardia
			Cryptosporidia
			Toxoplasma gondii
			Entamoeba histolytica
			d) Helminths
			Strongyloides stercoralis
			e) Bacteria
			Mycobacteria
			Listeria
			Nocardia asteroides
			Legionella pneumophilia
			Listeria monocytogenes
Partial immunodeficiencies	Ataxia telangiectasia	Autosomal recessive	Respiratory tract infections (viral and bacterial – not usually severe)
	Wiskott–Aldrich syndrome	Autosomal recessive	Burkitt's type lymphoma
	X-linked lymphoproliferative syndrome	X-linked	Fulminant EBV infection

studies in my own laboratory showed that the viability and morphology of human circulating monocytes incubated with the PNP inhibitor 8-aminoguanosine was normal over a 7-day period. PNP deficiency may not be entirely selective for T cells, as about half of affected patients have spastic paresis of the extremities and trunk, and some have megaloblastic changes in the bone marrow. Changes in the central nervous system may precede the onset of infections by many years, supporting the view that this is due to the metabolic defect and not to infection with an unknown neurotropic virus.

The susceptibility to infection varies between patients: some develop recurrent upper and lower respiratory tract bacterial infections, while others remain essentially healthy for long periods. However, PNP-deficient patients are prone to severe and sometimes fatal viral infections, particularly with varicella zoster, measles, cytomegalovirus and vaccinia viruses. However one PNP-deficient patient was documented to recover from both polio virus and hepatitis B virus infection, suggesting that these viruses are eliminated by T cell-independent mechanisms. Patients have a tendency to autoimmune phenomena, including haemolytic anaemia and systemic lupus erythematosus-like disease, which supports current theories involving T cell suppression of autoreactive B cell clones.

Thymic dysplasia (Di George syndrome)

Developmental defects of the third and fourth pharyngeal pouch in the fetus may lead to complete or partial absence of the thymus and parathyroid glands, as well as midline defects in the upper lip, hard palate and larynx, and anomalies of the great vessels of the thorax and heart[34]. Neonates with the most severe defects are unlikely to survive because of heart failure. Survivors usually have some residual thymic tissue, although there may be very few T cells in the circulation at birth, and only tiny foci of T cells in the paracortical regions of the lymph nodes. Nevertheless, many affected infants and young children remain healthy despite these defects, and there is usually a gradual expansion of T cell numbers in the circulation over the first few years of life[35]. Susceptibility to infection varies and may be influenced by associated factors such as hypocalcaemia and laryngeal and cardiac abnormalities. However, many patients have an increased susceptibility to upper and lower respiratory tract bacterial infections, *Pneumocystis carini* pneumonia, mucosal candidiasis and diarrhoea caused by a variety of organisms.

COMBINED IMMUNODEFICIENCIES

T, B and accessory cell defects (Table 2)

A variety of inherited defects affect all three main cell types involved in the immune response, and cause severe combined immunodeficiency (SCID).

The mechanism in three of these conditions is partly understood.

Adenosine deaminase (ADA) deficiency is an autosomal recessive disorder due to inheritance of two abnormal alleles on chromosome 20. This leads to an accumulation of deoxyadenosine, which is toxic to both T and B cells, although the mechanism is unclear[36]. Culturing normal monocytes/macrophages *in vitro* with inhibitors of ADA causes rounding of the cells within 6 h, followed by death[37]. Affected patients lack cellular immunity, are unable to make antibody and suffer from a variety of bacterial, viral, fungal and protozoal infections[38].

Failure to express major histocompatibility (MHC) Class II molecules on the surface of lymphocytes causes very severe combined immunodeficiency, and affected infants do not survive without a successful bone marrow transplant. This rare autosomal recessive disease is caused by mutations in factors which regulate the transcription of the Class II genes[39]. Unlike other types of SCID, patients usually have normal numbers of circulating lymphocytes which proliferate *in vitro* with mitogens, but not with antigens. Failure to express Class I antigens on lymphocytes has been described but it is compatible with relatively normal health.

A third type of SCID is caused by inherited defects in the gene on the X chromosome which codes for the γ chain of the interleukin-2 (IL-2) receptor[40]. At least two infants have been described with apparent failure to produce IL-2, although no defect in the coding gene has yet been documented. IL-2 will correct the *in vitro* proliferative defect in lymphocytes and was useful in treating one patient.

It is worth highlighting some infections which are particularly common in SCID patients. *Pneumocystis carinii* pneumonia used to occur in nearly all affected infants, and it is now common practice to prevent this with co-trimoxazole. However, the infants usually fail to thrive due to chronic diarrhoea and malabsorption associated with protozoal infections such as giardiasis and cryptosporidiosis, and a variety of enteric viruses. Nowadays, most affected infants are diagnosed early and are given a bone marrow transplant, with a success rate of >70% if the donor is a histocompatible normal sibling[41]. Graft versus host disease can occur if bone marrow from an unrelated donor is used, and this itself can cause a severe combined immunodeficiency state, leading to death from infection.

SYNDROMES ASSOCIATED WITH PARTIAL IMMUNODEFICIENCY (Table 2)

Ataxia telangiectasia

This autosomal recessive condition is caused by a defect in the repair of DNA damage caused by ionizing radiation. Although the main clinical problem is progressive central nervous system disease, there are subtle abnormalities in lymphocyte function[42]. More than half of all affected patients have selective IgA deficiency, sometimes in association with IgG$_2$ and/or IgE deficiency. There is thymic atrophy and a variety of functional defects in the circulating T cells, such as poor lymphocyte blastogenesis and failure to generate antigen-specific MHC-restricted T cell cytotoxicity to viruses. Delayed hypersensitivity skin tests are often depressed. There is a markedly raised incidence of malignant tumours, particularly lymphomas. There is no evidence that this is due to chronic infection with potentially oncogenic viruses, and can be explained by the increased rate of chromosomal breaks and translocations, which in the case of T cells frequently involve genes coding for the T cell receptor complex on chromosomes 7 and 14. A failure to repair DNA during the early phases of lymphocyte activation may underlie the immunodeficiency, although a further understanding of the mechanism will have to await the cloning of the relevant gene(s) on chromosome 11[43].

Wiskott–Aldrich syndrome

This X-linked disorder is characterized by severe thrombocytopenia, eczema and a high incidence of Epstein–Barr virus (EBV)-related B cell lymphomas. Patients are unable to generate IgM antibodies to polysaccharides, with raised levels of serum IgA and IgE, the latter being responsible for the atopy[44].

There is usually a gradual decline in T cell numbers and function with time. Some patients are prone to recurrent respiratory tract infections. The basic defect is not known, but there is altered expression of sialophorin (CD43) on lymphocytes, apparently due to post-translational abnormalities of glycosylation which may lead to partial failure of lymphocyte adhesion (to ICAM-1) following activation[45,46]. It is not clear why these patients are prone to Burkitt's type lymphomas, a finding which suggests some similarity with X-linked lymphoproliferative syndrome (see below).

X-linked lymphoproliferative syndrome (XLPS)

This was first described in the Duncan family, where affected males either died of fulminating infectious mononucleosis with liver necrosis, or developed hypogammaglobulinaemia or lymphomas[47]. Experience with this and similar families shows that affected males are healthy until they contract a primary EBV infection; there is then a gradual deterioration in T cell numbers and function in those that survive. The patients make normal antibodies to EBV, showing elevated titres of antibodies to viral capsid antigen (VCA) and early antigen. Interestingly, the heterozygote mothers tend to have high levels of anti-VCA antibodies, which some claim can be useful in identifying carriers[48]. The precise nature of the defect in XLPS is still unclear, but the evidence suggests a dysregulation in the control of CD8 cytotoxic/suppressor cells which may cause organ necrosis in the acute stage and immunodeficiency in the long term[49]. A greater understanding of the mechanism will have to await the cloning of the XLPS gene.

Chronic papilloma virus warts

Virus-associated warts are a feature of patients with a variety of known inherited or acquired defects in T cell function, although only a minority of such patients develop this complication. However, clinical immunologists have become aware of a significant number of patients, usually adults, who present with multiple recurring cutaneous warts which fail to respond to traditional therapy. These patients are otherwise healthy and investigations of immunity usually fail to show any significant defect. Some patients respond to systemic therapy with IFN-α, although there is no evidence that these patients have a specific defect in producing interferons. In others the management remains unsatisfactory, and further work is now needed to test the hypothesis that such patients have developed a disorder of immune regulation specifically affecting the ability of T cells to eliminate papilloma virus-infected cells.

DEFECTS IN NATURAL KILLER (NK) CELL CYTOTOXICITY

NK activity is severely depressed in the Chediak–Higashi syndrome, and this may be responsible for the predisposition to chronic viral infections and the terminal pancytopenic phase. Although patients have phenotypically recognizable NK cells, these show defective killing of target cells *in vitro*, although interaction with the target does stimulate oxidative metabolism[50]. There is also decreased NK activity in the Wiskott–Aldrich syndrome (see above) and it is argued that this may be partly responsible for the uncontrolled EBV replication[51]. However, a critical role for NK cells is still in doubt as they do not appear to be necessary for survival.

ACQUIRED IMMUNE DEFICIENCY SYNDROME (AIDS)

The spectrum of infection in AIDS is much broader than that seen in patients with selective T cell deficiency such as thymic aplasia, and it was this that prompted immunologists to suggest that HIV compromised monocytes/macrophages and was not selective for T cells. In fact, infections seen in AIDS are similar to those seen in the primary severe combined immunodeficiencies of infancy, where HIV infection now has to be considered in the differential diagnosis. The study of patients with AIDS has dramatically expanded our knowledge on the types and treatment of opportunistic infections associated with severe defects in cellular immunity. Such studies are not usually possible in SCID infants since they either succumb during the first severe infection or receive a bone marrow transplant soon after diagnosis. Table 2 lists the infections commonly seen in AIDS; detailed clinical aspects of these infections have been reviewed elsewhere[52]. There is still controversy over the immuno-pathological mechanisms in AIDS, although there is a growing consensus that the immunodeficiency is caused by disorganization of the central lymphoid system by a substantial reservoir of human immunodeficiency virus (HIV)

Table 3 Antibody and complement deficiency

Type	Inheritance	Characteristic infections
Agammaglobulinaemia	X-linked (XLA)	*Haemophilus influenzae* (non-typable) upper and lower respiratory infections
Common varied immunodeficiency (CVID)	? Autosomal dominant polygenic	Staphylococcal skin infections *Campylobacter* enteritis Giardiasis *Mycoplasma* arthritis Enterovirus CNS and muscle disease
Early complement component defects	Autosomal recessive	Pneumococcal septicaemia
C3 deficiency	Autosomal recessive	Multiple severe bacterial infections
Late component defects	Autosomal recessive	Gonococcal and meningococcal septicaemia
Properdin deficiency	X-linked	Meningococcal and pneumococcal septicaemia

in the follicular dendritic cells and macrophages. The immunodeficiency is further compounded by viral stimulation of T_{H2} immune response in those individuals with a genetic predisposition to this type of reaction. This leads to a predominance of subsets of lymphocytes which cannot secrete adequate levels of IL-2 or IFN-γ[53], which in turn explains the *in vitro* findings of deficient intracellular killing of *Toxoplasma* by macrophages from patients with AIDS, and the enhancement seen when IFN-γ is added to cultures[54].

HIV stimulates antibody production by an unknown mechanism, causing hypergammaglobulinaemia and adequate protection against the pathogens characteristically associated with antibody deficiency, such as *Haemophilus influenzae* and pneumococci. However, there is some failure of antibody production as the disease progresses, and this may explain the apparent increased susceptibility to systemic spread of *Mycoplasma fermentans* in AIDS, an organism that is normally confined to the upper respiratory mucosa[55].

COMPLEMENT DEFICIENCIES (Table 3)

Classical pathway – early component defects

Inherited deficiencies of C1, C4 and C2 are associated with systemic and discoid lupus-like syndromes, the common theme being immune complex-mediated inflammation in the skin and small vessels[56]. However, the defect is only one factor in the disease process, since the defects are compatible with normal health. The pattern of inheritance is autosomal recessive and the proximity of the genes for C2 and C4 with the histocompatibility Class II genes suggests that other factors, coded by genes within this complex, might also contribute to the mechanism of systemic lupus erythematosus (SLE). Deficiencies in these early components do predispose to life-threatening infection, particularly septicaemia and meningitis due to pneumococci, and to a lesser extent meningococci[57]. This is most obvious in C2 deficiency, possibly because this is the most common of the complement deficiencies, occurring in about 1 in 10 000 of the population, with over 50 kindreds being described. There is no predisposition to common viral infection, but there is a slightly raised incidence of Hodgkin's disease, suggesting a defect in the control of potentially oncogenic lymphotropic viruses.

Pneumococci are not phagocytosed efficiently by neutrophils in the absence of activated complement, although theoretically this could be achieved *in vivo* via the alternate pathway[58]. The issue probably depends upon the speed at which activated C3b can be generated for opsonization. This, together with the speed at which specific antibody can be generated, probably determines whether the initial infection is contained. Children with C2 deficiency are particularly prone to pneumococcal septicaemia, and it is sensible to administer pneumococcal vaccines and prophylactic penicillin.

C3 component

This is the most important component of complement, since it is activated by both the classical and alternate pathways, and produces functional fragments which mediate immune adherence and inflammation. Very few patients with inherited complete C3 deficiency have been described and most have died of infection within a few years, despite regular plasma transfusions[59]. Affected individuals are prone to infection with a variety of pyogenic bacteria, particularly pneumococci, group B *Haemophilus influenzae*, *Neisseria* and staphylococci; they are also prone to SLE-like disease. Theoretically, C4-mediated immune adherence can be achieved in the presence of specific antibody, and there is some support for this from *in vitro* studies of phagocytosis in the presence of C3-deficient serum[60]. As expected, there is a defect in the early mobilization of neutrophils to sites of inflammation, presumably due to the lack of chemotactic C5a produced, but the ability to produce a leucocytosis during infections varies between patients[61]. Antibody production is also compromised in C3-deficient patients due to inadequate fixation of immune complexes on antigen-presenting follicular dendritic cells. These combinations of defects explain why affected patients tend to have a worse prognosis than those with X-linked agammaglobulinaemia.

Late component defects

Between 15 and 30 patients have been described with a defect in each of C5, C6, C7 and C8. These patients all have a susceptibility to recurrent neisserial infections: Patients presenting with *N. meningitidis* meningitis or gonococcal arthritis should undergo routine assay of total serum haemolytic complement so that prophylactic penicillin can be considered and advice given on avoiding gonococcal infection. C5 is important because one of its cleavage products, C5a, is a potent chemoattractant for neutrophils; the other, C5b, initiates the membrane attack complex which is important for killing encapsulated organisms[62]. Not all individuals with C5 deficiency are prone to neisserial infection[57]. It is not clear whether this is due to residual C5 activity or the presence of an efficient compensatory mechanism.

Deficiency of C6, C7 and C8 is associated with recurrent infection by *Neisseria*, but not by other gram-negative organisms, such as *E. coli* and *Klebsiella* species, presumably because these are taken up and efficiently killed by phagocytes[63,64]. These patients characteristically present with a clinically mild meningitis, recover quickly following antibiotic treatment and then present again with a recurrence.

C9 deficiency, which is relatively common in Japan, is compatible with normal health, although a few patients suffer from neisserial infection[65]. C9-deficient serum will kill *Neisseria in vitro*, although less efficiently than normal serum, whereas the organisms survive if the serum lacks any of the other terminal components.

It is not clear why the classical pathway, and in particular the terminal components (except C9), are important for protection against *Neisseria*, particularly since some gonococci isolated from affected individuals are not killed *in vitro* by normal serum. However, this phenomenon is sometimes due to the presence of bound antibodies which block the activation of complement[66]. It is likely that the intact complement pathway is needed to both opsonize *Neisseria* for phagocytosis and to damage the organism's membrane, this combined effect preventing the growth of organisms during the initial infection. If the organisms persist then other factors, including blocking antibodies, may be generated and allow the infection to disseminate.

Deficiencies of regulatory proteins in the complement pathway

Inherited deficiency of C1 inhibitor (C1-INH) is not associated with a predisposition to infection. A few patients with factor I (C3b inactivator) deficiency have been reported and have a marked predisposition to infection by pyogenic organisms[67]. The one patient described with factor H deficiency had haemolytic uraemic syndrome. Deficiencies of both factor I and H lead to continuous consumption of C3, with low C3 levels and depressed total haemolytic complement activity.

Properdin is another regulator of C3 consumption, coded for by a gene on the X chromosome. Affected males with complete or partial properdin deficiency are susceptible to meningococcal meningitis and, to a lesser extent, pneumococcal septicaemia or pneumonia[64]. Unlike patients with terminal complement component defects, the infections may be severe and fulminant. Classical pathway haemolytic complement activity is normal, and assay for alternate pathway activity or serum properdin levels is required to diagnose the defect.

ANTIBODY DEFICIENCY (Table 3)

There has been a considerable advance in the past decade in our understanding of the critical role of antibodies in defence against infection. This has come from the study of X-linked agammaglobulinaemia (XLA) which is caused by mutations/deletions in a gene coding for a tyrosine kinase critical for B cell development[68]. T cell, monocyte/macrophage and antigen presenting cell function is normal. The more common non-familial form of hypogammaglobulinaemia (common varied immunodeficiency – CVID) is heterogeneous, many patients having clear evidence of subtle defects in T cells and antigen-presenting cells. In general, these patients suffer from the same spectrum of infections as those with XLA, but they are also prone to additional complications which may be related to unusual infections[69,70] (Figure 3).

X-linked agammaglobulinaemia

Bacterial infections

The over-riding problem in these patients is recurrent infection of the upper and lower respiratory tract with *Haemophilus influenzae* (Figure 4). Infants and children are also prone to chronic respiratory infection with *Branhamella catarrhalis*. *H. influenzae* isolated from sputum is usually non-typable and sensitive to a variety of commonly used antibiotics. Non-typable *H. influenzae* is considered to be a low-grade pathogen, although in the past there was debate as to whether it caused significant disease[71]. These organisms are ubiquitous in the environment and characteristically colonize the sinuses and bronchial tree after common respiratory viral infections. The middle ear is also often involved in young children. In the past, chronic infection with *H. influenzae* frequently led to bronchiectasis in children with XLA. However, the introduction of high dose intravenous immunoglobulin therapy (IVIG), which contains a range of specific IgG antibodies to the outer membrane proteins of *H. influenzae*[72], has had a major impact on the management of these children, and many now have long periods free from respiratory infection. Despite the fact that relatively little of the specific IgG infused intravenously reaches the respiratory mucosa (McIntosh & Webster – unpublished data), this demonstrates that IgG antibodies play a role in controlling the growth of *H. influenzae* on mucosal surfaces, although it does not tell us whether this isotype is more or less efficient than IgA. Nevertheless, despite high dose IVIG therapy, about one-third of XLA patients continue to suffer from symptoms of chronic bronchitis caused by *H. influenzae*, indicating that other mechanisms may be involved in the control of this organism. This seems likely in view of the few documented individuals with severe hypogammaglobulinaemia who remain healthy without treatment. Hypogammaglobulinaemic patients do tend to have low serum C1q levels[73], but we found no correlation between these levels and susceptibility to infection.

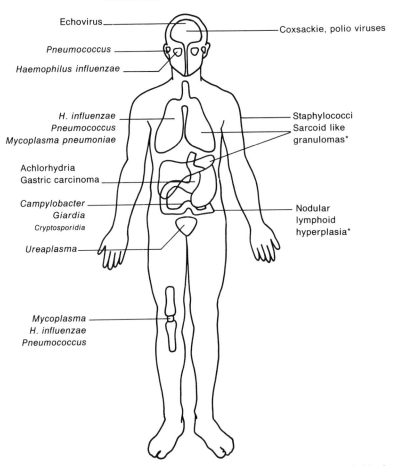

Echovirus

Coxsackie, polio viruses

Pneumococcus

Haemophilus influenzae

H. influenzae
Pneumococcus
Mycoplasma pneumoniae

Staphylococci
Sarcoid like
granulomas*

Achlorhydria
Gastric carcinoma

Campylobacter
Giardia
Cryptosporidia

Nodular
lymphoid
hyperplasia*

Ureaplasma

Mycoplasma
H. influenzae
Pneumococcus

Figure 3 Infections in hypogammaglobulinaemic patients. *These conditions are probably due to chronic infection with unknown organisms

1. Pneumococci

Agammaglobulinaemic patients are prone to pneumococcal pneumonia, septicaemia and meningitis which rarely occurs after the administration of low-dose intramuscular gammaglobulin (IMIG) replacement therapy. This suggests that relatively low levels of specific antibodies are adequate to protect against pneumococcal septicaemia, presumably by promoting opsonization of the first few invading organisms for phagocytosis in the spleen. However, despite IMIG treatment, there is a high risk of fulminant pneumococcal septicaemia in hypogammaglobulinaemic patients whose spleens have been surgically removed for hypersplenism or other reasons. Higher dose IVIG therapy protects against this complication. Although meningococcal meningitis and septicaemia have been described in antibody-

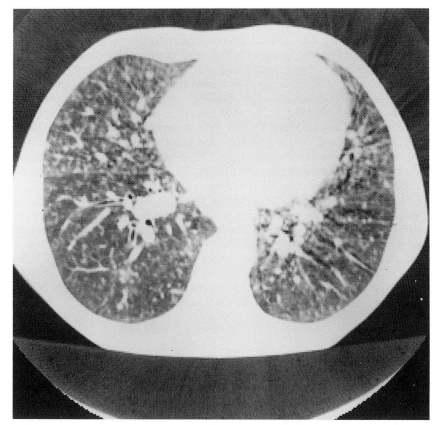

Figure 4 Computed tomography (CT) scan of the basal lung segments of an adult patient with hypogammaglobulinaemia. There is extensive bilateral bronchiectasis, with bronchial wall thickening and cystic changes

deficient patients, this complication is surprisingly rare, in contrast to the situation in patients with complement deficiencies.

2. Campylobacter and Helicobacter

Acute and chronic *Campylobacter jejuni* colitis is a recognized cause of acute and chronic diarrhoea in hypogammaglobulinaemic patients[74]. In normal individuals this is usually a mild and self-limiting infection. The organisms are not invasive but there is often superficial ulceration of the mucosa with inflammatory foci. Infection is less common in patients receiving IVIG therapy, although the mechanism of protection by IgG antibodies is not known. One possibility is that IgG neutralizes *Campylobacter* toxins, which some workers believe may cause the gut lesions[75]. IgG antibodies are also efficient at opsonizing these organisms for phagocytosis[76].

Although *Helicobacter pylori* is associated with chronic gastritis and

179

duodenal ulcer in immunocompetent patients[77], it is rarely found in the gastritis which commonly occurs in patients with common varied immuno-deficiency (CVID). This gastritis characteristically involves all areas of the stomach, sometimes with achlorhydria, and is probably a major factor in the high incidence of gastric carcinoma in this group of patients[69]. Investi-gations on gastric biopsies and juice from these patients show a moderate growth of mixed flora, although numbers and types of bacteria are very similar to those found in immunocompetent achlorhydric patients with classical pernicious anaemia[78]. The mechanism underlying the gastritis in CVID is unknown, but is probably due to an exaggerated inflammatory response to minor bacterial infection. Other types of chronic inflammatory bowel disease, such as gluten enteropathy, Crohn's disease and chronic low-grade colitis, also occur in CVID.

The rarity of *Helicobacter pylori* in the stomachs of antibody-deficient patients with gastritis is unlikely to be explained by the fact that these patients tend to take frequent courses of antibiotics. A more interesting possibility is that *H. pylori* cannot thrive in the stomach unless it is coated and protected by non-complement fixing antibodies, particularly IgA[79]. We have shown that *H. pylori* will spontaneously activate the classical comple-ment pathway, suggesting that the organism can be opsonized for phago-cytosis or lysed by complement in the absence of antibody[76].

Parasites

1. Giardia

Giardiasis is common and some agammaglobulinaemic patients invariably become chronically infected after visiting endemic areas. There is a strong impression that IVIG protects against infection, suggesting that IgG by itself is effective and raising the possibilility of the presence of 'blocking' IgA antibodies in those immunocompetent individuals who develop chronic giardiasis. These clinical observations are in accord with recent experiments in mice showing that IgG antibodies will immobilize *Giardia* trophozoites and lyse them in the presence of complement[80]. It is suggested that patients who have an inherited tendency to produce an aggressive mucosal inflammatory response to infection are more likely to clear *Giardia* because of increased leakage of IgG into the microenvironment. There is evidence that many CVID patients are in this category, particularly since they are prone to a variety of inflammatory conditions such as chronic gastritis, gluten enteropathy, Crohn's disease and low-grade colitis[69]. Such a mechanism could explain why giardiasis is now uncommon in CVID patients receiving IVIG therapy.

2. Cryptosporidia

Intestinal infestation with this protozoan is a recognized complication in patients with AIDS and in infants with severe combined immunodeficiency, indicating that cellular immunity is important for defence. However, some of the first descriptions of chronic cryptosporidiosis were in hypogamma-globulinaemic children, suggesting that antibodies are also involved in protection[81]. Nevertheless, cryptosporidiosis is an extremely rare complication in both XLA and CVID patients, and may only occur when such patients are debilitated by other chronic infections. Furthermore, some of these early patients probably suffered from the X-linked hyper-IgM syndrome[82], a condition characterized by antibody deficiency, neutropenia and variable T cell defects. However, antibodies probably play some part in protection, since orally administered bovine colostrum apparently cured chronic *Cryptosporidium*-associated diarrhoea in a patient with AIDS[83].

3. Mycoplasmas

These eukaryotic organisms can survive and multiply in the extracellular environment using cellular products such as urea and arginine as nutrients[84]. Some strains, such as *M. salivarium* and *M. hominis* are ubiquitous and can be considered as commensals in the respiratory and urogenital tracts. Others are more pathogenic, such as *Ureaplasma urealyticum* which is associated with recurrent urethritis in men and recurrent abortions in women. *Mycoplasma pneumoniae* is a recognized pathogen in the respiratory tract and characteristically causes an insidious pneumonitis in normal people.

Antibody-deficient patients are prone to severe infection with these organisms, with systemic spread to the joints causing a chronic destructive septic arthritis[85] (Figure 5). Awareness of this complication and prompt treatment with tetracyclines can prevent considerable morbidity. A variety of *Mycoplasma* strains have been shown to bind and activate the first component of complement, thereby triggering the pathway to generate activated C3b, which binds to receptors on neutrophils[86] (Figure 6). However, this is likely to be a disadvantage to the host since organisms remain viable after phagocytosis and could theoretically be disseminated by neutrophils in the circulation. It is not clear why mycoplasmas have a predilection for large joints in humans, but there is some clinical evidence that minor damage to joints or tissues predisposes to mycoplasma infection, probably because 'infected' neutrophils are attracted to these areas. Specific antibody of the IgG class inhibits the growth of mycoplasmas *in vitro*, probably through aggregation of the organisms and interference with the supply of nutrients. The importance of antibody in eradicating *Mycoplasma* infections has been convincingly demonstrated in two of our XLA patients who recovered from chronic multiple joint infection following repeated intravenous infusions of hyperimmune goat antiserum.

Enteroviruses

1. Echoviruses

There are more than 30 different serotypes of this RNA virus, which usually causes a self-limiting enteritis or mild meningitis in immunocompetent people, particularly children. Mild epidemics caused by a particular serotype tend

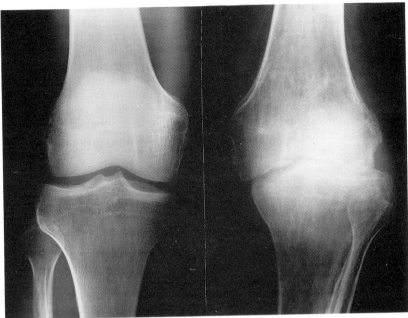

Figure 5 Radiograph showing destruction of left knee following a chronic *Ureaplasma urealyticum* arthritis of 2 years' duration in an adult with X-linked agammaglobulinaemia. The organism was unresponsive to all antibiotics tried, but was eliminated with hyperimmune goat serum

to spread through the community at intervals. Antibody-deficient patients, particularly those with XLA, are prone to a chronic echovirus infection of the central nervous system and muscles which is usually fatal, although patients have survived for up to 8 years[87]. Some patients develop a mild vasculitis affecting the muscles and subcutaneous tissues, with the gradual development of fibrosis between the muscle bundles, and eventual destruction of the muscle itself. This produces a characteristic 'wooden' sensation on palpation[88]. The central nervous system shows widespread chronic meningo-encephalitis, sometimes with massive thickening of the meninges due to chronic inflammation. This is associated with convulsions, headaches, eighth nerve deafness and, ultimately, failure of vital centres in the brain stem and death. Virus can be isolated from the muscle or cerebrospinal fluid, although in some cases the infection seems to be localized to the CNS. Different echovirus serotypes have been isolated from muscle and CNS in a few patients; it is not clear whether this is due to frequent spontaneous mutations in the envelope genes of these RNA viruses, or to primary infection with more than one strain.

Chronic echovirus meningo-encephalitis appears to be unique to patients with antibody deficiency. The critical role of antibody in controlling this virus can be demonstrated *in vivo* by improvement in the patient's condition after regular treatment with specific antibody given intravenously or intra-

Antibody

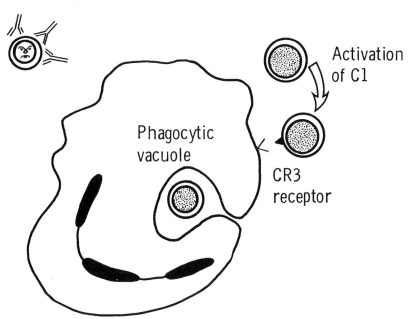

Figure 6 Phagocytosis of mycoplasmas in the absence of antibody. The organisms remain viable within the phagocytic vacuole. Antibodies inhibit the growth of these organisms

thecally, although most patients relapse if the treatment is discontinued[89]. This appears to be the only well documented viral infection which requires antibody for its resolution, although the mechanism has not been well studied. Spread of echoviruses from cell to cell may be particularly sensitive to inhibition by antibodies: in their absence, gradual dissemination of the infection occurs within the microenvironment of small blood vessels and capillaries, possibly in the endothelial cells. Antibodies may also be required to mediate antibody-dependent cytotoxicity against virus-infected cells. Recent work has demonstrated the importance of the traffic and interaction between lymphocytes in the CSF and locally draining lymph nodes[90]. Resident B lymphocytes are important for antibody production in the CNS, and the total lack of such cells in most XLA patients probably explains why they are particularly prone to echovirus disease.

These patients are probably also prone to chronic infections by other enteroviruses, particularly coxsackie viruses. Using the polymerase chain reaction with nucleotide primers from conserved regions of many different enteroviral genomes, we have demonstrated enteroviral RNA in the CSF from antibody-deficient patients presenting with a variety of CNS symptoms, particularly ataxia and dementia[91]. These CSFs were negative when cultured for viruses. Some of these patients were receiving regular IVIG therapy, and this may have partially neutralized echoviruses in the CNS; it is also possible that their disease was due to other enteroviruses which are difficult to culture. Poliovirus has caused paralytic disease in patients with severe combined immunodeficiency and occasionally following routine vaccination in XLA patients, who are known to have prolonged faecal excretion of vaccine strains following oral immunization[92]. It is interesting that there is no record of a parent or sibling with known primary immunodeficiency developing clinical poliomyelitis following routine immunization of an infant or child in the same family, despite the fact that potentially paralytic strains are known to be excreted following oral immunization. Since most patients with primary immunodeficiency are treated with IVIG, it is likely that enough specific IgG reaches the oropharynx via the crevicular fluid to neutralize such viruses following faecal–oral transmission.

2. Herpes and varicella viruses

In general, hypogammaglobulinaemic patients are not susceptible to infections with herpesviruses such as herpes simplex, cytomegalovirus and Epstein–Barr virus. However patients with common varied immunodeficiency (CVID) are prone to varicella zoster (shingles). The infection is usually not severe, is limited to a dermatome and resolves spontaneously[69]. Reactivation is very uncommon after starting replacement immunoglobulin therapy, although a few patients have severe recurring infection which requires long term treatment with acyclovir. These observations suggest that antibodies play a role in protection against reactivation of this virus, but against this is the rarity of cutaneous zoster in XLA patients. CVID patients commonly have low numbers of circulating CD4$^+$ T cells and poor T cell function, and this probably explains why varicella zoster reactivation is a common presenting feature.

Selective immunoglobulin class deficiencies

IgA deficiency occurs in about 1:700 of the UK population, and is clearly compatible with normal health in the Western World. Population surveys are needed in the Third World to show whether IgA is an important defence factor in less hygienic environments. There is a weak association with a predisposition to respiratory tract infections, which may be more marked in individuals with both IgA and IgG2 deficiency[93]. The clinical significance of selective IgG subclass deficiencies is becoming clearer, but redundancy in this system means that other IgG subclasses can compensate. IgG2 antibodies are mainly directed against bacterial polysaccharides, and a deficiency of this isotype is relatively common, possibly occurring in about 1:2000 of the UK population. Delayed IgG2 maturation may predispose young children to respiratory infections. IgG1 and IgG3 antibodies are primarily directed against protein antigens, IgG1 particularly against toxins such as tetanus toxin and IgG3 against viral proteins[93]. Partial IgG3 deficiency has recently been linked to chronic and recurring rhinosinusitis[94], although a better definition of these patients is awaited. Selective IgM deficiency is usually of no clinical significance: it is rarely inherited and usually occurs secondary to lymphoma. Studies on the effect of IgG replacement therapy in XLA have clearly demonstrated that IgG antibodies compensate for a lack of both IgM and IgA in serum and secretions.

References

1. Levinsky RJ, Tiedeman K. Successful bone marrow transplantation for reticular dysgenesis. Lancet. 1983; i: 671–673.
2. Perry VH, Gordon S. Macrophages and microglia in the nervous system. Trends Neurosci. 1988; 11: 273–277.
3. Dale DC, DuPont G, Wewerka JR, Bull JM, Chusid MJ. Chronic neutropenia. Medicine. 1979; 58: 128–144.
4. Medical Research Council Working Party on Leukaemia in Childhood. Analysis of treatment in childhood leukaemia. I. Prolonged predisposition to drug-induced neutropenia following craniospinal irradiation. Br Med J. 1975; 3: 563–566.
5. Hitzig WH. Familiare neutropenie mit dominanten erbgang und hypergammaglobulinamie. Helv Med Acta. 1959; 26: 779–784.
6. Asherson GL, Webster ADB. Diagnosis and treatment of immunodeficiency diseases. Oxford: Blackwell Scientific, 1980: 301–302.
7. Segal A, Walport M. Neutrophil and complement defects: recent advances. In Webster ADB, ed. Immunodeficiency and Disease. London: Kluwer Academic Publishers, 1988: 149–179.
8. Roos D. The molecular basis of chronic granulomatous disease. In: Gupta S, Griscelli C, eds. New Concepts of Immunodeficiency Diseases. Chichester: John Wiley, 1993: 311–352.
9. Nauseff WM, Root RK, Maleck HL. Biochemical and immunologic analysis of hereditary myeloperoxidase deficiency. J Clin Invest. 1983; 71: 1297–1307.
10. Parry MF, Root RK, Metcalf JA, Delaney KK, Kaplow LS, Richar WT. Myeloperoxidase deficiency. Prevalence and clinical significance. Ann Intern Med. 1981; 95: 293–301.
11. Root RK, Rosenthal AS, Balestra DJ. Abnormal bactericidal, metabolic and lysosomal functions of Chediak–Higashi syndrome. J Clin Invest. 1972; 51: 649–665.
12. Geha RS, Leung DYM. Hyper immunoglobulin E syndrome. In: Rosen FS, Seligmann M, eds. Immunodeficiencies. Philadelphia, PA: Harwood Academic, 1993: 571–583.
13. Gallin JI, Fischer A, Lisowska-Grospierre B, Anderson DC, Springer TA. Leukocyte adhesion deficiency: molecular basis and functional consequences. Immunodeficiency Rev. 1988; 1: 38–54.
14. Davies KA, Toothill VJ, Savill J, Hotchin N, Peters AM, Pearson JD, Haslett C, Burke M, Law SKA, Mercer NFG, Walport MJ, Webster ADB. A 19-year-old man with leucocyte adhesion deficiency. *In vitro* and *in vivo* studies of leucocyte function. Clin Exp Immunol. 1991; 84: 223–231.
15. Hosea SW, Brown EJ, Hamburger MI, Frank MM. Opsonic requirements for intravascular clearance after splenectomy. N Engl J Med. 1981; 304: 245–250.
16. Hosea SW, Burch CG, Brown EG, Berg RA, Frank MM. Impaired immune response in splenectomised patients to polyvalent pneumococcal vaccine. Lancet. 1981; i: 804–807.
17. Ceuppens JL, Baroja ML, van Vaek F, Anderson CL. Defect in the membrane expression of high affinity 72-kD Fcγ receptors on phagocytic cells in four healthy subjects. J Clin Invest. 1988; 82: 571–578.
18. Bernichou G, Kanellopoulos JM, Wallow C, Bove F, Defraissy JF. Interferon-γ restores T lymphocyte proliferation of non-responders to IgG₁ anti-CD3 via the induction of Fcγ₁ receptors on monocytes. Eur J Immunol. 1987; 17: 1175–1181.
19. Qualman SJ, Gupta PK, Mendelsohn G. Intracellular *Escherichia coli* in urinary malakoplakia. A reservoir of infection and its therapeutic implications. Am J Clin Pathol. 1984; 81: 35–42.
20. Abdou NI, Na Pombejara C, Sayawa A, Ragland C, Stechscwulte DJ, Nilsson U, Gourley W, Wattanabe I, Lindsey NJ, Allen MS. Malokoplakia: evidence for monocyte lysosomal abnormality correctable by cholinergic agonist *in vitro* and *in vivo*. New Engl J Med. 1977; 297: 1413–1419.

21. Komiyama A, Ichikawa M, Kanda H, Aoyama K, Yasui K, Yamazaki M, Kawai H, Miyagawa Y, Akabane T. Defective interleukin-1 production in a familial monocyte disorder with a combined abnormality of mobility and phagocytosis-killing. Clin Exp Immunol. 1988; 73: 500–504.
22. Dobbins WO. Whipple's disease: an historical perspective. Q J Med. 1985; 56: 523–531.
23. Dobbins WO. Is there an immune deficit in Whipple's disease? Dig Dis Sci. 1981; 26: 247–252.
24. Bjerknes R, Laerum OP, Oegaards S. Impaired bacterial degradation by monocytes and macrophages from a patient with treated Whipple's disease. Gastroenterology. 1985; 89: 1139–1151.
25. Feurle GH, Dörken B, Schöpf E, Lenhard V. HLA-B27 and defects in the T-cell system in Whipples disease. Eur J Clin Invest. 1979; 9: 385–389.
26. Nathan CF, Murray HW, Wiebe ME, Ruben BY. Identification of interferon-γ as the lymphokine that activates human macrophage oxidative metabolism and antimicrobial activity. J Exp Med. 1983; 158: 670–689.
27. Nathan CF, Kaplan G, Levis WR, Nusra A, Witmer MD, Sherwin SA, Job CK, Horowitz CR, Steinman RM, Cohn ZA. Local and systemic effects of intradermal recombinant interferon-γ in patients with lepromatous leprosy. N Engl J Med. 1986; 315: 6–15.
28. Denis M, Forget A, Pelletier M, Skamene E. Pleiotropic effects of the *Bcg* gene. III. Respiratory burst in Bcg-congenic macrophages. Clin Exp Immunol. 1988; 73: 370–375.
29. Winston DJ, Terito MC, Ho WG, Miller MJ. Gale RP, Golde DW. Alveolar macrophage dysfunction in human bone marrow transplant recipients. Am J Med. 1982; 73: 859–866.
30. Murray HW, Rubin BY. Masur H, Roberts RB. Impaired production of lymphokines and immune (gamma) interferon in the acquired immunodeficiency syndrome. N Engl J Med. 1984; 310: 883–887.
31. Murray HW, Gellene RA, Libby DM, Rothermel CD, Rubin BY. Activation of tissue macrophages from AIDS patients: *in vitro* response of AIDS alveolar macrophages to lymphokines and interferon-gamma. J Immunol. 1985; 135: 2374–2377.
32. Amman AJ. Immunological aberrations in purine nucleoside phosphorylase deficiencies. In: Enzyme Defects and Immune Dysfunction. Ciba Foundation Symposium Series, 68. Amsterdam: Elsevier, 1979: 55–69.
33. Zegers BJM, Stoop JW. Metabolic causes of immune deficiency: mechanisms and treatment. In: Webster ADB, ed. Immunodeficiency and Disease. London: Kluwer Academic, 1988: 113–131.
34. Hong R. The DiGeorge anomaly. In: Rosen FS, Seligmann M, eds. Immunodeficiencies. Philadelphia, PA: Harwood Academic, 1993: 167–176.
35. Barrett DJ, Amman AJ, Wara DW, Cowan MJ, Fisher TJ, Stiehm ER. The clinical and immunologic spectrum of the DiGeorge syndrome. J Clin Lab Immunol. 1981; 6: 1–6.
36. Webster ADB. Lymphocyte disorders in immunodeficiency. In: Peters TJ, ed. Subcellular Pathology of Systemic Disease. London: Chapman and Hall Medical, 1987: 304–320.
37. Fisher D, Martin B, van der Weyden R, Snyderman R, Kelley WN. A role for adenosine deaminase in human monocyte maturation. J Clin Invest. 1976; 58: 399–407.
38. Morgan G, Levinsky RJ, Hugh-Jones K, Fairbanks LD, Morris GS, Simmonds A. Heterogeneity in biochemical, clinical and immunological parameters in severe combined immunodeficiency due to adenosine deaminase deficiency. Clin Exp Immunol. 1987; 70: 491–499.
39. Griscelli C, Lisowska-Grospierre B. Combined immunodeficiency with defective expression in MHC class II genes. In: Gupta S, Griscelli C, eds. New Concepts of Immunodeficiency Diseases. Chichester: John Wiley, 1993: 177–190.
40. Noguchi M, Rosenblatt HM, Adelstein S, McBride OW, Leonard WJ. Interleukin-2 receptor γ chain mutation results in X-linked severe combined immunodeficiency in humans. Cell. 1993; 73: 147–157.
41. Fischer A, Griscelli C, Friedrich W, Kubanek B, Levinsky R, Morgan G, Vossen J, Wagemaker G, Landais P. Bone marrow transplantation for immunodeficiencies and osteopetrosis. European Survey 1968–1985. Lancet. 1986; ii: 1080–1083.
42. Waldmann TA. Ataxia telangiectasia. A multi-system hereditary disease with immunodeficiency, impaired organ maturation, X-ray hypersensitivity, and a high incidence of neoplasia. Ann Intern Med. 1983; 99: 367–379.

43. Gatti RA. Ataxia-telangiectasia: genetic studies. In: Gupta S, Griscelli C, eds. New Concepts of Immunodeficiency Diseases. Chichester: John Wiley, 1993: 203–229.

44. Blaese RM, Strober W, Waldmann TA. Immunodeficiency in the Wiskott Aldrich syndrome. In: Bergsma D, Good RA, Finstad J, Paul NW, eds. Immunodeficiency in Man and Animals. Sunderland, USA: Sinauer, 1975: 250–254.

45. Rosenstein Y, Park JK, Bierer BE, Burakoff SJ. The Wiskott-Aldrich syndrome: An immunodeficiency associated with defects of the CD43 molecule. In: Gupta S, Griscelli C, eds. New Concepts of Immunodeficiency Diseases. Chichester: John Wiley, 1993: 249–268.

46. Remold-O'Donnell E, Kenney DM, Parkman R, Cairns L, Savage B, Rosen FS. Characterization of a human lymphocyte surface sialoglycoprotein that is defective in Wiskott Aldrich syndrome. J Exp Med. 1984; 159: 1705–1723.

47. Purtilo DT, Cassel CK, Young JP, Harper R, Stephenson SR, Landing BH, Jawter GF. X-linked recessive progressive combined variable immunodeficiency (Duncan's disease). Lancet. 1975; i: 935–940.

48. Sakamoto K, Freed HJ, Purtilo DT. Antibody responses to Epstein-Barr virus in families with the X-linked lymphoproliferative syndrome. J Immunol. 1980; 125: 921–925.

49. Sullivan JL, Woda BA. X-linked lymphoproliferative syndrome. In: Rosen FS, Seligman M, eds. Immunodeficiencies. Harwood Academic, 1993: 585–600.

50. Grossi CE, Crist WM, Abo T, Velardi A, Cooper MD. Expression of the Chediak Higashi lysosomal abnormality in human peripheral blood lymphocyte populations. Blood. 1985; 65: 837–844.

51. Vilmer E, Lenoir GM, Virelizier JL, Griscelli C. Epstein-Barr serology in immunodeficiencies: an attempt to correlate immune abnormalities in Wiskott Aldrich and Chediak Higashi syndromes and ataxia telangiectasia. Clin Exp Immunol. 1984; 55: 249–256.

52. Pinching AJ, ed. AIDS and HIV infection. Clin Immunol Allergy. London: WB Saunders; 1986; 6: 467–558.

53. Clerici M, Shearer GM. A $T_H1 \to T_H2$ switch is a critical step in the etiology of HIV infection. Immunol Today. 1993; 14: 107–111.

54. Eales LJ, Moshteal O, Pinching AJ. Microbicidal activity of monocyte derived macrophages in AIDS and related disorders. Clin Exp Immunol. 1987; 67: 227–235.

55. Hawkins RE, Rickman LS, Vermund SH, Carl M. Association of mycoplasma and human immunodeficiency virus infection: detection of amplified Mycoplasma fermentans DNA in blood. J Infect Dis. 1992; 165: 581–585.

56. Lachmann PJ. Complement. In: McGee JO'D, Isaacson PG, Wright NA, eds. Oxford Textbook of Pathology. Vol. 1. Oxford: Oxford University Press, 1993: 259–266.

57. Rother K. Summary of reported deficiencies. In: Rother K, Rother U, eds. Hereditary and Acquired Complement Deficiencies in Animals and Man. Basel: Karger, 1986: 202–211.

58. Winkelstein JA, Shin HS, Wood WB Jr. Heat labile opsonins to pneumococcus. III. The participation of immunoglobulin and of the alternate pathway of C3 activation. J Immunol. 1972; 108: 1681–1689.

59. Lambris JD. The multi-functional role of C3, the third component of complement. Immunol Today. 1988; 9: 387–393.

60. Cooper NR. Immune adherence by the fourth component of complement. Science. 1969; 165: 396–398.

61. Ward PA, Cochrane CG, Müller-Eberhard NJ. The role of serum complement in chemotaxis of leukocytes in vitro. J Exp Med. 1965; 122: 327–346.

62. Würzner R, Orren A, Lachmann PJ. Inherited deficiencies of the terminal components of human complement. In: Rosen FS, Seligmann M, eds. Immunodeficiencies. Harwood Academic, 1993: 295–312.

63. Haeney MR, Thompson RA, Faulkner J, Mackintosh P, Ball AP. Recurrent bacterial meningitis in patients with genetic defects of terminal complement components. Clin Exp Immunol. 1980; 40: 16–24.

64. Levy J, Schlesinger M. Complement deficiency: C7, C8 and properdin. In: Gupta S, Griscelli C, eds. New Concepts in Immunodeficiency Diseases. Chichester: John Wiley, 1993: 269–292.

65. Lint TF, Gewurz H. Component deficiencies – the ninth component. In Rother K, Rother U, eds. Hereditary and Acquired Complement Deficiencies in Animals and Man. Basel: Karger, 1986: 307–310.

66. Griffiss JM, Bertram MA. Immunoepidemiology of meningococcal disease in military recruits. II. Blocking of serum bactericidal activity by circulating IgA early in the course of invasive disease. J Infect Dis. 1977; 136: 733–739.
67. Thompson RA, Lachmann PJ. A second case of human C3b inhibitor (KAF) deficiency. Clin Exp Immunol. 1977; 27: 23–39.
68. Vetrie DF, Vorechovsky I, Sideras P, Holland J, Davies A, Flinter F, Hammarström, Kinnon C, Levinsky R, Bobrow M, Smith CIE, Bentley DR. The gene involved in X-linked agammaglobulinaemia is a member of the src family of protein-tyrosine kinases. Nature. 1993; 361: 226–233.
69. Hermaszewski RA, Webster ADB. Primary hypogammaglobulinaemia: a survey of clinical manifestations and complications. Q J Med. 1993; 86: 31–42.
70. Spickett GP, Webster ADB, Farrant J. Cellular abnormalities in common variable immunodeficiency. In: Rosen FS, Seligmann M, eds. Immunodeficiencies. Philadelphia, PA: Harwood Academic, 1993: 111–126.
71. Murphy TF, Apicella MA. Nontypable Haemophilus influenzae: a review of clinical aspects, surface antigens and the human immune response to infection. Rev Infect Dis. 1987; 9: 1–15.
72. Lever AML, Gross J, Webster ADB. Serum factors for opsoniozation of non-typable H. influenzae. J Clin Microbiol. 1985; 20: 33–38.
73. Stroud RM, Nagaki K, Pickering RJ, Gewurz H, Good RA, Cooper MD. Sub-units of the first complement component in immunologic deficiency syndromes. Independence of C1s and C1q. Clin Exp Immunol. 1970; 7: 133–137.
74. Ahnen DJ, Brown WR. Campylobacter enteritis in immune-deficient patients. Ann Intern Med. 1982; 96: 187–188.
75. Klipstein FA, Engert RF, Short H, Schenk EA. Pathogenic properties of Campylobacter jejuni: assay and correlation with clinical manifestations. Infect Immunity. 1985; 50: 43–49.
76. Bernatowska E, Jose P, Davies H, Stephenson M, Webster D. Interaction of campylobacter species with antibody, complement and phagocytes. Gut. 1989; 30: 906–911.
77. Goodwin CS, Worsley B. Peptic ulcer disease and Helicobacter pylori infection. Curr Opin Gastroenterol. 1992; 8: 122–127.
78. Forsythe SJ, Dolby JM, Webster ADB, Cole JA. Nitrate- and nitrite-reducing bacteria in the achlorhydric stomach. J Med Microbiol. 1988; 25: 253–259.
79. Griffiss JM. Biologic function of the serum IgA system: modulation of complement mediated affector mechanisms and conservation of antigenic mass. Ann NY Acad Sci. 1983; 409: 697–707.
80. Belosevic M, Faubert GM, Dharampaul S. Antimicrobial action of antibodies against Giardia muris trophozoites. Clin Exp Immunol. 1994; 95: 485–489.
81. Sloper KS, Dourmashkin PR, Bird RB, Slavin G, Webster ADB. Chronic malabsorption due to cryptosporidiosis in a child with immunoglobulin deficiency. Gut. 1982; 23: 80–82.
82. Korthäuer U, Graf D, Mages HW, Brière F, Munoreedevi P, Malcolm S, Ugazio AG, Notarangelo LD, Levinsky RJ, Kroczek RA. Defective expression of T-cell CD40 ligand causes X-linked immunodeficiency with hyper-IgM. Nature. 1993; 361: 539–543.
83. Unger BLP, Ward DJ, Fayer R, Quinn CA. Cessation of cryptosporidium associated diarrhoea in an acquired immunodeficiency syndrome patient after treatment with hyperimmune colostrum. Gastroenterology. 1990; 58: 2962–2965.
84. Taylor-Robinson D, McCormack WM. The genital mycoplasmas. N Engl J Med. 1980; 302: 1003–10, 1063–1067.
85. Roifman CM, Rao CP, Lederman HM, Lavi S, Quinn P, Gelfand EW. Increased susceptibility to mycoplasma infection in patients with hypogammaglobulinaemia. Am J Med. 1986; 80: 590–594.
86. Webster ADB, Furr PM, Hughes-Jones NC, Gorick BD, Taylor-Robinson D. Critical dependence on antibody for defence against mycoplasmas. Clin Exp Immunol. 1988; 71: 383–387.
87. McKinney RE Jr, Katz SL, Wilfert CM. Chronic enteroviral meningoencephalitis in agammaglobulinemic patients. Rev Infect Dis. 1987; 9: 334–356.
88. Webster ADB. Echovirus disease in hypogammaglobulinaemia patients. Clin Rheum Dis. 1984; 10: 189–203.
89. Erlendsson K, Swartz T, Dwyer JM. Successful reversal of echovirus encephalitis in X-

linked hypogammaglobulinaemia by intraventricular administration of immunoglobulin. N Engl J Med. 1985; 312: 351–353.
90. Cserr HF, Knopf PM. Cervical lymphatics, the blood–brain barrier and the immunoreactivity of the brain; a new view. Immunol Today. 1992; 13: 507–512.
91. Webster ADB, Rotbart HA, Warner T, Rudge P, Hyman N. Diagnosis of enterovirus brain disease in hypogammaglobulinemic patients by polymerase chain reaction. Clin Infect Dis. 1993; 17: 657–661.
92. Wyatt HV. Poliomyelitis in hypogammaglobulinaemia. J Infect Dis. 1973; 128: 802–806.
93. Hanson LA, Björkander J, Söderström R, Söderström T. Clinical significance of IgG subclass and IgA deficiency. In: Webster ADB, ed. Immunodeficiency and Disease. London: Kluwer Academic, 1988: 99–111.
94. Scadding GK, Lund VJ, Darby YC, Navas-Romero J, Seymour N, Turner MW. IgG subclass levels in chronic rhinosinusitis. Rhinology. 1994; 32: 15–19.

9
Immunoprophylaxis and Immunotherapy of Gram-negative Bacterial Infections

J. D. BAUMGARTNER and M. P. GLAUSER

INTRODUCTION

Over the last decades the incidence of gram-negative bacterial infections has risen markedly in most medical centres[1,2]. At the Boston City Hospital, the incidence of gram-negative bacteraemia increased from 0.9/1000 admissions in 1935 to 11.2/1000 admissions in 1972[3]. In the USA it was estimated that approximately 71 000 episodes of documented gram-negative septicaemia occurred annually, and an unknown, perhaps even higher, number of potentially lethal gram-negative infections occurred in the presence of sterile blood cultures[4]. During the last decade, the rise seems to have plateaued. At the present time, half of all cases of sepsis and septic shock are due to endotoxin-containing micro-organisms, the rest occur during gram-positive bacterial infections, and infrequently during fungal and even viral infections. Overall, despite adequate treatment of infection and supportive care in intensive care unit, sepsis kills an estimated 100 000 people a year in the United States[5]. The mortality associated with gram-negative bacteraemias is still in the range 20–35%[3,4,6–9], and 50% or more of those developing gram-negative septic shock (20–30% of patients with gram-negative bacteremia) die[10–13]. The development of a new effective treatment is thus a major challenge of modern medicine.

The current understanding of the pathogenesis of sepsis and septic shock is that bacteria release substances which overstimulate systemic inflammatory mediators and cells, leading to hypotension and progressive multiple organ failure[14]. The major toxic mediator of gram-negative sepsis is the lipopolysaccharide (LPS, also called endotoxin), a component of the outer bacterial membrane. Antibiotics are unable to prevent the effects of LPS, and may even promote the release of LPS from bacteria[15]. Various therapeutic approaches have been investigated. Despite successes in experimental animal models, well designed clinical trials have failed to demonstrate the utility high doses of corticosteroids or opiate antagonists in patients with septic shock[10-12,16]. Other approaches being studied at the present time include administrations of detoxified analogues of lipid A (the toxic part of LPS), inhibitors of cytokines (antibodies against tumour necrosis factor or interleukin-1 receptor antagonist), inhibitors of coagulation disorders (such as protein C) and inhibitors of some prostaglandin derivatives.

Administration of anti-endotoxin antibodies has also been used in an attempt to improve the outcome of gram-negative infections. A review of the present knowledge of the biological activity of LPS is beyond the scope of this chapter. However, LPS can induce the full picture of septic shock when injected in adequate amounts to animals. The activity of LPS depends on the dose administered and on the animal species. In rabbits, $0.1\,\mu g$ of native, purified LPS causes fever and $100\,\mu g$ induces severe haemodynamic disturbances. Man appears to be even more sensitive to the pyrogenic action of LPS: 10 times less LPS is required to produce the same febrile response in man than is required in rabbits[17]. LPS is extremely immunogenic, and antibodies to LPS demonstrate a better protective potency *in vivo* than antibodies directed at other antigenic determinants of gram-negative bacteria.

The conditions associated with a high risk of severe gram-negative infection, such as admission to intensive care units or immunosuppression, are often acute or unexpected. Therefore, active immunization may be too slow or may not promote an adequate humoral immune response, and research has focused mainly on passive immunotherapy.

STRUCTURE OF ENDOTOXIN

LPS is composed of three major parts. The innermost part, lipid A, comprises fatty acids linked to a diglucosamine and is the structure responsible for the toxic effects of LPS. Attached to the lipid A by a saccharide molecule called 3-deoxy-D-manno-2-octulo-sonate (KDO) is the core region, which is composed of a few sugars, phosphate and ethanolamine. The outer part of LPS, the side-chain (O polysaccharide or O antigens) consists of repeating units of oligosaccharides, which vary between different gram-negative strains and are responsible for antigenic specificity (serotypes). Several hundreds of serotypes of gram-negative bacteria may be responsible for infections in humans. The structure of lipid A and the core region is more conserved between strains than are the side-chains, although the core structure is also subject to significant inter- and intraspecies variability[18-21]. Antibodies can be elicited against any of these three endotoxin parts.

O SEROTYPE-SPECIFIC ANTIBODIES

Immunization with gram-negative bacilli that possess a complete LPS molecule on their surface induces anti-LPS antibodies directed against the immunodominant, species-specific O antigens. Studies in animals have shown that these specific antibodies are highly protective against infections caused by the immunizing bacterial strain[22,23], but do not afford protection against challenges with antigenically different strains. This specificity of protection precludes the broad use of antibodies to O antigens for passive immunotherapy in patients with gram-negative infections, since hundreds of serotypes exist. Two approaches have been attempted however to circumvent the problem of the high diversity of serotypes.

The first approach is to administer polyvalent purified immunoglobulins. The purified immunoglobulin fraction contains the antibodies present in the pool of plasma from which it is extracted. Since plasma from thousands of donors is pooled for preparing purified immunoglobulins, these may contain antibodies against a large number of bacteria. Since the 1940s, cold ethanol precipitation has been used for separating the immunoglobulin fraction of plasma. The original preparations had to be injected by the intramuscular route and did not prove useful in the management of bacterial infections in patients with normal immunoglobulin levels, perhaps because the maximum dose that could be administered by this route was small. New techniques now allow intravenous administration of immunoglobulin so that high doses may be administered with immediate bioavailability. Intravenous immunoglobulins (IVIG) have a good opsonic activity against various bacteria and have been shown to protect against various infections in animals. These data have produced renewed interest in the use of immunoglobulins for the prophylaxis and treatment of bacterial infections.

The great diversity of bacterial serotypes remains a major problem, however. If a given antibody is present only in a fraction of the donors, it will be diluted in the pool and its relative concentration will be low. The maximum volume of IVIG that can be administered during one infusion contains 15–25 g of IgG, which represents only 15–25% of the total body IgG levels. The amount of a specific antibody may therefore remain insufficient to confer protection. It is possible to administer very high doses of IVIG over several days, but, in addition to the expense, such doses of IVIG may block the reticuloendothelial system, a property that has been used to reduce the clearance of circulating platelets in idiopathic thrombocytopenia. In patients with infections, such a blockade could be detrimental.

For these reasons, carefully planned clinical trials appear mandatory for exploring the efficacy and the cost-effectiveness of IVIG in bacterial infections. Studies of the prophylaxis of infections in intensive care unit patients and in neonates have suggested some efficacy of IVIG[24–28]. However, none of these studies has demonstrated an impact on mortality, and cost-effectiveness analysis is lacking. Precise recommendations for the prophylactic use of IVIG in this setting cannot therefore be made. Some studies have reported some benefit from the use of IVIG in patients with established infections[29–33]. Unfortunately, the results of some of these trials are subject to criticism because of problems in study design, such as non-blinded evaluations, small numbers of cases or insufficient documentation of infections. In addition, the protection was apparent only in some subgroups of patients or in some special types of infections that might have been analysed separately a posteriori. Currently, the role of IVIG in the management of bacterial infections is still largely controversial[34].

The second approach is to focus on bacteria with only a few different LPS serotypes, such as *Pseudomonas aeruginosa*. While active immunization with *P. aeruginosa* has been studied for almost 20 years with some success[35], passive transfer of *P. aeruginosa* LPS-specific antibodies by the intramuscular administration of hyperimmune immunoglobulins has given conflicting results in burn patients[35,36]. Although in the early studies the amount of antibodies administered was limited by the intramuscular route of administration, *P. aeruginosa* hyperimmune IVIG preparations have shown good immunological and opsonic activity *in vitro* and were protective in animal experiments[37-41]. However, there have been no reports of clinical trials with such preparations. Recently, murine or human type-specific anti-*P. aeruginosa* monoclonal antibodies of various subclasses have also been shown to be protective in animal models[42]. The administration of a mixture of type-specific monoclonal antibodies is a feasible and interesting alternative, but even if this approach is effective, this expensive serotype-specific passive immunotherapy will apply only to a minority of patients with microbiologically documented *P. aeruginosa* infections. Since a delay of 24–48 h is often necessary before the cause of a bacterial infection can be diagnosed, a major problem in this type of approach is the need for rapid identification of the infecting pathogen.

ANTIBODIES TO THE LPS CORE

Rough mutants of gram-negative bacilli are characterized by enzymatic deficiencies that prevent the attachment of the O polysaccharide side-chains to the central LPS core. The term 'rough' applies to the macroscopic appearance of colonies of these organisms on agar plate, the roughness being due to the hydrophobicity of the lipid part of the LPS that is exposed at the surface of the mutant bacteria, while the smoothness is related to the hydrophilicity of the O side chains on the surface of normal strains. These mutants expose on their surface various parts of the core region which are normally hidden by the O side chains and are therefore poorly accessible to immunological reactions. Since the core LPS might share structures which are common to all gram-negative bacilli, a working hypothesis formulated during the 1960s was that core LPS antibodies might cross-react between various gram-negative bacteria, and might possibly be protective against a wide range of gram-negative bacteria. The administration of anti-core LPS antibodies was therefore considered an attractive alternative to the administration of specific antibodies in the management of patients with gram-negative infections. However, the precise epitope specificity of the postulated cross-reactive antibodies remains unclear at the present time. Indeed, several core types have been described[19,43]. In addition, the mutations leading to rough forms may involve different steps in core synthesis, so that complete or incomplete core structures are produced[19,43] (Figure 1). Each rough mutant induces predominantly a strain-specific antibody response[44]

R mutants of *S.minnesota*

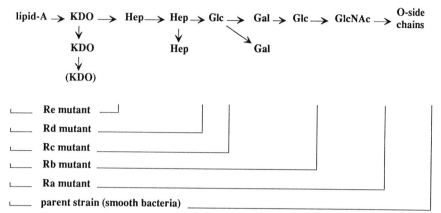

Figure 1 Schematic representation of the sugar composition of the LPS of *Salmonella minnesota* S128 and its main rough mutants (adapted from refs 19, 43). LPS is a major cell wall antigen of gram-negative bacteria, anchored to the outer cell membrane by the lipid A, which is composed of fatty acids linked to a diglucosamine. The core region, attached to the lipid A by a saccharide molecule, 3-deoxy-D-manno-2-octulo-sonate (KDO), is composed of a few sugars (heptose, glucose, galactose, N-acetyl-glucosamine), phosphate and ethanolamine. Lipid A and the core region are relatively conserved among gram-negative bacteria. In contrast, there are several hundreds of serotypes of O antigens (side-chains), which are hydrophilic polymers composed of a variable number of repeating units of oligosaccharides. The degree of polymerization of O antigens is variable (the number of oligosaccharide units varies from 1 to >40). In enzyme-deficient rough mutants, O antigens are lacking and the core region is exposed at the surface. The hydrophobicity of lipid A is responsible for the rough appearance of these mutants on agar plates. Core LPS antibodies are produced after immunization with rough mutants. In *Salmonella minnesota*, the roughest form is called Re mutant (its LPS is composed only of lipid A, KDO, phosphate and ethanolamine) and the smoothest is called Ra mutant. The Rc mutant is deficient in the enzyme UDP-galactose-epimerase, and cannot incorporate galactose in the core. The J5 mutant of *E. coli* 0111:B4 has an incomplete R3 core, which is one of several core types found in the species *E. coli*. Like the Rc mutant, it is deficient in UDP-galactose-epimerase, but the precise chemical composition of its endotoxin is only partially known

and the characterization of cross-reactive antibodies has been exceedingly difficult. A major problem has been the lack of reproducibility of many published experiments. LPS and lipid A are difficult to use as antigens in serological tests due to their lipidic and hydrophobic nature. Some immunoglobulins, especially of the IgM type, might bind non-specifically to hydrophobic substances and might therefore be misinterpreted as cross-reactive antibodies to lipid A or to rough LPS forms[45]. While some groups have reported observations suggesting that various polyclonal or monoclonal core LPS antibodies might be cross-reactive, other attempts have revealed little or no cross-reactivity.

The concept of cross-protection afforded by core LPS antibodies was supported mainly by three lines of arguments. First, by results of experimental studies of passive immunotherapy with antisera from rabbits immunized with rough mutants[46–48]. The first successful animal studies were published 20 years ago and although some subsequent experiments gave similar results several investigators were not able to reproduce these results. Second, by retrospective studies in humans which have suggested that high titres of antibodies to core LPS correlate with improved survival of patients with gram-negative bacteraemia[19,49–51]. Third, by prospective clinical trials which have shown that the survival of patients with gram-negative bacteraemia who received serum of humans immunized with rough mutant of gram-negative bacteria was improved, and that similar serum might prevent gram-negative shock in high-risk surgical patients[13,52].

In vitro studies of anti-core LPS antibodies

The concept of cross-protection afforded by antisera to rough mutants or by monoclonal antibodies to the core LPS implies the existence of antibodies which recognize the core LPS of smooth gram-negative bacteria. However, two difficulties arise with this concept of cross-reaction. First, in smooth strains, O side-chains are linked covalently to the core region. Such linkage induces conformational changes which might lead to differences in antigenic specificities or might prevent access of antibodies to the core region. In other words, even if chemical analogies can be demonstrated among core LPS from different gram-negative bacteria, it remains to be established whether these chemical analogies correspond to common antigenic structures. Of note is the observation that immunization with smooth bacteria does not elicit detectable antibodies against core LPS determinants, suggesting that core LPS determinants might not be available on the LPS of smooth strains. Second, it must be emphasized that significant inter- and intraspecies variability of the core region has been shown among smooth gram-negative bacteria. Both of these observations might explain the fact that broad cross-reactions between anti-core LPS antibodies and LPS from smooth strains have not been unequivocally and directly demonstrated so far.

Immunofluorescent tests using whole smooth bacteria as antigens have indirectly suggested the existence of cross-reactive antibodies, because absorption of antiserum to the rough Re mutant of *Salmonella minnesota* with the Re LPS eliminated fluorescence[53,59]. Indirect evidence came from the observation that extensive absorption of antiserum to the rough J5 mutant of *Escherichia coli* 0111 with various smooth bacteria decreased the levels of core LPS antibodies[55]. Antibodies to J5 LPS have also been reported to cross-react to a greater extent with smooth *E. coli* strains grown in the presence of sub-inhibitory concentrations of a β-lactam antibiotic[56], or with smooth LPS when it had been extracted from exponentially growing bacteria[52]. These findings might explain some discrepancies between the apparent cross-protection afforded *in vivo* and the lack of *in vitro* cross-reactivity with LPS extracted from stationary phase bacteria. The use of purified LPS as an antigen in direct or indirect haemagglutination tests, complement-dependent haemolysis assays, precipitin tests in agar gel, radioimmunoassays, enzyme-linked immunosorbent assays (ELISA) and immunoblot assays have revealed little cross-reative antibody in antisera to rough mutants[45,47,58-62].

Several groups have studied the *in vitro* cross-reactivity of anti-core LPS monoclonal antibodies. In common with the polyclonal antibodies, the results obtained have been controversial. Some authors have found monoclonal antibodies, usually with specificity for lipid A, to cross-react with smooth gram-negative bacteria and, to a lesser extent, with LPS extracted from these bacteria[63-68]. However, others have been unable to demonstrate cross-reactivity with intact smooth bacteria or LPS. Cross-reactivity appeared only after acid hydrolysis of the smooth LPS, suggesting that the side-chains might restrict the access of antibodies to antigenic sites on the inner core[20,69-71].

These discrepancies might be explained by the fact that LPS structures, particularly the core and lipid A, are hydrophobic. This hydrophobic nature is responsible for non-specific sticking of immunoglobulins, especially IgM, which may lead to artefactual apparent cross-reactivity[45]. Thus, depending on the serologic methods used, non-specific binding may or may not be observed.

Experimental models of protection with anti-core LPS antibodies

In addition to the difficulties encountered in demonstrating *in vitro* cross-reactivity, the mechanisms by which antibodies to core LPS protect against infection have not been established. Rabbit anti-core LPS antiserum is apparently not bacteriolytic in the presence of complement, and it increases only weakly the opsonization and phagocytosis of gram-negative bacteria and the intravascular clearance of LPS[72-74]. Moreover, immunization of mice with Rd and Re mutants results in the formation of bactericidal plaque-forming cells directed against both mutants and their parental strains, but not against other gram-negative strains[75]. The protection found experimentally by some authors therefore has to be explained by other mechanisms, possibly by neutralization of LPS. However, a direct neutralization of LPS by anti-core LPS antibodies *in vitro* has not yet been demonstrated.

The first studies suggesting that antisera directed against rough mutants of gram-negative bacteria might protect against unrelated smooth strains or endotoxins were published 20 years ago[46,48] and subsequent experiments from the same researchers gave similar results. However, none of these experiments clearly demonstrated that the protection observed with antisera to rough mutants was mediated by antibodies directed against the core LPS. The precise epitope(s) of the core LPS and the type of immunoglobulin (IgG, IgM or both) hypothetically involved in cross-protection remained controversial[76-79]. Controversies have also emerged as to the very existence of the cross-protection afforded by antisera to rough mutants. Several investigators have been unable to demonstrate that core LPS antisera were protective in animal models of gram-negative sepsis[40,80-95,134,135]. Similar contradictory results were also found with monoclonal antibodies against core LPS.

Table 1 Ineffectiveness of rabbit J5 antiserum in models of peritonitis or endotoxaemia in mice

Model	LPS or bacterial challenge	Rabbit serum*		
		Homologous	Anti-J5	Non-immune
Endotoxaemia	J5 LPS	–	214	1.6
	0111 LPS	500	20	20
Peritonitis	E. coli 0111	3.0×10^5	1.3×10^5	1.7×10^5
	P. aeruginosa #3	>1200	<12	<12

Adapted from ref. 95.
*0.5 ml iv/mouse injected 1 h before i.p. challenge with a mixture of LPS + galactosamine (endotoxaemic lethality model) or with a mixture of bacteria + mucin + haemoglobin (peritonitis model). The results are expressed as LD_{50} (ng LPS/mouse or CFU/mouse, respectively).

One explanation for the discrepant observations regarding protection afforded by anti-core LPS antibodies might reside in the type of animal models and in the bacterial strains that have been chosen for testing. A criticism often raised against the negative studies was that they used animal models given high inocula of bacteria or high levels of endotoxin, which might have prevented the demonstration of an effect by anti-core LPS antibodies, which are believed to possess a weaker, although much broader, protective power, than homologous antibodies[96]. Using very small inocula to induce endotoxaemia or bacteraemia in compromised mice, we nevertheless failed to demonstrate a protective effect of rabbit anti-core LPS antiserum, whereas homologous antisera were protective (Table 1)[95].

Another explanation for contradictory observations resides in the fact that endotoxin contamination of antibody preparations or of antisera to be tested might give false apparent protection. As little as 4 ng of LPS/kg of body weight given prophylactically may induce a state of tolerance in mice, and is protective against lethal challenge with gram-negative bacteria[97–99]. Since in most of the studies of antibodies the test preparation is administered before LPS or bacterial challenge, and since antibody preparations are easily contaminated with small amounts of LPS, apparent protection in animal models might have been due to tolerance induced by minute amounts of LPS contained in the preparations tested. Another difficulty in evaluating the data observed with monoclonal antibodies has been that they were often used either as ascitic fluid or as tissue culture supernatant, raising the possibility that factors other than the specific antibody might be responsible for the protection. Such an example was recently reported. A monoclonal antibody against core LPS was previously found to be highly protective in a murine model of E. coli sepsis when tested in culture supernatant. After the antibody was fully purified, the protection could no longer be shown[100]. Experimental data obtained with incompletely purified antibodies are therefore difficult to interpret.

Retrospective studies in humans relating outcome of gram-negative bacteraemias to anti-core LPS antibody levels

In humans, the importance of anti-endotoxin antibodies in the defence against gram-negative infections has been suggested clinically by retrospective

Table 2 Relationship between survival and titres of antibody to core LPS in patients with gram-negative bacteraemia

Reference	Antibody measured (method of detection)	Antibody levels	Percent survival	p
51, 101[a]	Anti-Re LPS (indirect haemagglutination)	<1:80	40	<0.01
		>1:80	85	
49[b]	Anti-J5 LPS (ELISA)			
	IgG antibody	<10	14	<0.001
		>10	79	
	IgM antibody	<30	44	0.01
		>30	81	

[a]Antibody levels (titres), were measured in 175 patients with gram-negative bacteraemia.
[b]Antibody levels (μg/ml) were determined in 43 patients with *P. aeruginosa* bacteraemia.

studies relating the outcome of patients to levels of antibodies against core LPS at the onset of bacteraemia due to various gram-negative bacilli[51,101] or due to *P. aeruginosa*[49]. Two rough strains were used as antigens to detect core LPS antibodies in patients: the Re mutant of *S. minnesota*[51,101] and the J5 mutant of *E. coli* 0111[49]. Both studies (Table 2) showed that the survival of patients with gram-negative bacteraemia was related to levels of anti-core LPS antibodies measured by indirect haemagglutination or ELISA, and this correlation appeared to be independent of the levels of O side-chain-specific antibodies. Both IgG and IgM core glycolipid antibodies were associated with a lower mortality. Although these studies did not demonstrate a causal relationship between high levels of anti-core LPS antibodies and survival, they suggested that these antibodies, as well as those directed against O side-chains, might play a role in the defence of patients against gram-negative bacteraemias.

However, the role of antibodies to core LPS was challenged in a study in which intravenous immunoglobulins were administered to septic shock patients[78]. During this trial, serum samples were collected from patients at entry to the study and antibodies to J5 LPS, to Re LPS, to lipid A and to a mixture of seven smooth LPS were measured. There was no correlation between high levels of any of these antibodies and an improved outcome of the patients (Table 3)[102]. The only significant correlation was that non-survivors had a median level of anti-lipid A IgM higher than survivors, a finding which is not supportive for a protective role for anti-lipid A IgM. Therefore, the findings of this prospective study did not confirm the findings of the retrospective studies of McCabe *et al.*[51,101] and Pollack *et al.*[49].

Clinical studies with antiserum or hyperimmune purified intravenous immunoglobulins directed against rough mutants

The urgent need for a new treatment of sepsis prompted investigators to perform clinical studies with polyclonal anti-core LPS antibodies without knowledge of the epitope responsible for cross-protection and despite the

Table 3 Relationship between survival and levels of antibody to core LPS in patients with gram-negative septic shock[102]

Antigens[a]	Immunoglobulin class	Median antibody levels (μg/ml)		p
		Survivors (n = 30)	Non-survivors (n = 28)	
J5 LPS	IgG	1.8	2.3	NS
	IgM	2.0	1.9	NS
Re LPS	IgG	4.8	6.0	NS
	IgM	0.6	0.5	NS
Lipid A	IgG	<0.5	0.5	NS
	IgM	<0.5	1.0	<0.01
Smooth LPS	IgG	10.7	8.7	NS
	IgM	3.6	4.1	NS

NS = not significant
[a]Coated on ELISA plates as complexes with high density lipoproteins.

many controversies remaining in the field. Four studies have used human serum or plasma collected from volunteers after immunization with the J5 mutant of *E. coli* 0111 (J5 antiserum), one study used anti-J5 immune globuline and one study used globulin enriched in antibodies against the Re mutant of *S. minnesota* S128.

Clinical studies with J5 antiserum

Only two of the four clinical studies of J5 antiserum (Table 4) were successful. In two studies, the antiserum was administered for the treatment of gram-negative bacteraemias or septic shock. In the first and well-known therapeutic study, 304 patients with a septic syndrome received a single intravenous infusion of either *E. coli* J5 antiserum or pre-immune (control) serum, near the onset of illness[13]. Among the 212 patients with gram-negative bacteraemia, the mortality rate was significantly reduced in J5 antiserum recipients, especially in those with shock at entry (from 77% to 44%, respectively). However, this study suffered from the absence of evaluation of the severity of illnesses among the patients at entry other than by listing underlying diseases. Moreover, there was an unusually high mortality in the control group of patients with septic shock (77%). In a second therapeutic study, *E. coli* J5 immune plasma was compared to pre-immune plasma for the treatment of fulminant meningococcaemia in children. J5 immune plasma was prepared from volunteers immunized with a vaccine provided by E.J. Ziegler, with a schedule similar to that in the previous study[13]. The trial was prematurely discontinued after 73 children had been enrolled, because the intermediate analysis revealed no survival improvement in the J5 plasma recipients. Although the objective of randomizing 100 patients was not obtained, this study suggested nevertheless that a major impact of J5 immune plasma on the mortality of meningococcaemia was unlikely[103].

In two other studies, J5 antiserum was administered for the prophylaxis of systemic gram-negative infections in high-risk patients (Table 4). In surgical

Table 4 Clinical studies with human J5 antiserum in the treatment or prevention of gram-negative infections

Study (reference)	Control group	J5 group	p
Therapeutic studies			
Patients with gram-negative bacteraemia (131)			
Mortality			
All patients	42/109 (39%)	23/103 (22%)	0.011
Patients in shock	30/33 (77%)	18/41 (44%)	0.003
Children with purpura fulminans (50)			
Mortality (all patients)	12/33 (36%)	10/40 (25%)[a]	N.S.
Prophylactic studies			
Neutropenic patients (67)			
Febrile days/days of observation	517/964 (54%)	516/917 (56%)	N.S.
Gram-negative sepsis	7/57 (12%)	8/52 (15%)	N.S.
Mortality	1/57 (2%)	4/52 (8%)	N.S.
High risk surgical patients (6)			
Septic shocks	15/136 (11%)	6/126 (5%)	0.049[b]
Subsequent deaths	9/136 (7%)	2/126 (2%)	0.033[b]

[a]This trend disappeared after correction for unbalances in risk factors at randomization using a logistic regression model.
[b]These p values were obtained with one-tailed Fisher's tests. The p values obtained with the χ^2 test are 0.10 for the difference in the incidence of gram-negative shock and 0.08 for the associated mortality.

patients at high risk of developing gram-negative infections[52], repeated doses of J5 immune plasma did not prevent the acquisition of new focal gram-negative infections, but seemed to prevent the development of gram-negative septic shock and its fatal outcome. However, the study should be analysed with caution because the number of patients developing septic shock was small and because statistical evaluation was performed with one-tailed tests, and the results are not significant with two-tailed tests. In another prophylactic study, 150–200 ml of J5 antiserum was administered at the onset of neutropenia in 100 patients with 109 episodes of prolonged neutropenia (mean 17 days)[104]. When compared to control serum, J5 antiserum did not reduce the number of febrile days, the number of gram-negative bacteraemic episodes, or deaths from these infections. This inability to demonstrate a beneficial effect was attributed to the insufficient amount of antibody administered, because most febrile episodes occurred 1 week or more after the administration of one single plasma unit.

Clinical studies with hyperimmune purified intravenous globulins

Two studies with hyperimmune intravenous IgG (IVIG) have been performed (Table 5). The first study investigated the protective efficacy of a purified anti-*E. coli* J5 IgG preparation (J5-IVIG) obtained from volunteers immunized with J5 vaccine. In this multicentre study[78], 70 patients with established gram-negative septic shock were blindly allocated to receive either a single dose of 200 mg/kg body weight of either control IVIG (Sandoglobulin®) or

Table 5 Clinical studies with core LPS intravenous immunoglobulins (IVIG)

Study	Control group	Core LPS IVIG group	p
Therapeutic study in patients with gram-negative septic shock[78]			
Duration of shock (h)	10 (3–144)	12 (2–36)	N.S.
Mortality	1/41 (49%)	15/30 (50%)	N.S.
Prophylactic study in high risk post-surgical patients[28]			
Rate of infection/100 patient-days	3.84	3.61	N.S.
Rate of gram-negative sepsis/100 patient-days	0.32	0.40	N.S.
Mortality	22/112 (20%)	20/108 (19%)	N.S.

In the therapeutic study[78], a standard preparation of IVIG (control) was compared to hyperimmune anti-*E. coli* J5 IVIG. In the prophylactic study[28], an intravenous preparation of albumin (control) was compared to hyperimmune anti-Re LPS IVIG.

of J5-IVIG. Mortality from gram-negative septic shock was identical in the two groups. In addition, J5-IVIG did not reduce the number of systemic complications of shock and did not delay the occurrence of death. This study suggested, therefore, that anti-J5 LPS IgG was not effective in the treatment of gram-negative septic shock.

The second study was a prophylactic study in surgical patients at high-risk of developing infections. Patients were randomized to receive intravenously either a standard human IVIG preparation (Gammagard®), or an IVIG preparation enriched in anti-Re LPS antibodies (core-LPS IVIG), or albumin as placebo. In the 329 evaluable patients, the number of acquired infections was significantly lower in patients treated with the standard IVIG than in those receiving core-LPS IVIG or albumin. No difference in the occurrence of focal or systemic gram-negative infections was observed between core-LPS IVIG and albumin (Table 5). The mortality due to infections was not significantly different between the three groups. Therefore, anti-Re LPS IgG did not have a detectable impact on the prevention of gram-negative infections or on their systemic complications[28].

The failure of hyperimmune IVIG cannot be explained by an insufficient amount of anti-J5 LPS IgG or anti-Re LPS IgG (respectively) administered to the patients, since they received a far greater amount than was administered through the infusion of antiserum or plasma in the two successful studies[13,52]. One possible explanation for the effectiveness of core LPS IVIG is therefore that IgM antibodies, which were absent from the IVIG preparations, might be necessary for protection. However, since the mode of action of anti-core LPS antibodies is unknown, there is no solid basis for such a claim. Although some experimental data suggested that IgM-enriched serum fractions are more effective than IgG-enriched fractions[79] other studies have found IgG antibodies to be as effective or even more effective than IgM[51,105].

Investigations of the factor responsible for protection during the two successful clinical studies using J5 antiserum in humans

In the two apparently successful clinical trials[13,52], the mechanism of the postulated cross-protection was not established. Indeed, there was no

Table 6 Effects of vaccination of humans with *E. coli* J5 on antibodies to LPS

Antigen[a]	Median IgG levels (μg/ml)			Median IgM levels (μg/ml)		
	Pre-immune	Immune	Fold increase	Pre-immune	Immune	Fold increase
J5 LPS	4	13	3.25	3	9	3
Re LPS	5	5	1	1	1	1
Lipid A	3	3	1	<0.5	<0.5	1
0111 LPS	<0.5	<0.5	1	1	1	1
Smooth LPS[b]	21	26	1.24	4	4	1

Adapted from ref. 106.
[a]Coated on ELISA plates as complexes with high density lipoproteins.
[b]Mixture of LPS from seven smooth bacterial strains.

significant relationship between anti-J5 LPS antibody levels administered to the patients and the improved outcome[13] (and personal unpublished data). In addition, immunopurified anti-J5 LPS polyclonal antibodies did not cross-react with other smooth or rough LPS types[50], suggesting therefore that anti-J5 LPS antibodies were not the factors responsible for protection in J5 antiserum. However, the J5 LPS is a complex structure with a core composed of several sugars and lipid A. Thus, it might be that immunization with *E. coli* J5 can elicit a mixture of antibodies directed at different epitopes such as terminal core sugars, as well as deeper structures of the lipid A or the lipid A-KDO region. According to this hypothesis, antibodies to the terminal core sugars might be predominant and J5-specific, whereas antibodies to lipid A or lipid A-KDO might be less abundant but cross-reactive. To investigate whether the protective factor in J5 antiserum could be antibodies directed at other LPS epitopes, we measured in 70 healthy volunteers the antibody response to various LPS epitopes after vaccination with *E. coli* J5[106]. Such vaccination produced only a three-fold median increase in IgG or IgM antibodies to J5 LPS, contrasting with a several hundred-fold increase observed in rabbits. There was no significant increase in antibodies to other rough structures (lipid A and lipid A-KDO) or to smooth structures (LPS from *E. coli* 0111, the parent strain of J5 mutant, and a mixture of LPS from seven smooth bacterial strains) (Table 6). Therefore, as far as immunogenicity is concerned, it seems that rough mutants behave in a similar way to smooth bacteria: despite the fact that the chemical structure of the inner core is similar between these bacteria, the addition of sugars to lipid A during the synthesis of LPS might obscure the immunogenic conformation of the inner core, so that no antibody to the common deeper structures are elicited.

Conclusions of the clinical studies with polyclonal core LPS antibodies

The message that can be globally drawn from these studies is limited. Two of the studies with antiserum against whole *E. coli* J5 bacteria suggested a possible benefit[13,52]. However, the epitope responsible for the protective effect could not be determined. Two other studies with the same antiserum could not demonstrate a protective effect[103,104]. Finally, no benefit could be shown when anti-J5 or anti-Re intravenous immune globulin was used[28,78]. Although some of these studies were sometimes cited as indirect evidence for the effectiveness of anti-lipid A antibodies, it should be stressed that immunization of volunteers with *E. coli* J5 vaccine induced an increase only in IgG and IgM type-specific anti-J5 LPS antibodies, which are not cross-reactive, but no increase in antibodies directed against other epitopes of the core LPS, or against lipid A[106]. This disappointing observation underscores the need for a more precise knowledge of the immunochemistry of LPS and of the mechanisms by which anti-LPS antibodies afford protection.

ANTI-LIPID A ANTIBODIES

A critical review of the past experimental data does not strongly support a cross-protective power of antibodies to lipid A for at least three reasons. First, although the lipid A is chemically the more conserved region of the molecule, its availability as a common epitope on LPS has never been demonstrated and thus remains hypothetical[107]. It should be stressed that isolated lipid A does not exist in nature because even in the roughest mutant, LPS is composed of lipid A with covalent binding to at least one core sugar. No known enzyme is able to hydrolyse this covalent binding. Second, polyclonal antibodies against lipid A do not appear to be protective[59,82,87,108–110]. Third, the mechanism of protection of human J5 antiserum cannot be attributed to anti-lipid A antibodies, as discussed above.

However, interest in anti-lipid A antibodies was renewed when two monoclonal antibodies, HA-1A and E5, were reported to cross-protect against wild-type LPS in animal models. Although these studies should have been interpreted with caution because they were performed with ascitic or hybridoma fluids, not with purified antibodies[111,112], monoclonal antibodies against the lipid A part of endotoxins were once considered as the leading candidates for an effective new treatment of sepsis. Results of initial clinical trials appeared promising. There was a surge of enthusiasm among physicians and investors when HA-1A was made commercially available in some European countries and an advisory panel of the FDA recommended its approval in USA in September 1991. However, for reasons outlined below a second trial of HA-1A was requested by the FDA. A few months later, this trial was abruptly stopped and sales in Europe were suspended because interim analysis revealed an increased mortality in HA-1A-treated patients. Since the marketing campaign had been very active and said nothing about the scientific controversies in the field, many people had a distorted knowledge about these antibodies. The failure of HA-1A was thus largely unforseen. The next paragraphs are an attempt to describe objectively the story of these antibodies, whose usefulness is now in doubt.

The first clinical trials of anti-lipid A monoclonal antibodies

Tested as a crude hybridoma supernatant, HA-1A antibody was reported to broadly cross-react with various unrelated LPS or whole gram-negative bacteria and to protect against LPS in the dermal Shwartzman reaction in rabbits and against lethal gram-negative bacteraemia in mice[111]. Based on these promising data, a licence to develop this antibody for clinical use was purchased by two pharmaceutical companies. One company (Centocor Inc., Malvern, PA) decided to proceed immediately into clinical trials, whereas the other (Mérieux, Lyon, France) decided to reinvestigate the antibody experimentally after purification. Unexpectedly, researchers in this latter company were unable to demonstrate protection in animals. This antibody was also studied in detail by our group. We found that HA-1A bound non-specifically to hydrophobic molecules such as gram-negative and gram-positive bacterial membranes, yeasts, high-density lipoproteins and cardiolipin. In our hands, it bound only very weakly to lipid A with an affinity constant lower than $10^4/M$[113]. Moreover, we could not reproduce the results obtained with the experimental animal models reported in the first publication[114]. In addition, HA-1A did not decrease levels of tumour necrosis factor (TNF) and interleukin-6 induced in mice by LPS injections, suggesting that it did not prevent LPS reaching its target on macrophages[114].

While these disappointing laboratory results were being generated, HA-1A was being studied in patients with a presumptive diagnosis of gram-negative infection, gram-negative sepsis or gram-negative bacteraemia. HA-1A did not reduce the mortality in the overall population, nor in patients with microbiologically documented gram-negative infections. However, there was a significant decrease in mortality among patients with gram-negative bacteraemia[115]. When the results were analysed in detail, in contrast with the erroneous statement in the original article[115], it appeared that the difference was virtually limited to patients who were in shock at entry to the study (Table 7)[116].

In parallel, another anti-lipid A antibody, E5 (Xoma Corp.), was also studied in patients. This trial was designed to investigate whether this antibody would improve the survival of patients with documented gram-negative infection plus a systemic response. No decrease in mortality was observed in the whole group; however, when subgroups were analysed there appeared to be a decrease in mortality in the patients without shock at study entry, whereas patients in shock were not protected (Table 7)[117].

The second clinical trials of anti-lipid A monoclonal antibodies

A second study of E5 was clearly necessary since protection was observed only in a subgroup of patients which had not been defined prospectively. The new hypothesis was put forward that E5 was effective only in patients without shock, and the second trial, designed specifically to test this hypothesis, included about 835 patients with a sepsis syndrome without shock. Two-thirds of the cases proved to be due to gram-negative infections. The results were disappointing because, although there was apparently some

Table 7 Mortality in patients with gram-negative sepsis according to the presence or absence of shock in the first clinical studies of anti-lipid A monoclonal antibodies (mAb) HA-1A and E5

Study	Mortality at 14 days (patients dead/all patients)		p
	Placebo	Anti-lipid A mAb	
HA-1A monoclonal antibody[115,116]			
All patients with gram-negative bacteraemia[a]	32/95 (34%)	25/105 (24%)	0.12
Patients in shock	23/48 (48%)	13/54 (24%)	0.012
Patients not in shock	9/47 (19%)	12/51 (24%)	0.60
E5 monoclonal antibody[117]			
All patients with gram-negative sepsis	42/152 (28%)	41/164 (25%)	0.60
Patients in shock	28/89 (32%)	32/90 (36%)	0.56
Patients not in shock[b]	14/63 (23%)	8/74 (11%)	0.07

[a]No difference was observed when all patients with gram-negative sepsis (bacteraemic and non-bacteraemic) were analysed.
[b]Analysis of the Kaplan–Meier curves showed a statistically significant survival advantage in the E5 group ($p = 0.01$). A trend for improved survival was observed in both bacteraemic and non-bacteraemic patients.

improvement in morbidity, the study failed to confirm that E5 could reduce the mortality among patients with gram-negative sepsis and no shock[118].

At first glance, the results for HA-1A appeared clearer because the protection was observed in one of the prospectively defined subgroups. Despite the controversies and unknowns remaining, Centocor succeeded in obtaining a licence to release HA-1A on the market in several European countries. In the USA however, the HA-1A trial was reanalysed by independent experts according to the data presented by Centocor at a FDA meeting on September 4, 1991, obtained through the Freedom of Information Act[116]. This second-look analysis discovered that the publication of the study[110] had been unduly optimistic. First, the statistical results were found to be marginal because a significant difference was observed in only one of many overlapping subgroups. In addition, when deaths unrelated to sepsis were discarded, the results were no longer significant (Table 8). Second, more patients in the placebo arm than in the HA-1A arm received inadequate or unknown antibiotics and the former had more end-organ failure at study entry than the latter. Third, a protective effect was seen only at six study sites whereas there was a slight advantage of placebo in the 16 other sites. Therefore, it was suggested that the null hypothesis was not convincingly rejected. In addition, the FDA learned that Centocor had changed some of the study endpoints after reviewing interim results, possibly skewing the outcome[119]. A second trial was ordered by the FDA. A few months later, Centocor abruptly halted this second study and withdrew the drug from the 10 European countries where it had been approved, because the death rate was higher among a group of patients who had received the drug than among patients in the placebo group[120].

Although the disappointing results of the second clinical study of HA-1A were not totally unexpected owing to the lack of reproducibility of the

Table 8 Mortality due to sepsis and all causes in the HA-1A trial, according to patient subgroup

| Subgroup[b] | Mortality at 14 days due to sepsis and all causes[a] (patients dead/all patients (%)) | | p at day 14[c] | p at 28 days[c] | |
	Placebo	Ha-1A		Mortality due to sepsis	all causes
Gram-negative bacteraemia	32/95 (34)	25/105 (24)	0.12	0.039	0.014
Gram-negative sepsis	47/145 (32)	40/137 (29)	0.56	0.29	0.18
Gram-negative infection	61/207 (29)	56/194 (29)	0.89	0.47	0.30

Adapted from ref. 116.

[a]Mortality due to sepsis equalled mortality due to all causes at 14 days.

[b]The three overlapping subgroups were patients with 'gram-negative bacteraemia' who had positive blood cultures for gram-negative bacteria, whether or not they had positive cultures for other microbes; patients with 'gram-negative sepsis' who had documented infection with gram-negative organisms (with or without bacteraemia) but no infection with other microbes; patients with 'gram-negative infection' who consisted of all patients with gram-negative disease, regardless of other kinds of ongoing infection.

[c]In addition to three subgroups, two categories of mortality (due to sepsis and due to all causes) were analysed for two times after infusion (at 14 days and over a 28-day period). The FDA analysts suggested that because multiple comparisons were made, the level of statistical significance should be adjusted: the p value should be below a level that was somewhere between 0.01 and 0.03.

preclinical data, Wall Street was stunned by Centocor's announcement that it had prematurely stopped the study. Millions of dollars were lost. Many people asked themselves how a drug whose usefulness is now in doubt could raise such high and unfounded expectations. The answer lies in a tale of highly touted scientific data that could not be replicated and of too much faith placed in the results of a single, overinterpreted, clinical study, while warnings from a few researchers went largely unheeded by many financial analysts and physicians.

FUTURE AREA OF RESEARCH

Following the ill-fated story of HA-1A, research has moved away from the field of immunotherapy against endotoxin and focused on the host mediators involved in the pathophysiology of sepsis. This approach is potentially interesting because host mediators seem fairly similar in gram-negative and in gram-positive sepsis, thus possibly avoiding the need to establish an early microbiological diagnosis before treating the patients. Interactions with the cytokine network using monoclonal antibodies against TNF or using a recombinant interleukin-1 receptor antagonist (IL-1ra) were clearly successful in animal models of endotoxaemia or acute shock, in which a bolus of endotoxins or bacteria was injected. It must be stressed, however, that these models do not mimic closely the situation in patients, in whom the systemic syndrome is often a complication of a progressive bacterial proliferation within tissues[121]. Both approaches are now being studied in humans. Intermediate analysis of the results of clinical studies was considered disappointing because only modest reductions in mortality were reported in subgroups of patients[122]. We must wait until the detailed results of the clinical studies are available in order to know whether the blockade of one of many overlapping cytokines will be able to down-regulate the inflammation cascade in the clinical setting.

At the present time, in the absence of successful alternative approaches, endotoxin remains an important target for therapies of septic shock. Anti-endotoxin antibodies which have nothing in common with HA-1A are now under study. Recently, a new class of monoclonal antibodies with a cross-reactivity pattern intermediate between the narrow range of type-specific antibodies and the 'broad range' of anti-lipid A antibodies has been described. For instance, the antibody WN1 222-5 recognizes a well-defined epitope of the core R3 of *E. coli* and cross-reacts with all the tested serotypes of *E. coli*, *Salmonella* spp. and *Shigella* spp.[123,124]. *In vivo*, it afforded cross-protection against the LPS strains that it recognized *in vitro*[123]. However, it did not react with *Pseudomonas* spp., *Klebsiella* spp. and some other gram-negative strains. Therefore, the administration of a mixture of a few antibodies with a complementary spectrum might be worth study.

Substantial progress has been made recently in the understanding of how LPS can trigger the immune system. Two members of a family of proteins possessing LPS binding sites, LPS-binding protein (LBP) and bactericidal permeability-increasing protein (BPI)[125-131] have been recognized. These proteins have a striking homology in DNA sequence, but they have different functions. LPS forms a high affinity complex with LBP in blood. This complex binds to CD14 on monocytic cells and on primed neutrophils, resulting in increased expression of LPS-inducible genes. LBP was first described as an acute phase reactant, but it is now clear that LBP is present in normal serum in sufficient amounts to respond to minute concentrations of LPS. In contrast to LBP, BPI inhibits the LPS-induced triggering of macrophages. BPI is present predominantly, if not solely, in neutrophil granules. However, BPI may be released in small amounts during degranulation of activated neutrophils, which might represent a possible negative feedback mechanism of LPS-mediated events. The biological roles of LBP, BPI and CD14 are now being actively investigated, as is their modulation by soluble receptors[132] and antibodies[133].

CONCLUSIONS

At the present time, the treatment of the gram-negative septic syndrome with antibodies directed against lipid A or other epitopes of the core LPS should still be considered as investigational. None of the investigated preparations has yet emerged as an established therapeutic modality that can be administered routinely to patients with septic syndrome or septic shock. Clearly, additional basic experiments are warranted to improve our understanding of the mediators of sepsis and to establish the fundamental scientific knowledge that would be mandatory before new clinical trials can be instituted.

References

1. Kreger BE, Craven DE, Carling PC, *et al.* Gram-negative bacteremia. III. Reassessment of etiology, epidemiology and ecology in 612 patients. Am J Med. 1980; 68: 332–343.
2. McCabe WR, Jackson GG. Gram-negative bacteremia. I. Etiology and ecology. Arch Intern Med. 1962; 110: 845–855.
3. McGowan JE Jr, Barnes MW, Finland M. Bacteremia at Boston City Hospital: occurrence and mortality during 12 selected years (1935–1972) with special reference to hospital-acquired cases. J Infect Dis. 1975; 132: 326–341.
4. Wolff SD, Bennett JV. Gram-negative-rod bacteremia. N Engl J Med. 1974; 291: 733–734.
5. Increase in National Hospital Discharge Survey rates for septicemia – United States, 1979–1987. MMWR. 1990; 39; 31–34.
6. Bryan CS, Reynolds KL, Brenner ER. Analysis of 1,186 episodes of Gram-negative bacteremia in non-university hospitals: the effects of antimicrobial therapy. Rev Infect Dis. 1983; 5: 629–638.
7. Felty AR, Keefer CS. Bacillus coli sepsis. A clinical study of 28 cases of bloodstream infection by the colon bacillus. JAMA. 1924; 82: 1430–1433.
8. Kreger BE, Craven DE, Carling PC, *et al.* Gram-negative bacteremia. IV. Reevaluation of clinical features and treatment in 612 patients. Am J Med. 1980; 68: 344–355.
9. Shenep JL, Morgan KA. Kinetics of endotoxin release during antibiotic therapy for experimental gram-negative bacterial sepsis. J Infect Dis. 1984; 150: 380–388.
10. Bone RG, Fisher CJ, Clemmer TP. A controlled clinical trial of high-dose methylprednisolone in the treatment of severe sepsis and septic shock. N Engl J Med. 1987; 317: 653–658.
11. Sprung CL, Caralis PV, Marcial EH, *et al.* The effects of high-dose corticosteroids in patients with septic shock: a prospective, controlled study. N Engl J Med. 1984; 311: 1137–1143.
12. The Veterans Administration Systemic Sepsis Cooperative Study Group. Effect of high-dose glucocorticoid therapy on mortality in patients with clinical signs of systemic sepsis. N Engl J Med. 1987; 317: 659–665.
13. Ziegler EJ, McCutchan JA, Fierer J, *et al.* Treatment of Gram-negative bacteremia and shock with human antiserum to a mutant *Escherichia coli.* N Engl J Med. 1982; 307: 1225–1230.
14. Glauser MP, Zanetti G, Baumgartner JD, *et al.* Septic shock: pathogenesis. Lancet. 1991; 338: 732–736.
15. Jacob L. Ueber allgemain Infektion durch Bacterium coli commune. DAKMM. 1909; 97: 303–307.
16. De Maria A, Craven DE, Heffernan JJ, *et al.* Naloxone versus placebo in treatment of septic shock. Lancet. 1985; i: 1363–1365.
17. Wolff SM. Biological effects of bacterial endotoxins in man. J Infect Dis. 1973; 128: 259S–264S.
18. Fuller NA, Wu MC, Wilkinson RG, *et al.* The biosynthesis of cell wall lipopolysaccharide in *Escherichia coli.* VII. Characterization of heterogenous 'core' oligosaccharide structures. J Biol Chem. 1973; 248: 7938–7950.
19. Jansson PE, Lindberg AA, Lindberg B, *et al.* Structural studies on the hexose region of the core in lipopolysaccharides from enterobacteraceae. Eur J Biochem. 1981; 115: 571–577.
20. Pollack M, Chia JKS, Koles NL, *et al.* Specificity and cross-reactivity of monoclonal antibodies reactive with the core and lipid A regions of bacterial lipopolysaccharide. J Infect Dis. 1989; 159: 168–188.
21. Rietschel ET, Wollenweber HW, Brade H, *et al.* Structure and conformation of the lipid A component of lipopolysaccharides. In: Proctor RA, Rietschel ET, eds. Handbook of endotoxin. Volume 1: Chemistry of endotoxin. Amsterdam: Elsevier, 1984: 187–220.
22. Pfeiffer R, Kolle W. Ueber di spezifische Immunitaets-reaktion der Typhus-bacillen. Z Hyg Infektionskr. 1896; 21: 203–246.
23. Tate WJ, Douglas H, Braude AI. Protection against lethality of E. coli endotoxin with 'O' antiserum. Ann NY Acad Sci. 1966; 133: 746–762.
24. Baker CJ, Melish ME, Hall RT, *et al.* Intravenous immune globulin for the prevention of nosocomial infection in low-birth-weight neonates. N Engl J Med. 1992; 327: 213–219.

25. Chirico G, Rondini G, Piebani S, et al. Intravenous immunoglobulin therapy for prophylaxis of infection in high-risk neonates. J Pediatr. 1987; 110: 437–442.
26. Glinz W, Grob JP, Nydegger UE, et al. Polyvalent immunoglobulins for prophylaxis of bacterial infections in patients with multiple trauma. Intensive Care Med. 1985; 11: 288–294.
27. Haque KN, Zaidi MH, Haque SK, et al. Intravenous immunoglobulin for prevention of sepsis in preterm and low birth weight infants. Pediatr Infect Dis. 1986; 5: 622–625.
28. The Intravenous Immunoglobulin Collaborative Study Group. Prophylactic intravenous administration of standard immune globulin as compared with core-lipopolysaccharide immune globulin in patients at high risk of postsurgical infection. N Engl J Med. 1992; 327: 234–240.
29. Dominioni L, Dionigi R, Zanello M, et al. Effects of high-dose IgG on survival of surgical patients with sepsis scores of 20 or greater. Arch Surg. 1991; 126: 236–240.
30. Duswald KH, Müller K, Seifert J, et al. Wirksamkeit von i.v. Gammaglobulin gegen backterielle Infektionen chirurgischer Patienten. Muench Med Wschr. 1980; 122: 832–836.
31. Just HM, Metzger M, Vogel W, et al. Einfluss einter adjuvanten immunoglobulintherapie auf Infectionen bei Patienten einer opertiven Intensive-Therapie-Station. Klin Wochenschr. 1986; 64: 245–256.
33. Sidiropoulos D, Böhme U, Von Muralt G, et al. Immunoglobulinsubstitution bei der Behandlung der neonatalen Sepsis. Schweiz Med Wochenschr. 1981; 111: 1649–1655.
34. Zanetti G, Glauser MP, Baumgartner JD. Use of immunoglobulins in prevention and treatment of infections in critically-ill patients: review and critique. Rev Infect Dis. 1991; 13: 985–992.
35. Young LS. Immunoprophylaxis and serotherapy of bacterial infections. Am J Med. 1984; 76: 664–671.
36. Baumgartner JD, Glauser MP. Controversies in the passive immunotherapy of bacterial infections in the critically-ill patients. Rev Infect Dis. 1987; 9: 194–205.
37. Collins MS, Dorsey JH. Comparative anti-*Pseudomonas aeruginosa* activity of chemically modified and native immunoglobulins G (human), and potentiation of antibiotic protection against *Pseudomonas aeruginosa* and group B *Streptococcus in vivo.* Am J Med. 1984; 76: 155–160.
38. Collins MS, Roby RE. Protective activity of an intravenous immune globulin (human) enriched in antibody against lipopolysaccharide antigens of *Pseudomonas aeruginosa.* Am J Med. 1984; 76: 168–174.
39. Holder IA, Naglich JG. Experimental studies of the pathogenesis of infections due to *Pseudomonas aeruginosa.* Treatment with intravenous immune globulin. Am J Med. 1984; 76: 161–167.
40. Pennington JE, Menkes E. Type-specific versus cross-protective vaccination for gram-negative pneumonia. J Infect Dis. 1981; 144: 599–603.
41. Pollack M. Antibody activity against *Pseudomonas aeruginosa* in immune globulins prepared for intravenous use in humans. J Infect Dis. 1983; 147: 1090–1098.
42. Pennington JE. Impact of molecular biology on *Pseudomonas aeruginosa* immunization. J Hosp Infect. 1988; 11 (Suppl.): 96–102.
43. Westphal O, Jann K, Himmelspach K. Chemistry and immunochemistry of bacterial lipopolysaccharides as cell wall antigens and endotoxins. Prog Allergy. 1983; 33: 9–39.
44. Nixdorff KK, Schlecht SS. Heterogeneity of the haemagglutinin responses to *Salmonella minnesota* R-antigens in rabbits. J Gen Microbiol. 1972; 71: 425–440.
45. Heumann D, Baumgartner JD, Jacot-Guillarmod H, et al. Antibodies to core lipopolysaccharide determinants: absence of cross-reactivity with heterologous lipopolysaccharides. J Infect Dis. 1991; 163: 762–768.
46. Braude AI, Douglas H. Passive immunization against the local Schwartzman reaction. J Immunol. 1972; 108: 505–512.
47. Chedid L, Parant M, Parant F, et al. A proposed mechanism for natural immunity to enterobacterial pathogens. J Immunol. 1968; 100: 292–301 .
48. McCabe WR. Immunization with R mutants of *S. minnesota.* I. Protection against challenge with heterologous gram-negative bacilli. J Immunol. 1972; 108: 601–610.
49. Pollack M, Huang AI, Prescott RK, et al. Enhanced survival in *Pseudomonas aeruginosa* septicemia associated with high levels of circulating antibody to *Escherichia coli* endotoxin

core. J Clin Invest. 1983; 72: 1874–1881.

50. Pollack M, Young LS. Protective activity of antibodies to exotoxin A and lipopolysaccharide at the onset of *Pseudomonas aeruginosa* septicaemia in man. J Clin Invest. 1979; 63: 276–286.

51. Zinner SH, McCabe WR. Effects of IgM and IgG antibody in patients with bacteremia due to gram-negative bacilli. J Infect Dis. 1976; 133: 37–45.

52. Baumgartner JD, Glauser MP, McCutchan JA, *et al.* Prevention of Gram-negative shock and death in surgical patients by prophylactic antibody to endotoxin core glycolipid. Lancet. 1985; ii: 59–63.

53. Eskenazy M, Konstantinov G, Ivanova R, *et al.* Detection by immunofluorescence of common antigenic determinants in unrelated Gram-negative bacteria and their lipopolysaccharides. J Infect Dis. 1977; 135: 965–969.

54. Young LS, Hoffman KR, Stevens P. Core glycolipid of enterobacteriaceae: immunofluorescent detection of antigen and antibody. Proc Soc Biol Med. 1975; 149: 389–396.

55. Baumgartner JD, O'Brien TX, Kirkland TN, *et al.* Demonstration of cross-reactive antibodies to smooth Gram-negative bacteria in *Escherichia coli* J5 antiserum. J Infect Dis. 1987; 156: 136–143.

56. Overbeck BP, Schellekens JFP, Lippe W, *et al.* Carumonam enhances reactivity of *Escherichia coli* with mono- and polyclonal antisera to rough mutant *Escherichia coli* J5. J Clin Microbiol. 1987; 156: 136–143.

57. McCallus DE, Norcross NL. Antibody specific for *Escherichia coli* J5 crossreacts to various degrees with an *Escherichia coli* clinical isolates grown for different lengths of time. Infect Immun. 1987; 55: 1042–1046.

58. De Jongh-Leuvenik J, Vreede RW, Marcelis JH, *et al.* Detection of antibodies against lipopolysaccharides of *Escherichia coli* and *Salmonella* R and S strains by immunoblotting. Infect Immun. 1985; 50: 716–720.

59. Johns MA, Bruins SC, McCabe WR. Immunization with R mutants of *Salmonella minnesota.* II. Serological response to lipid A and the lipopolysaccharide of Re mutants. Infect Immun. 1977; 17: 9–15.

60. Ng AK, Chen CLH, Chang CM, *et al.* Relationship of structure to function in bacterial endotoxins: serologically cross-reactive components and their effect on protection of mice against some Gram-negative infections. J Gen Microbiol. 1976; 94: 107–116.

61. Schwartzer TA, Alcid DV, Numsuwan V, *et al.* Immunochemical specificity of human antibodies to lipopolysaccharide from the J5 rough mutant of *Escherichia coli* O111:B4. J Infect Dis. 1989; 159: 35–42.

62. Siber GR, Kania SA, Warren HS. Cross-reactivity of rabbit antibodies to lipopolysaccharide of *Escherichia coli* and other gram-negative bacteria. J Infect Dis. 1985; 152: 954–964.

63. Bogard WC Jr, Dunn DL, Abernethy K, *et al.* Isolation and characterization of murine monoclonal antibodies specific for gram-negative bacterial lipopolysaccharide: association of cross-genus reactivity with lipid A specificity. Infect Immun. 1986; 55: 899–908.

64. Dunn DL, Bogard WC Jr, Cerra FB. Efficacy of type-specific and cross-reactive murine monoclonal antibodies directed against endotoxin during experimental sepsis. Surgery. 1985; 98: 283–289.

65. Kirkland TN, Colwell DE, Michalek SM, *et al.* Analysis of the fine specificity and cross-reactivity of monoclonal anti-lipid A antibodies. J Immunol. 1986; 137: 3614–3619.

66. Miner KM, Manyak CL, Williams E. Characterization of murine monoclonal antibodies to *Escherichia coli* J5. Infect Immun. 1986; 52: 56–62.

67. Mutharia LM, Crockford G, Bogard WC Jr, *et al.* Monoclonal antibodies specific for *Escherichia coli* J5 lipopolysaccharide: cross-reaction with other gram-negative bacterial species. Infect Immun. 1984; 45: 631–636.

68. Nelles MJ, Niswander CA. Mouse monoclonal antibodies reactive with J5 lipopolysaccharide exhibit extensive serological cross-reactivity with a variety of Gram-negative bacteria. Infect Immun. 1984; 46: 677–681.

69. Gigliotti F, Shenep JL. Failure of monoclonal antibodies to core glycolipid to bind intact strains of *Escherichia coli.* J Infect Dis. 1985; 151: 1005–1011.

70. Pollack M, Raubitschek AA, Larrick JW. Human monoclonal antibodies that recognize conserved epitopes in the core-lipid A region lipopolysaccharides. J Clin Invest. 1987; 79: 1421–1430.

71. Shenep JL, Gigliotti F, Davis DS, et al. Reactivity of antibodies to core glycolipid with gram-negative bacteria. Rev Infect Dis. 198 7; 9(Suppl.): S639–S643.

72. Young LS, Stevens P. Cross-protective immunity to gram-negative bacilli: studies with core glycolipid of Salmonella minnesota and antigens of Streptococcus pneumoniae. J Infect Dis. 1977; 136: 174S–180S.

73. Young LS, Stevens P, Ingram J. Functional role of antibody against 'core' glycolipid of enterobacteriaceae. J Clin Invest. 1975; 56: 850–861.

74. Ziegler EJ, Douglas H, Sherman JE, et al. Treatment of E. coli and Klebsiella bacteremia in agranulocytic animals with antiserum to a UDP-Gal epimerase-deficient mutant. J Immunol. 1973; 111: 433–438.

75. Michael JG, Mallah I. Immune response to parental and rough mutant strains of Salmonella minnesota. Infect Immun. 1981; 33: 784–787.

76. Baumgartner JD, Glauser MP. Immunotherapy of endotoxemia and septicemia. Immunobiology. 1993; 187: 464–477.

77. Baumgartner JD, Wu MM, Glauser MP. Interpretation of data regarding the protection afforded by serum, IgG or IgM antibodies after immunization with the rough mutant R595 of Salmonella minnesota. J Infect Dis. 1989; 160: 347–348.

78. Calandra T, Glauser MP, Schellekens J, et al. Treatment of gram-negative septic shock with human IgG antibody to Escherichia coli J5: A prospective, double blind, randomized study. J Infect Dis. 1988; 158: 312–319.

79. McCabe WR, DeMaria A Jr, Berberich H, et al. Immunization with rough mutants of Salmonella minnesota: Protective activity of IgM and IgG antibody to the R595 (Re chemotype) mutant. J Infect Dis. 1988; 158: 291–300.

80. Greisman SE. Experimental gram-negative bacterial sepsis: optimal methylprednisolone requirements for prevention of mortality not preventable by antibiotics alone. Proc Soc Biol Med. 1982; 170: 436–442.

81. Greisman SE, Johnston CA. Failure of antisera to J5 and R595 rough mutants to reduce endotoxemic lethality. J Infect Dis. 1987; 157: 54–64.

82. Hodgin LA, Drews J. Effect of active and passive immunizations with lipid A and Salmonella minnesota Re 595 on gram-negative infections in mice. Infection. 1976; 4: 5–10.

83. Martinez D, Callahan LT III. Prophylaxis of Pseudomonas aeruginosa infections in leukopenia mice by a combination of active and passive immunization. Eur J Clin Microbiol. 1985; 4: 186–189.

84. Morris DD, Bottoms GD, Whitlock RH, et al. Endotoxin-induced changes in plasma concentrations of thromboxane and prostacyclin in neonatal calves given antiserum to a mutant Escherichia coli (J5). Am J Vet Res. 1986; 47: 2520–2524.

85. Morris DD, Cullor JS, Whitlock RH, et al. Endotoxemia in neonatal calves given an antiserum to a mutant Escherichia coli (J5). Am J Vet Res. 1986; 47: 2554–2565.

86. Morris DD, Whitlock RH, Merryman GS, et al. Endotoxin-induced changes in the hemostatic system in neonatal calves: the effect of antiserum to mutant Escherichia coli (J5). Am J Vet Res. 1986; 47: 2514–2519.

87. Mullan NA, Newsome PM, Cunnington PG, et al. Protection against gram-negative infections with antiserum to lipid A from Salmonella minnesota R595. Infect Immun. 1974; 10: 1195–1201.

88. Peter G, Chernow M, Keating MH, et al. Limited protective effect of rough mutant antisera in murine Escherichia coli bacteremia. Infection. 1982; 10: 228–232.

89. Sadoff JC, Futrovsky SL, Sidberry HF, et al. Detoxified lipopolysaccharide-protein conjugates. Semin Infect Dis. 1982; 4: 346–354 .

90. Straube E, Naumann G, Broschewitz U. Effect of immunization with Escherichia coli endotoxin with 'O' antiserum. Ann NY Acad Sci. 1966; 133: 746–762.

91. Trautmann M, Hahn H. Antiserum against Escherichia coli J5: A re-evaluation of its in vitro and in vivo activity against heterologous gram-negative bacteria. Infection. 1985; 13: 140–145.

92. Van Dick WC, Verbrugh HA, Van Erne-van der Tol ME, et al. Escherichia coli antibodies in opsonisation and protection against infection. J Med Microbiol. 1981; 14: 381–389.

93. Vuopio-Varkila J. Experimental Escherichia coli peritonitis in immunosuppressed mice: the role of specific and non-specific immunity. J Med Microbiol. 1988; 25: 33–39.

94. Vuopio-Varkila J, Karvonen M, Saxen H. Protective capacity of antibodies to outer-

membrane components of *Escherichia coli* in a systemic mouse peritonitis model. J Med Microbiol. 1988; 25: 77–84.

95. Weinbreck P, Baumgartner JD, Cometta A, *et al*. Failure of passive immunization with rabbit antiserum to *E. coli* J5 in bacteremia and endotoxemic lethality in mice. Abstract 622: in Programme and Abstracts of the 28th Interscience Conference on Antimicrobial Agents and Chemotherapy, Los Angeles. Washington: American Society for Microbiology, 1988: 218.

96. Ziegler EJ. Protective antibody to endotoxin core: the emperor's new clothes? J Infect Dis. 1988; 158: 286–290.

97. Chong KT, Huston M. Implications of endotoxin contamination in the evaluation of antibodies to lipopolysaccharides in a murine model of gram-negative sepsis. J Infect Dis. 1987; 156: 713–719.

98. Urbaschek B, Ditter B, Becker KP, *et al*. Protective effects and role of endotoxin in experimental septicemia. Circ Shock. 1984; 14: 209–222.

99. Woods JP, Black JR, Barritt DS, *et al*. Resistance to meningococcemia apparently conferred by anti-H.8 monoclonal antibody is due to contaminating endotoxin and not to specific immunoprotection. Infect Immun. 1987; 55: 1927–1928.

100. Silva AT, Appelmelk BJ, Cohen J. Purified monoclonal antibody to endotoxin core fails to protect mice from experimental gram-negative sepsis. J Infect Dis. 1993; 168: 256–257.

101. McCabe WR, Kreger BE, Johns M. Type-specific and cross-reactive antibodies in gram-negative bacteremia. N Engl J Med. 1972; 287: 261–267.

102. Baumgartner JD, Heumann D, Calandra T, *et al*. Antibodies to core LPS in patients with Gram-negative septic shock: Absence of correlation with outcome. In: Program and Abstracts of the 29th Interscience Conference on Antimicrobial Agents and Chemotherapy, Houston, Washington: American Society for Microbiology, 1989: 175.

103. J5 Study Group. Treatment of severe infectious purpura in children with human plasma from donors immunized with *Escherichia coli* J5: A prospective double-blind study. J Infect Dis. 1992; 165: 695–701.

104. McCutchan JA, Wolf JL, Ziegler EJ, *et al*. Ineffectiveness of single-dose human antiserum to core glycolipid (*E. coli* J5) for prophylaxis of bacteremic, gram-negative infection in patients with prolonged neutropenia. Schweiz Med Wschr. 1983; 113 (Suppl. 14): 40–45.

105. Davis CE, Ziegler EJ, Arnold K. Neutralization of meningococcal endotoxin by antibody to core glycolipid. J Exp Med. 1978; 147: 1007–1017.

106. Baumgartner JD, Heumann D, Calandra T, *et al*. Antibodies to lipopolysaccharides after immunization of humans with the rough mutant *Escherichia coli* J5. J Infect Dis. 1991; 163: 769–772.

107. Baumgartner JD. Immunotherapy with antibodies to core LPS: a critical appraisal. Infect Dis Clin North Am. 1991; 5: 915–927.

108. Bruins SC, Stumacher R, Johns MA, *et al*. Immunization with R mutants of *Salmonella minnesota*. III. Comparison of the protective effect of immunization with lipid A and the Re mutant. Infect Immun. 1977; 17: 16–20.

109. Galanos C, Luederitz O, Westphal O. Preparation and properties of antisera against the lipid-A component of bacterial lipopolysaccharides. Eur J Biochem. 1971; 24: 116–122.

110. Mattsby-Baltzer I, Kaijser B. Lipid A and anti-lipid A. Infect Immun. 1979; 23: 758–763.

111. Teng NNH, Kaplan HS, Hebert JM. Protection against Gram-negative bacteremia and endotoxemia with human monoclonal IgM antibodies. Proc Natl Acad Sci USA. 1985; 82: 1790–1794.

112. Young LS, Gascon R, Alam S, *et al*. Monoclonal antibodies for treatment of gram-negative infections. Rev Infect Dis. 1989; 11 (Suppl.7): S1564–S1571.

113. Baumgartner JD, Heumann D, Glauser MP. The HA-1A monoclonal antibody for gram-negative sepsis. N Engl J Med. 1991; 325: 281–282.

114. Baumgartner JD, Heumann D, Gerain J, *et al*. Association between protective efficacy of anti-lipopolysaccharide (LPS) antibodies and suppression of LPS-induced tumor necrosis factor α and interleukin 6. Comparison of O side chain-specific antibodies with core LPS antibodies. J Exp Med. 1990; 171: 889–896.

115. Ziegler EJ, Fisher CJ, Sprung CL, *et al*. Treatment of gram-negative bacteremia and septic shock with HA-1A human monoclonal antibody against endotoxin. A randomized, double-blind, placebo-controlled trial. N Engl J Med. 1991; 324: 429–436.

116. Warren HS, Danner RL, Munford RS. Anti-endotoxin monoclonal antibodies. N Engl J Med. 1992; 326: 1153–1157.
117. Greenman RL, Schein RMH, Martin MA, et al. A controlled clinical trial of E5 murine monoclonal IgM antibody to endotoxin in the treatment of gram-negative sepsis. JAMA. 1991; 266: 1097–1102.
118. Wenzel R, Bone R, Fein A, et al. Results of a second double-blind, randomized, controlled trial of antiendotoxin antibody ES in gram-negative sepsis. In: Program and abstracts of the 31st Interscience Conference on Antimicrobial Agents and Chemotherapy. Washington, DC: American Society for Microbiology; 1991: 234.
119. Winslow R. Effectiveness of new drug against septic infections is questioned by agency. Wall Street Journal, 1992; Apr 16: B5.
120. Fisher LM. Investors punish Centocor for more bad news. New York Times. 1993; Jan 19: D1.
121. Zanetti G, Heumann D, Gerain J, et al. Cytokine production after intravenous or peritoneal gram negative bacterial challenge in mice. Comparative protective efficacy of antibodies to TNFα and to LPS. J Immunol. 1992; 148: 1890–1897.
122. Piercey L. Star-crossed lovers – is biotech bad for science? Biopeople. 1993; 4: 20–27.
123. Di Padova FE, Barclay R, Liehl E, et al. Widely cross-reactive anti-LPS core monoclonal antibodies have LPS neutralizing properties. Abstract CB404. J Cell Biochem. 1992: Suppl. 16C: 170.
124. Saxen H, Vuopio-Varkila J, Luk J, et al. Detection of enterobacterial lipopolysaccharides and experimental endotoxemia by means of an immunolimulus assay using both serotype-specific and cross-reactive antibodies. J Infect Dis. 1993; 168: 393–399.
125. Heumann D, Gallay P, Betz-Corradin S, et al. Competition between bactericidal/permeability-increasing protein and lipopolysaccharide-binding protein for lipopolysaccharide binding to monocytes. J Infect Dis. 1993; 167: 1351–1357.
126. Marra MN, Snable JL, Scott RW, et al. Bactericidal/permeability-increasing protein: a naturally occurring lipopolysaccharide antagonist. Circ Shock. 1991; 34: 47.
127. Ooi CE, Weiss J, Doerfler ME, et al. Endotoxin-neutralizing properties of the 24 kD N-terminal fragment and a newly isolated 30 kD C-terminal fragment of the 55–60 kD bactericidal/permeability-increasing protein of human neutrophils. J Exp Med. 1991; 174: 649–655.
128. Schumann RR, Leong SR, Flaggs GW, et al. Structure and function of lipopolysaccharide binding protein. Science. 1990; 249: 1429–1431.
129. Tobias PS, Mathison JC, Ulevitch RJ. A family of lipopolysaccharide binding proteins involved in responses to gram-negative sepsis. J Biol Chem. 1988; 263: 13479–13481.
130. Tobias PS, Soldau K, Ulevitch RJ. Isolation of a lipopolysaccharide-binding acute phase reactant from rabbit serum. J Exp Med. 1986; 164: 777–793.
131. Wright SD, Ramos RA, Tobias PS, et al. CD14, a receptor for complexes of lipopolysaccharide (LPS) and LPS binding protein. Science. 1990; 249: 1431–1433.
132. Bazil V, Strominger JL. Shedding as a mechanism of down-modulation of CD14 on stimulated human monocytes. J Immunol. 1991; 147: 1567–1574.
133. Heumann D, Gallay P, Barras C, et al. Control of LPS binding and LPS-induced TNF secretion in human peripheral blood monocytes. J Immunol. 1992; 148: 3505–3512.
134. Greisman SE, DuBuy JB, Woodward CL. Experimental gram-negative bacterial sepsis: reevaluation of the ability of rough mutant antisera to protect mice. Proc Soc Biol Med. 1978; 158: 482–490.
135. Greisman SE, DuBuy JB, Woodward CL. Experimental gram-negative bacterial sepsis: prevention of mortality not preventable by antibiotics alone. Infect Immun. 1979; 25: 538–557.

10
Current and Future Approaches to Vaccination Against Virus Diseases

C. R. HOWARD

INTRODUCTION

The control of infectious diseases by vaccination has been applied to an ever-increasing number of veterinary and human viral pathogens since Jenner's observation that smallpox can be prevented by prior inoculation of individuals with cowpox. The eradication of smallpox over a decade ago is the most notable example of a successful vaccination programme, achieved by employing a stable product and a well-coordinated programme of delivery and surveillance. Particular reasons for this success include the probable absence of an animal reservoir, absence of multiple serotypes and ease of vaccine delivery. This is not always the case, however. For example, zoonotic infections (those with a natural host species other than man) can be controlled at best, and cannot be effectively eliminated. Rabies is a good example: Pasteur's use of formaldehyde for the inactivation of live rabies virus was a novel approach that is still widely used in vaccine production (Table 1). Another good example of a virus that cannot be eliminated is yellow fever: continuing vigilance for the emergence of infections from the natural monkey host is required. Here the approach has been to develop strains by passage *in vitro* to a degree whereby growth is restricted to non-target organs and tissues. Vaccination strategies are often hampered, however, by the tendency of viruses to undergo rapid antigenic variations in response to increasing levels of herd immunity (e.g. influenza), by the stability of existing vaccine materials (e.g. measles virus) or by changes in social behaviour e.g. hepatitis B, human immunodeficiency virus (HIV).

Thus infectious diseases remain major causes of morbidity and mortality in both industrialized and developing countries, despite the overall general reduction in deaths due to improved standards of living and better health care. Many of these diseases take their toll in childhood, and for this reason

Table 1 Currently available virus vaccines

Disease	Vaccine type
Widely used	
Poliomyelitis	Live attenuated/inactivated
Measles	Live attenuated
Mumps	Live attenuated
Rubella	Live attenuated
Hepatitis B	Subunit
Restricted use	
Smallpox	Live heterologous virus (vaccinia)
Yellow fever	Live attenuated
Influenza	Subunit
Rabies	Inactivated
Adenovirus	Live attenuated
Japanese B	Inactivated
Varicella	Live attenuated

the World Health Organisation has been at the forefront through its Expanded Programme on Immunisation (EPI) in encouraging the implementation of vaccines against childhood diseases, using existing products. However, the deficiencies of presently available vaccines have yet to be overcome; for this reason, the Children's Vaccine Initiative was established in 1991. This serves to stimulate not only the development of improved vaccines to overcome the difficulties of stability, delivery and antigenic variation, but also to ensure their economic availability and effective use. It is against this background that this chapter reviews the current status in the availability of viral vaccines and how the application of new technology may help overcome difficulties in the control of virus infections and the rational design of newer vaccines.

THE REQUIREMENTS OF A SUCCESSFUL VACCINE

The objective of vaccination is to provide effective immunity — this often means the establishment of adequate levels of antibody — and a primed population of immune cells which can expand rapidly on renewed contact with antigen. A vaccine also has to be safe yet effective in over 90% of recipients. Other necessary attributes of a successful vaccine include good stability and an adequate supply of immunogen, the cost of which is economically feasible for large-scale use. Present vaccines fulfil many of these criteria (Table 2), yet have been developed in a manner that owes more to serendipity than rational design. It is important to be aware that vaccination does not always result in total immunity against a subsequent exposure to the virus. Protection is sufficient, however, to prevent clinical disease in the target organ. The efficiency and time of delivery is also important; if delivered at the correct time, a small but significant number of individuals may remain susceptible, yet increasing levels of herd immunity may be adequate to prevent further circulation of virus in the community. In this context it

Table 2 The requirements of a successful vaccine

Biological
  Induce protective immune responses in over 90% of recipients
  Stimulate immunological memory
  Give protection against all serotypes
  Effective in infants
  Safe and heat-stable

Other
  Economically feasible for use
  Epidemiological criteria established for effective use

---

cannot be over-emphasized that effective vaccination strategies require good surveillance and rapid epidemiological investigation of outbreaks immediately they occur.

The identification of protective antigens is a first step in the rational design of vaccines. These have been identified for a wide range of viruses, and in some cases correlated with the structure of the virus particle[1]. In the case of enveloped viruses, these antigens are principally located on surface glycoproteins that are presented to the immune system both as whole virus and also on the surface of infected cells. Additional components not present in virus particles may also be important. An example is the NS1 glycoprotein expressed on the surface of yellow fever virus-infected cells; passive immunization of mice with NS1 antibodies will protect mice against lethal disease and purified NS1 protein will protect monkeys[2].

The presence of neutralizing antibody is often taken as a correlate of immunity in hosts vaccinated against diseases where antibody is of prime importance, e.g. foot-and-mouth disease and hepatitis B. However, evidence that neutralization plays a major role *in vivo* has not been unequivocally shown for most virus vaccines. The immunogenicity of the protective protein depends upon the genetic haplotype of the host, the available repertoire of T and B cells, the functioning of the idiotypic network and the method of antigen presentation. Macromolecules express a large number of potential epitopes on their surface, but not all are immunogenic. The specificity of the immune response is restricted to immunodominant areas of the viral protein, as exemplified by the influenza haemagglutinin molecule: studies with monoclonal antibodies and synthetic peptides have shown clearly that antibody binds to one or more of five major antigenic domains[3]. Not all individuals respond equally to all sites, and reinfection may lead to a broadening of the response; this means that immunization may only give partial protection and that repeated doses are necessary to achieve a sufficiently broad protective B cell response. Antiviral antibodies may not always be beneficial, however. For example, it has been suggested that heterotypic antibody plays a role in the development of dengue haemorrhagic fever by enhancing the level of replication by a second dengue virus of different subtype[4]. This phenomenon of antibody-mediated enhancement is common among the flaviviruses and alphaviruses; it has also been suggested to occur in HIV infections[5].

The identification of T helper sites is important for the induction of antibody to T-dependent antigens, including the majority of viral proteins. The commonly held view that T cells recognize short sequences of proteins and, in contrast to B cells, that the tertiary structure of the protein is unimportant has been challenged, as has the concept that T and B cell epitopes are located on discrete parts of the molecule. In the case of influenza virus, both B and T cells recognize the same determinants[6]. There is also evidence to suggest that T helper cell epitopes in the internal matrix and nucleoprotein polypeptides may provide help to haemagglutinin-specific B cells, thus augmenting the antibody response to protective antigens[7].

WHOLE VIRUS VACCINES

A glance at those virus vaccines in widespread use shows that the majority represent live virus strains that have been attenuated by passage of wild-type virus in cell culture (Table 2). The resulting virus has lost its ability to infect target organs while retaining a restricted capacity for replication in other organs and tissues close to the portal of entry. This limited replication tends to stimulate longer-lasting B cell responses as well as cellular immunity. There are substantial advantages in the use of attenuated vaccines: the restricted replication of virus in host tissues produces a much larger dose of stimulating antigen, the immune response takes place largely at the site of infection, and, in the case of budding viruses, infected cells stimulate good levels of cytotoxic T cells.

Considerable experience has been obtained with attenuated strains of yellow fever, polio, measles and rubella viruses. However, there still remains a risk associated with the use of these, for example encephalitis may follow measles immunization. In many countries, almost all cases of poliomyelitis can be ascribed to the reversion of vaccine shed by vaccinated individuals. Despite the high levels of herd immunity that can be achieved in a target population by the use of the live attenuated vaccine, reduction of poliovirus infection below a certain level in the developed world may require revision of vaccination strategies to include the use of both attenuated and inactivated poliovirus vaccines. However, the recent remarkable nearly complete elimination of poliomyelitis from South and Central America was accomplished entirely by use of attenuated vaccine; the number of cases fell by 99% in 6 years, from 721 in 1985 to 7 in 1991[8]. In contrast, outbreaks continue to occur in Europe, particularly among individuals in religious groups who decline to be vaccinated. This occurred recently in the Netherlands, a country which uses inactivated vaccine exclusively.

Drawbacks to the use of attenuated vaccines include the risk of other adventitious agents present as contaminants of the cell substrates used for growth: until recently yellow fever vaccine grown in chick embryos was frequently contaminated with avian leucosis virus. More important, attenuated vaccines are inherently less stable and require expensive 'cold-chain' facilities in order to prevent loss of potency prior to delivery. Additionally, attenuated vaccines cannot be given immediately after birth as maternal antibodies may restrict or prevent replication of the attenuated vaccine. The use of live vaccines is also not possible for children with immune deficiency states, patients being treated with immunosuppressive agents, and those with lymphomas and leukaemia.

The concept of live attenuated vaccines is based on the fact that such virus strains do not differ significantly from wild-type virus in regions of the viral proteins responsible for the induction of protective immunity. The process of passaging virus *in vitro* in order to accumulate the necessary genetic mutations is unpredictable: for example, it has not been possible to repeat the process whereby the 17D vaccine strain of yellow fever virus was developed by successive passage in chick embryo cells[9]. Critical to the process of attenuation is the identification of genetic markers. Temperature sensitivity is often useful, e.g. for poliovirus[10] and rubella[11]. The lack of a corresponding marker for hepatitis A, however, is hampering the development of attenuated hepatitis A vaccines, and several candidate immunogens have become over-attenuated[12]. These attempts have been largely superceded by the finding that inactivated hepatitis A virus particles are particularly good human immunogens[13].

The molecular basis of attenuation is poorly understood, although some progress is now being made to unravel the complexities of nucleotide changes which occur in the poliovirus genome. Studies of type 3 virus have shown 10 nucleotide changes, only three of which result in changes of amino acid. Two are located in the 5'-non-coding region at positions 220 and 472; revertant viruses that have regained some neurovirulence have been found to have a back mutation at position 472, suggesting that RNA folding in this region may be important in determining host tissue tropism[14].

The introduction of the inactivated Salk poliovirus vaccine in the USA in the 1950s produced a sharp decline in the number of cases of poliomyelitis. However, inactivated poliovirus vaccine has a number of specific disadvantages, the most important being that it fails to prevent gastrointestinal infection. Although the individual is protected, the absence of vaccine replication in the gut means that the vaccine virus cannot be disseminated in the community in the same way as attenuated vaccines, and it is therefore less efficient in controlling spread in endemic areas. Booster doses are required, and although such vaccines generally stimulate good levels of circulating antibody they are generally considered less efficient in stimulating T cell responses and immunological memory. There are also associated problems in manufacture; considerably more antigenic material is required for an immunizing dose, leading to an increase in cost. There is also a requirement for an adjuvant.

Inactivated vaccines are prepared from whole virus that has been chemically treated, usually by a low concentration of formaldehyde, in order to prevent further infectivity. Considerable care needs to be exercised, however, in order that the immunogenic potential of the viral protein is not impaired and that the virus is monodisperse at the time of treatment. Rigorous methods for detecting residual infectivity are also necessary. Problems occur rarely, the most publicized case being the occurrence of paralytic disease in some recipients of early batches of poliovirus vaccine due to failure of chemical inactivation[15]. Problems can also arise with the potency of individual subtypes in the vaccine. This is well-illustrated by the outbreak of poliomyelitis in Finland in 1984–1985, a country that has only used inactivated poliovirus vaccine. A drop in the potency of type 3 (less than 305 of vaccinees had anti-type 3 antibodies) led to a large number of infections from an imported wild-type 3 virus[16].

Inactivated vaccines may also have a deleterious effect on vaccinees subsequently exposed to wild-type virus. A formalin-inactivated measles vaccine gave short-lived immunity in children, and on exposure to infectious virus these individuals developed a clinically more serious illness[17]. This appeared due to the fact that the immunogenicity of the fusion protein (F) in the measles vaccine was markedly reduced as a result of the inactivation process compared to the more resistant haemagglutinin, or H protein. This meant that the recipients responded quickly to the H protein on exposure to wild-type virus, leading to an accentuation of the immunopathology of the disease not held in check by effective immunity to the F protein as a result of its absence from the vaccine. Similar difficulties have also been experienced with the development of an inactivated vaccine against another paramyxovirus, the respiratory syncytial virus (RSV). In a clinical trial among children conducted in the 1960s, an inactivated RSV vaccine failed to induce protection despite the presence of neutralizing antibodies. More serious was a higher frequency of severe lower respiratory tract disease in vaccine recipients[18]. Once again, the selective abolition of an important immunogenic component primed the host such that on infection an accelerated immune response to non-protective antigens developed, leading to an enhanced immunopathology.

HEPATITIS B: AN EXAMPLE OF A SUCCESSFUL SUBUNIT VACCINE

Hepatitis B is a global public health problem, with an estimated 300 million asymptomatic carriers world-wide. This reservoir of infection is maintained largely by the transmission of the hepatitis B virus (HBV) to infants born to carrier mothers. Unusually for virus infections, HBV produces a vast excess of envelope protein in the liver; this is assembled into 22 nm surface antigen-positive (HBsAg) particles. The implications of this are two-fold. First, because of shared antigenic determinants the presence of HBV can be detected by serological tests. Second, plasma from asymptomatic carriers can be used as a source of immunogen. The virtual absence of *in vitro* culture systems for HBV stimulated the exploitation of native antigen proteins as human vaccines. These 'first generation' hepatitis B vaccines are prepared by the initial separation of HBsAg particles from virions present in plasma and then by rigorous chemical treatment to ensure the biological safety of the final product. These have been largely replaced, however, by HBsAg particles expressed in yeast, representing the first human vaccine product that has become widely available as a result of gene cloning technology (Figure 1).

Protection against HBV correlates, at least in part, with the appearance

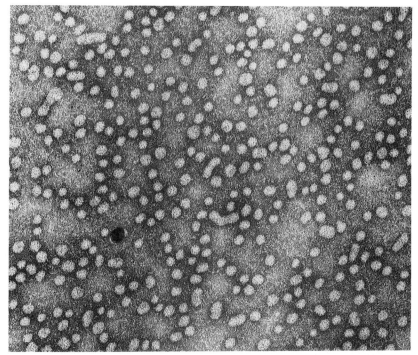

Figure 1 Electron micrograph of hepatitis B surface antigen (HBsAg), the major constituent of hepatitis B vaccines. These 22 nm particles bear protective antigens that are also present on hepatitis B virus particles, and may be expressed in yeast and other expression systems (micrograph courtesy of Dr PR Young)

of antibody to HBsAg (anti-HBs), the major constituent being the S protein (molecular weight 25 400) and its glycosylated form (molecular weight 30 000) cross-linked via disulphide bonds. Antibodies to the *a* determinants confers protection, whereas antibodies to the subtype determinants do not. A model of the predicted secondary structure of the S protein is shown in Figure 2.

The collective experience since 1976 in over 30 million recipients of hepatitis B vaccine has highlighted some general features relevant to the potential use of other recombinant products. For example, subunit vaccines are highly immunogenic in man if correctly presented to the immune system, and protection may last as long as 10 years[19]. In common with inactivated vaccines, full immunity requires multiple injections over a period as long as 6 months, and individuals with natural or acquired immunodeficiency states respond poorly. Contrary to early expectations of induced tolerance, it is clear that such vaccines can be administered in the first few days of life. This is an important observation, as subunit vaccines could be used in place of live attenuated vaccines against infections such as measles for immunization before the age of six months, when maternal antibody restricts the growth of live vaccines. Attempts to immunize infants at 6 months rather than at 9

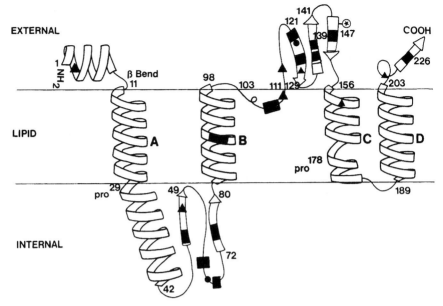

Figure 2 Predicted secondary structure of the major S protein of hepatitis B virus. The 226 amino acid protein has at least four transmembrane helices, with the protective antigens being located on hydrophilic regions between amino acids 120 and 150 (modified from Stirk et al[62])

months of age using a high-dose attenuated measles vaccine leads to an increase rather than a decrease in the risk of disease on exposure to wild-type virus.

Seroconversion rates to hepatitis B vaccines vary between 85% and 100% in healthy adults, declining thereafter with increasing age. Weight also appears to be a critical factor, with diminished responses in obese individuals under the age of 30. The longevity of the anti-HBs response is related to the level of antibodies present in the serum 4–6 weeks after the final vaccine dose: circulating antibody persists for 3 years or more in successfully vaccinated persons[20]. As there is a marked increase in antibody titre after the final dose, completion of the vaccination schedule is critical in order to confer full immunity, probably as the immune response matures over this period to conformational epitopes on HBsAg particles. The appearance of anti-HBs antibodies at a level of ⩾ 10 mIU/ml has long been regarded as a minimum level of protection. Extensive retrospective studies suggest that evidence of asymptomatic infection may occur in recipients with antibody levels < 20 mIU/ml; the need for a minimum level of antibody is reinforced by epidemiological data indicating that prevention of asymptomatic infections as opposed to clinical disease depends on a minimum titre of antibody. Some now argue that this is not important and may serve to stimulate an improved level of protection; however, epidemiological studies have shown that the chronic persistent carrier state develops more often from anicteric infections.

The predominant subclass of anti-HBs antibody in vaccine recipients is

IgG1 and this subclass shows the highest affinity for HBsAg[21]. However, there is a more even distribution of anti-Bs antibodies across the IgG subclasses in those naturally immune to HBV. In general terms, it is beginning to be appreciated that vaccines induce a somewhat different profile of IgG subclasses to that seen in natural immunity. The significance of this is unclear, although differences in the biological activities of the specific antibodies may be expected. Antibodies to envelope proteins of other viruses are predominantly IgG1, whereas other subclasses are more substantially represented in response to nucleocapsid proteins. The findings suggest that antibody subclass is controlled by the method of antigen presentation, which in turn depends upon the choice of adjuvant.

There is some suggestion that individuals with HLA-D7 and lacking D1 respond less well than others[22]. Few data are available, however, as to the nature of the deficiency in non-responding vaccine recipients — indeed the role of cellular immunity in generating both B and T cell protective responses is not clear. Approximately one-third of such individuals respond to a later booster dose, albeit with only low levels of antibody. This is in marked contrast to individuals who respond to the initial vaccination; these respond promptly to revaccination, producing levels of anti-HBs in excess of those obtained by primary immunization[23]. This boosting effect is observed even in persons whose antibody has waned below the level of detection for several years. This demonstrates the existence of immunological memory to the vaccine over this period and indicates that such persons will probably be protected from subsequent exposure to infection. However, a booster dose is advisable; apart from the reassurance of circulating antibodies, it is still not clear how long immunological memory lasts.

Non-responsiveness to hepatitis B vaccine is considerably more common in patients with acquired or inherited immunodeficiency states. In particular, seroconversion rates in patients on maintenance dialysis are <63% with many showing anti-HBs titres below the desired level for protection. The response rate may be improved considerably by the use of vaccine containing additional HBV pre-S antigenic specificities[24]. Individuals affected with HIV also respond poorly to the vaccine.

Infants born to mothers persistently infected with HBV have a ⩾90% risk of infection during the first year of life; more than 85% of these infections become persistent, and consequently add to the number of asymptomatic carriers in the population. Infants respond well to hepatitis B vaccines, and the vaccine is often administered with a specific immunoglobulin, with the result that the rate of chronic infection in these immunized infants falls to <10%. The reason for the apparent failure of prophylaxis in one-fifth of this group is not clear, but it is most likely that these infants were exposed to the virus prior to immunization, possibly having acquired the infection *in utero*. A small but significant number of HBV variants have appeared as a result of the combined use of vaccine and immunoglobulin, monoclonal antibodies, or vaccine alone. The majority have occurred in children and are associated with asymptomatic hepatitis B virus infection, which results from a change in amino acid composition at position 145 in the S gene. This amino acid substitution of a glycine for an arginine residue in the *a* determinant abrogates the protective effect of anti-HBs antibodies induced by the vaccine[25]. A second mutation of the immunodominant lysine at position 141 for glutamic acid has been found in approximately 8% of children receiving vaccine alone as part of a childhood immunization programme in The Gambia[26].

NEWER APPROACHES TO VACCINE DEVELOPMENT

The development of hepatitis B vaccines using recombinant DNA technology is now serving as a benchmark for the production of other genetically engineered vaccine products. The HBV S gene has now been expressed in a number of transfected cell types, in particular yeast (*Saccharomyces cerevisiae*). The expressed HBsAg particles elicit anti-HBs antibodies in man indistinguishable in specificity from those induced by the plasma-derived products. Drawbacks of this technology include the need to rupture the host cell in order to release antigen, its purification, and the need to constantly monitor the expression vector for any mutations that may affect the immunogenicity of the final product. This means that such recombinant vaccines are relatively expensive to produce. Expression systems using mammalian cells are under development for hepatitis B and other vaccines which circumvent some of the difficulties associated with expression in yeast. One particular advantage is that secreted antigens can be purified from the cell culture supernatant and the product is fully glycosylated where appropriate. The baculovirus system is an alternative source of antigens, having the advantage of greater yields of expressed protein per cell. This has been used to advantage for the production of HBsAg[27] and the gp120 protein of HIV[28,29].

Improved antigen presentation systems

Subunit vaccines, such as those against influenza and hepatitis B, require the use of immunological adjuvants. The only adjuvant accepted for human use at present is alum, although this is of limited effectiveness with influenza haemagglutinin and does not stimulate cell-mediated responses. Several alternative approaches have been explored. The first is the use of phospholipid vesicles (liposomes) whereby the immunogens become trapped within multi-lamellar structures[30]. Liposomes are biodegradable and non-toxic, with the added advantage that other substances with adjuvanting properties can be included, such as interleukin-2.

An alternative strategy is the use of saponins to form immune stimulating complexes (iscoms). These consist of quillaic acid in micelle form around which the immunogen becomes complexed[31]. Iscoms show remarkable properties compared to conventional vaccines. For example, HBsAg reformulated into iscoms and delivered in saline induces much greater levels of anti-HBs antibodies in mice than does conventional vaccine and these responses are sustained for considerably longer[32]. As with liposomes, iscoms can overcome genetic restriction of animals to mount an immune response.

Although it has long been thought that subunit vaccines cannot induce class I-restricted cellular responses, recent work with HIV iscoms has shown that gp160-iscoms elicit cytotoxic T cells in mice[33].

One of the major difficulties in the use of inactivated and subunit vaccines is the need for multiple doses in order to achieve and maintain effective levels of immunity. The development of so-called controlled release vaccines which enable all necessary doses to be delivered in a time-dependent fashion is now considered possible. Using polymers of lactic and glycolic acids, for example, it is possible to microencapsulate antigens for delivery such that the rate and time of release can be controlled by adjusting the ratio of the two polymers. Thus a single dose may contain several microencapsulation formulations designed to mimic primary and secondary immunizations[34].

The use of virus vaccine vectors

The introduction into carriers of genes coding for protective antigens is a natural extension of expression of such proteins by recombinant DNA technology. Work in this area falls into two general categories: first, the use of live vectors such as vaccinia and adenovirus, the genomes of which can accommodate substantial quantities of foreign DNA, and second, subunit vehicles consisting of heterologous epitopes expressed together with the carrier protein. Here among the two most promising vehicles are hepatitis B virus nucleocapsids and HBsAg particles.

Vaccinia virus has a large double-stranded DNA genome of about 185 kb, approximately 14% of which is non-essential for replication, and can be replaced with foreign genes under the control of vaccinia promoters. A plasmid containing the foreign gene, relevant promoters, a selectable marker, and flanking sequences homologous to the vaccinia genome can be introduced into cells infected with virus; double recombination is mediated by the flanking sequences of the plasmid with the result that the foreign gene is inserted precisely into the viral genome. A considerable range of viral and other foreign antigens have now been expressed in recombinant vaccinia virus[35]. The principal reservation regarding the use of vaccinia virus-based vaccines includes the frequency of complications, as high as 1 in 1000 with some strains, the restriction of their use to populations non-immune to vaccinia, and the probable single use of such a vaccine in each individual. The question of complications, however, is likely to yield to efforts designed to reduce the virulence of the most useful vaccinia virus strains. In addition to these concerns, laboratory studies in chimpanzees have shown that the level of immunity induced does not always give complete protection. Although the use of vaccine vectors can be argued for certain diseases, such as those associated with high mortality that affect a limited number of individuals, this approach is unlikely to be of value for diseases that can be effectively controlled by other vaccine candidates. However, a number of experimental veterinary vaccines using recombinant vaccinia have given remarkable results; recombinant vaccinia virus expressing the rabies glycoprotein has been given in fox bait[36] and extensive trials are underway in Africa to control rinderpest[37].

A similar strategy has been adopted for the insertion of foreign genes into adenovirus[38]. These viruses have been used for several decades to protect military recruits from respiratory disease; however, the virus used is not attenuated and must be delivered orally, contained within gelatin capsules. This limits the usefulness of the approach. There is also some concern regarding the role of the E1A gene which is known to act as a proto-oncogene in cellular transformation of cultured cells.

Several RNA viruses also offer promise as live vectors. Live attenuated strains of poliovirus have been used to make chimaeric particles containing neutralizing epitopes from heterologous serotypes of foreign linear determinants. This work is based on the finding that poliovirus cDNA is infectious in culture, and recombination is therefore possible by simultaneous transfection with appropriately constructed plasmids containing the sequence coding for the foreign antigen. Although many of the poliovirus-neutralizing epitopes are discontinuous, one region of the VP1 molecule forms a surface loop structure that can be replaced with heterologous epitopes[39]. In addition to the introduction of the respective type 3 sequence into the more stable type 1 particle[40], some success has also been achieved with introducing HIV sequences[41]. Other possibilities for vectors include yellow fever virus; again the prior demonstration of infectious cDNA is necessary[42].

Macromolecular carriers

There are a number of advantages in the use of short peptide fragments bearing B cell epitopes relevant for protection. However, these must often be linked to larger carrier molecules which provide T helper cell epitopes necessary for stimulating anti-peptide antibodies. Traditionally, the approach has been to link such peptides either by chemical means to carrier proteins such as tetanus toxoid, or to express these as fusion proteins contiguous with a larger molecule, such as *E. coli* β-galactosidase. It has become clear, however, that there are alternative carriers which give an enhanced level of immunogenicity. One of these is the inner core of HBV, serologically referred to as HBcAg.

Hepatitis B cores consist of a major polypeptide of molecular weight 22 000 which readily assembles into a 27 nm particle with a predicted tertiary structure similar to that of the picornaviruses[43]. The addition of a short segment representing residues 141–160 of the VP1 protein of foot-and-mouth disease virus at the amino terminus gave a 200-fold increase in antibody response on a weight for weight basis compared to the same sequence expressed as a fusion protein with β-galactosidase[44]. The core particles have a single immunodominant B cell antigenic determinant; replacement with a foreign epitope is possible, with the added advantage that the particles no longer elicit anti-HBc antibodies but retain the epitopes recognized by T helper cells.

Anti-idiotypes and synthetic peptides

Two further approaches to hepatitis B vaccination are of wider interest, both of which offer the opportunity to precisely manipulate the immune response in terms of enhancement or suppression. The first is the use of anti-idiotype antibodies bearing internal images of protective epitopes and the second, the use of short synthetic peptides mimicking similar epitopes on the virus surface. Both offer the opportunity to use molecules that represent single, defined epitopes that are able to substitute for antigen ('surrogate antigens'). A proportion of anti-idiotype antibodies contain within the hypervariable region an internal image that resembles a surface determinant on the original antigen with respect to recognition by antibody. Although internal image anti-idiotype antibodies may stimulate B cells of high affinity to HBsAg[45] these antibodies elicit a more restricted range of B cell responses than do synthetic peptides. Such a surrogate vaccine would consist of either a single peptide containing a number of B cell epitopes together with appropriate T helper cell sites or a cluster of monoclonal internal image anti-idiotypes.

Synthetic peptide analogues of protective antigens have a number of unique advantages as immunogens, in addition to safety and economic considerations. These include the ability to direct the immune response to very localized regions of the viral protein, particularly conserved regions of proteins which are 'immunosilent' in the native molecule, and the capacity to generate new peptide sequences as a consequence of changes in the viral proteins in the face of increasing herd immunity. Ideally, synthetic peptide vaccines should mimic the continuous or discontinuous epitopes that are important for the induction of an effective immune response and also contain a sequence that may act as an adjuvant[46]. It is this latter requirement that at present is hampering peptide vaccine development. Perhaps the best experimental example of an effective synthetic peptide immunogen is the immunization of cattle with a peptide analogue of residues 131–160 of the VP1 protein of foot-and-mouth disease virus[47]. The success achieved with this immunogen appears due to the extreme flexibility of this region of the virus VP1 polypeptide[48]. With short peptide sequences, however, there has been concern that a cross-reactive response against host tissues will be induced and that escape mutants could arise which are non-reactive owing to the restricted specificity of the anti-peptide antibodies for the native protein. These fears have been largely unfounded, although caution is still needed and animal experiments still need to be extended to human use by careful selection of adjuvants and carrier molecules.

PROSPECTS FOR HIV VACCINES

The development of an effective HIV vaccine for human use is perceived at present as being a major priority in vaccine research. The rational design of such a vaccine, however, is made more difficult by our failure to understand fully what constitutes protective immunity: unlike many viral diseases successfully controlled by immunization, the development of natural immunity in the course of HIV infection does not correlate with protection. Attenuated vaccines are not likely to be accepted and, as already indicated for flavivirus infections, there is evidence that induction of certain antibodies may actually be harmful, leading to a potentiation of virus growth. Vaccinologists are also confronted with a number of other problems; the inherent antigenic variability of HIV, even in the same infected individual, virus latency, cell-to-cell spread, and above all the propensity of HIV to infect cells of the immune system. Antibody to the envelope glycoprotein gp120 can lyse T cells or inhibit their function, and infection of CD4$^+$ T cells can trigger antibody-dependent cellular cytotoxicity against uninfected CD4$^+$ cells.

A number of sites on gp120 have been characterized as potential antigens for stimulating immunity, the most important of which is the so-called 'V3 loop'. This is a disulphide-bridged loop of 35 amino acids with a β-sheet and a conserved gly-pro-gly sequence at its centre[49]. This antigenic domain is known to induce neutralizing antibodies, the levels of which are lower in patients with terminal disease than in those with much longer expected survival times. Unfortunately, the amino acid sequence shows hypervariability on either side of the GPG tip and as a result antibody is strictly type-specific. One way round this problem may be to induce antibodies to conserved sequences elsewhere on gp120. However, such conserved domains are only weakly immunogenic in the native envelope structure[50]. This could be overcome either by the use of short synthetic peptide analogues of these regions or by inserting the conserved sequences into other protein carriers, such as hepatitis B core protein[44] or poliovirus[41], but neither have been tested in humans.

All of the experimental approaches outlined above have been explored in the production of possible HIV immunogens. Testing of candidate immunogens presents some difficulties: the chimpanzee is the only practical species for their evaluation, and this species does not develop an AIDS-like illness on infection with HIV. Nevertheless a number of products have been examined, including recombinant vaccinia, expressing gp120 protein and its precursor gp160, and synthetic peptide analogues of the V3 loop. Some success has been achieved with these preparations, although the dose of challenge appears critical, as does the need for the gp120 protein to be cleaved from its precursor. The high degree of sequence variation also poses problems. There are at least five variable regions in the gp120 envelope glycoprotein molecule including the V3 region. Not only do isolates from different geographical locations show variable amino acid sequences in these domains, but isolates from the same individual over a period of time may also show changes, albeit to a lesser extent. The presence of neutralizing antibodies does not prevent disease progression *in vivo*[51]. An effective vaccine may require, therefore, a more extensive repertoire of epitopes, particularly those dependent on conformation. Identifying features of the immune response that allow viruses to escape the immediate effects of neutralizing antibody is a major obstacle in designing vaccines against diseases such as HIV.

Recently, attention has turned to the use of the simian immunodeficiency virus (SIV), which is related to the HIV-2 found predominantly in West

Africa. The advantage of this model system is that SIV produces a disease in rhesus macaques that is very similar to that seen in humans[52]. Also the sequence in the V3 loop of SIV gp120 appears to undergo considerably less variation. There is some encouragement that an inactivated SIV vaccine may induce protection; experimental results range from a delay in infection and disease[53] to complete protection in the majority of immunized animals[54]. As with all vaccines, route of administration, antigenic dose and type of adjuvant are all factors that may determine the extent of protective efficacy.

Clinical trials in humans have proceeded with a number of candidate vaccines in advance of evidence of efficacy being obtained from animal studies. Most notable are the trials involving recombinant vaccinia virus vectors, but studies are also in progress with gp120/gp160 subunit preparations and peptides mimicking a region of the capsid protein *gag*. The parameters being quantified so far relate to the immunogenicity and safety of these preparations, particularly with respect to any possible immunosuppression. To date there has not been any cause for concern on these issues: the immunogens have been well tolerated and shown to induce anti-HIV antibodies. Although there have also been attempts to use vaccinia virus recombinants in HIV-positive individuals, it is clear that the development of HIV vaccines has to proceed in a rational and clearly defined manner, and the factors necessary for protection must first be defined in the macaque model.

INTRACELLULAR IMMUNIZATION

Strategies described so far assume that effective vaccines stimulate an immune response capable of either preventing the insertion of viral genomes into host cells or stimulating a class I-restricted cytotoxic T cell response to eliminate foci of established infection. The major challenge now is to control virus infections that have either become established prior to the development of an effective B cell response or that by their very nature diminish the efficacy of the host's cytotoxic T cells.

The term intracellular immunization was first coined by Baltimore[55], who proposed that cells could be infected with an altered virus that would interfere with the replication and spread of HIV. This could work by a number of ways, for example by introducing mutant viruses into cells that expressed altered trans-dominant proteins that would make new particles non-infectious: there is a precedence for this in that many RNA viruses produce defective interfering particles, particularly when the multiplicity of infection is high. These require help from the parental virus and their presence can reduce the number of standard virus particles produced. The effect of introducing interfering particles may have immunological as well as molecular benefits, for example influenza defective interfering particles modulate the specific humoral immune response[56].

Alternatively, designer RNA molecules can be introduced which bind viral nucleoproteins in preference to the native genome and which block assembly or bind in an anti-sense fashion to genome sequences, thus preventing gene expression and/or replication. The introduction of RNA that can cleave viral RNA (ribozymes) is an alternative approach that is particularly attractive in treatment of HIV[57] and other persistent virus infections[58].

Intracellular immunization using naked DNA is an alternative means of producing antigens without the need to express the protein *in vitro*. Wolff *et al.*[59] discovered that direct intramuscular immunization of mice with plasmid DNA containing a strong promoter of gene expression resulted in persistent expression of the gene in striated muscle at the site of injection. This initial work has been taken further with the observations that protective immunity to influenza haemagglutinin[60] and nucleoprotein[61] can be induced by direct inoculation of plasmid DNA into chickens and mice, respectively. The advantages are clear: there is no need to inoculate an infectious genome, plasmid DNA is stable, and probably most importantly of all, the expressed protein can provide a large array of potential epitopes for sampling by different MHC alleles. This would have considerable advantages over synthetic peptide-based vaccines, although fresh questions would then arise as to how long antigen expression would remain, the probability of induced immune dysregulation and regulatory concerns over the introduction of recombinant DNA molecules directly into the host.

A successful outcome will undoubtedly benefit vaccine research in many other areas and decrease the necessity of the serendipitous approach characteristic of vaccine development since the times of Jenner and Pasteur.

References

1. Minor PD, Evans DMA, Ferguson M, Schild GC, Westrop G, Almond JW. Principal and subsidiary antigenic sites of VP1 involved in the neutralisation of poliovirus type 3. J Gen Virol. 1985; 65: 1159–1165.
2. Schlesinger JJ, Brandriss MW, Cropp CB, Monath TP. Protection against yellow fever virus nonstructural protein NS1. J Virol. 1986; 60: 1153–1155.
3. Wiley DC, Skehel JJ. The structure and function of the haemagglutinin membrane glycoprotein of influenza virus. Annu Rev Biochem. 1987; 56: 365–394.
4. Halstead SB. Pathogenesis of dengue: challenges to molecular biology. Science. 1988; 239: 476–481.
5. Takeda A, Ennis FA, Sweet RA. Model for enhancement of HIV-1 infection by antibody. In: Brown F, Channock RM, Ginsberg HS, Lerner RA, eds. Vaccines 90: modern approaches to new vaccines including the prevention of AIDS. New York: Cold Spring Harbor, 1989: 333–337.
6. Hurwitz JL, Hackett CJ, McAndrew EC, Gerhard W. Murine Th response to influenza virus: Recognition of haemagglutinin, Neuraminidase, matrix and nucleoproteins. J Immunol. 1985; 134: 1994–1998.
7. Scherle PA, Gerhard W. Functional analysis of influenza-specific helper T cell clones *in vivo*: T cell specific for internal proteins provide cognate help for B cell responses to haemagglutinin. J Exp Med. 1986; 164: 1114–1128.
8. World Health Organisation. Status report on polio eradication. World Immunization News. 1992; 8: 16–17.
9. Theiler M. The virus. In: Strode GK, ed. Yellow fever. New York: McGraw-Hill, 1951: 39–137.
10. Nakano JH, Hatch MH, Thieme ML, Nottay B. Parameters for differentiating vaccine-derived and wild poliovirus strains. Prog Med Virol. 1978; 24: 178–206.
11. Linneman CC, Hutchinson L, Rotte TC, Hegg ME, Schiff GM. Stability of the rabbit immunogenic marker of RA 27/3 rubella vaccine virus after human passage. Infect Immun.

1974; 9: 547–549.

12. Provost PJ, Emini EA, Lewis JA, Gerety RJ. Progress towards the development of a hepatitis A vaccine. In: Zuckerman AJ, ed. Viral hepatitis and liver disease. New York: Alan R Liss, 1988: 83–86.

13. Purcell RH. Approaches to immunization against hepatitis A virus. In: Hollinger FB, Lemon SM, Margolis HS, eds. Viral hepatitis and liver disease. Baltimore: Williams and Wilkins, 1991: 41–46.

14. Evans DMA, Dunn G, Minor PD, Schild GC, Cann AJ, Stanway G, Almond JW, Currey K, Maizel JV. Increased neurovirulence associated with a single nucleotide change in a noncoding region of the Sabin type 3 poliovirus vaccine. Nature. 1985; 314: 548–550.

15. Nathanson N, Langmuir AD. The Cutter incident. Poliomyelitis following formaldehyde-inactivated poliovirus vaccination in the United States. Am J Hyg. 1963; 78: 16–28.

16. Hovi T, Huovilainen A, Kuronen T, Poyry T, Salama N, Cantell K, Kinnumen E, Lapinleimu K, Roivainen M, Stenvik M, Silander A, Thoden C-J, Salminen S, Weckstrom P. Outbreak of poliomyelitis in Finland: Widespread circulation of antigenically altered poliovirus type 3 in a vaccinated population. Lancet. 1986; i: 1427–1432.

17. Fulginiti VA, Eller JJ, Downie AW, Kempe CH. Atypical measles in children previously immunised with inactivated measles virus vaccine. JAMA. 1967; 202: 1075–1080.

18. Kapikian AZ, Mitchell RH, Chanock RM, Shvedoff RA, Stewart CE. An epidemiologic study of altered clinical reactivity to respiratory syncytial (RS) virus infection in children previously vaccinated with an inactivated RS virus vaccine. Am J Epidemiol. 1969; 89: 404–421.

19. Hadler SC, Francis DP, Maynard JE, Thompson SE, Judson FN, Echenberg DF, Ostrow DG, O'Malley PM, Penley KA, Altman NL, Braff E, Shipman GF, Coleman PJ, Madel EJ. Long-term immunogenicity and efficacy of hepatitis B vaccine in homosexual men. New Engl J Med. 1986; 315: 209–214.

20. Jilg W, Schmidt M, Deinhardt F. Decline of anti-HBs after hepatitis B vaccination and timing of revaccination. Lancet. 1990; 335: 173–174.

21. Persson MAA, Brown SE, Steward MW, Hammarstrom L, Smith CIE, Howard CR. Binding characteristics of human specific antibodies of the various IgG subclasses. J Immunol. 1988; 140: 3875–3879.

22. Dienstag JL. Immunologic mechanisms in chronic hepatitis. In: Vyas GN, Dienstag JL, Hoofnagle JH, eds. Viral hepatitis and liver disease. New York: Grune and Stratton, 1984: 135.

23. Jilg W, Schmidt M, Deinhardt F. Immune responses to hepatitis B vaccination. J Med Virol. 1988; 24: 377–384.

24. Coursaget P, Adamowicz P, Bourdil C, Yvonnet B, Buisson Y, Barres J-L, Saliou P, Chiron J-P, Mar ID. Anti-preS2 antibodies in natural hepatitis B virus infection and after immunisation. Vaccine. 1988; 6: 357–361.

25. Harrison TJ, Valliammai T, Hopes EA, Oor CJ, Zuckerman AJ. A hepatitis B virus antibody escape mutant from Singapore. J Gastroenterol Hepatol. 1993; 8: S80–S82.

26. Karthigesu V, Allison LMC, Fortuin M, Mendy M, Whittle HC, Howard CR. A novel hepatitis B variant in the sera of immunised children. J Gen Virol. 1994; 75: 443–448.

27. Lanford RE, Luckow V, Kennedy RC, Dreesman GR, Notvall L, Summers MD. Expression and characterisation of hepatitis B virus surface antigen polypeptides in insect cells with a baculovirus expression system. J Virol. 1989; 63: 1549–1557.

28. Hu S-L, Kosowski SG, Schaaf KF. Expression of envelope glycoproteins of human immunodeficiency virus by an insect virus vector. J Virol. 1987; 61: 3617–3620.

29. Rusche JR, Lynn DL, Robert-Guroff M, Langlois AJ, Lyerly HK, Carson H, Krohn K, Ranki A, Gallo RC, Bolognesi DP, Putney SD, Matthews TJ. Humoral response to the entire human immunodeficiency virus envelope glycoprotein made in insect cells. Proc Natl Acad Sci USA. 1987; 64: 6924–6928.

30. Gregoriados G. Immunological adjuvants: a role for liposomes. Immunol Today. 1990; 11: 89–97.

31. Höglund S, Dalsgaard K, Lövgren K, Sundquist B, Osterhaus A, Morein B. ISCOMs and immunostimulation with viral antigens. In: Harris JR, ed. Subcellular biochemistry, vol. 15: virally-infected cells. New York: Plenum, 1989: 39–68.

32. Howard CR, Frew A, Sundquist B, Morein B. Iscoms (immune-stimulating complexes) and

the presentation of synthetic peptides. In: Meheus A, Spier RA, eds. Vaccines for sexually-transmitted diseases. London: Butterworths, 1989: 134–138.

33. Takahashi H, Takeshita T, Morein B, Putney S, Germain RN, Berzofsky JA. Induction of CD8[+] cytotoxic T cells by immunisation with purified HIV-1 envelope protein in ISCOMS. Nature. 1990; 344: 873–875.

34. Eldridge JH, Staas JK, Meulbrook JA, McGhee JR, Tice TR, Gilley RM. Biodegradable microspheres as a vaccine delivery system. Mol Immunol. 1991; 28: 287–294.

35. Moss B, Flexner C. Vaccinia virus expression vectors. Annu Rev Immunol. 1987; 5: 305–324.

36. Blancou J, Kieny MP, Lathe R, Lecocq JP, Pastoret PP, Soulebat JP, Desmettre P. Oral vaccination of the fox against rabies using a live vaccinia virus. Nature. 1986; 322: 373–375.

37. Yilma T, Hsu D, Jones L, Owen S, Grubman M, Mebus C. Protection of cattle against rinderpest with vaccinia recombinants expressing the HA or F gene. Science. 1988; 242: 1058–1061.

38. Morin JE, Lubeck MD, Barton JE, Conley AJ, Davies AR, Hung PP. Recombinant adenovirus induces antibody response to hepatitis B surface antigen in hamsters. Proc Natl Acad Sci USA. 1987; 84: 4625–4630.

39. Stanway G, Hughes PJ, Westrop GD, Evans DMA, Dunn G, Minor PD, Schild GC, Almond JW. Construction of poliovirus intertypic recombinants by use of cDNA. J Virol. 1986; 57: 1187–1190.

40. Burke KL, Dunn G, Ferguson M, Minor PD, Almond JW. Antigen chimeras of poliovirus as potential new vaccines. Nature. 1988; 332: 81–82.

41. Evans D, Mckeating J, Meredith J, Burke KL, Matrak K, Johns A, Minor PD, Weiss RA. An engineered poliovirus chimaera with broadly reactive HIV-1 neutralising antibodies. Nature. 1989; 339: 385–387.

42. Rice CM, Grakoui A, Galler R, Chambers TJ. Transcription of infectious yellow fever virus RNA from full-length cDNA templates produced by *in vitro* ligation. New Biol. 1990; 1: 1–25.

43. Argos P, Fuller S. A model for the hepatitis B virus core protein: prediction of antigenic sites and relationship to RNA virus capsid proteins. EMBO J. 1988; 7: 819–824.

44. Clarke BE, Newton SE, Carroll AR, Francis MJ, Appleyard G, Syned AD, Highfield PE, Rowlands DJ, Brown F. Improved immunogenicity of a peptide epitope after fusion to hepatitis B core protein. Nature. 1987; 330: 81–82.

45. Thanavala YM, Brown SE, Howard CR, Roitt IM, Steward MW. A surrogate hepatitis B virus antigenic epitope represented by a synthetic peptide and an internal image anti-idiotype antibody. J Exp Med. 1986; 164: 227–236.

46. Steward MW, Howard CR. Synthetic peptides: a next generation of vaccines? Immunol Today. 1987; 8: 51–58.

47. Bittle JL, Houghton RA, Alexander H, Schinnick TM, Sutcliffe JG, Lerner RA, Rowlands DJ, Brown F. Protection against foot and mouth disease virus by immunisation with a chemically synthesised protein predicted from the viral nucleotide sequence. Nature. 1982; 298: 30–33.

48. Achaya R, Fry E, Stuart DI, Fox G, Rowlands DJ, Brown F. The three-dimensional structure of foot-and-mouth disease virus at 2.9Å. Nature. 1989; 337: 709–716.

49. LaRosa GJ, Davide JP, Weinhold K, Waterbury JA, Profy AT, Lewis JA, Langlois AJ, Dressman GR, Boswell RN, Shadduck P, Holley LH, Karplus M, Bolognesi DP, Matthews TJ, Emini EA, Putney SD. Conserved sequence and structural elements in HIV-1 principal neutralisation determinant. Science. 1990; 249: 932–935.

50. Guyander M, Emerman M, Sonigo P, Clavel F, Montagnier I, Alizon M. (1987). Genome and organisation and transactivation of the human immunodeficiency virus type 2. Nature. 1987; 326: 662–669.

51. von Gegerfelt A, Albert J, Morfeldt-Manson L, Broliden K, Fenyo EM. Isolate-specific neutralising antibodies in patients with progressive HIV-1 related disease. Virology. 1991; 185: 12–168.

52. Letvin N, Daniel M, Sehgal P, Desrosiers RC, Hunt RD, Waldron LM, Mackey JJ, Schmidt DK, Chalifoux LV, King NM. Induction of AIDS-like disease in Macaque monkeys with T-cell tropic retrovirus. STLV-III. Science. 1985; 230: 71–73.

53. Sutjipto S, Pederson NC, Gardner MB, Hanson CV, Gettie A, Jennings M, Higgins J, Marx PA. Inactivated simian immunodeficiency virus vaccine failed to protect rhesus macaques from intravenous or genital mucosal infection but delayed disease in intravenously exposed animals. J Virol. 1990; 64: 2290–2297.
54. Murphey-Corb M, Martin LN, Davidson-Fairburn B, Montelaro RC, Miller M, West M, Ohkawa S, Baskin GB, Zhang JY, Putney SD, Allison AC, Eppstein DA. A formalin-inactivated whole SIV vaccine confers protection in macaques. Science. 1987; 246: 1293–1297.
55. Baltimore D. Intracellular immunisation. Nature. 1988; 335: 395–396.
56. Marcus PI, Gaccione C. Interferon induction by viruses. XIX. Vesicular stomatitis virus-New Jersey: High multiplicity passages generate interferon-inducing, defective-interfering particles. Virology. 1989; 171: 630–633.
57. Sarver N, Cantin EM, Chang PS, Zaia JA, Ladne PA, Stephens DA, Rossi JJ. Ribozymes as potential anti-HIV1 therapeutic agents. Science. 1990; 247: 1222–1225.
58. Xing Z, Whitton JL. An anti-lymphocytic choriomeningitis virus ribozyme expressed in tissue culture cells diminishes viral RNA levels and leads to a reduction in infectious virus yield. J Virol. 1993; 67: 1840–1847.
59. Wolff JA, Malone P, Williams WCG, Acsadi A, Jani A, Felger PL. Direct gene transfer into mouse muscle in vivo. Science. 1990; 247: 1465–1468.
60. Robinson HL, Hunt LA, Webster RG. Protection against a lethal influenza virus challenge by immunization with a haemagglutinin-expressing plasmid DNA. Vaccine. 1993; 11: 957–960.
61. Ulmer JB, Donnelly JJ, Parker SE, Rhodes GH, Felger PL, Dwarki VJ, Gromkowski SH, Deck BR, DeWitt CM, Friedman A, Haw LA, Leander KR, Martinez D, Perry HC, Shiver JW, Montgomery DL, Liu MA. Heterologous protection against influenza by injection of DNA encoding a viral protein. Science. 1993; 259: 1745–1749.
62. Stirk HJ, Thornton J, Howard CR. A topological model of hepatitis B surface antigen. Intervirology. 1992; 33: 148–158.

Index

Immunology and Medicine Series

1. A.M. McGregor (ed.). *Immunology of Endocrine Diseases.* 1986
   ISBN: 0-85200-963-1
2. L. Ivanyi (ed.). *Immunological Aspects of Oral Diseases.* 1986 ISBN: 0-85200-961-5
3. M.A.H. French (ed.). *Immunoglobulins in Health and Disease.* 1986
   ISBN: 0-85200-962-3
4. K. Whaley (ed.). *Complement in Health and Disease.* 1987 ISBN: 0-85200-954-2
5. G.R.D. Catto (ed.). *Clinical Transplantation: Current Practice and Future Prospects.* 1987
   ISBN: 0-85200-960-7
6. V.S. Byers and R.W. Baldwin (ed.). *Immunology of Malignant Diseases.* 1987
   ISBN: 0-85200-964-X
7. S.T. Holgate (ed.). *Mast Cells, Mediators and Disease.* 1988 ISBN: 0-85200-968-2
8. D.J.M. Wright (ed.). *Immunology of Sexually Transmitted Diseases.* 1988
   ISBN: 0-74620-087-0
9. A.D.B. Webster (ed.). *Immunodeficiency and Disease.* 1988 ISBN: 0-85200-688-8
10. C. Stern (ed.). *Immunology of Pregnancy and its Disorders.* 1989
    ISBN: 0-7462-0065-X
11. M.S. Klempner, B. Styrt and J. Ho (ed.). *Phagocytes and Disease.* 1989
    ISBN: 0-85200-842-2
12. A.J. Zuckerman (ed.). *Recent Developments in Prophylactic Immunization.* 1989
    ISBN: 0-7923-8910-7
13. S. Lightman (ed.). *Immunology of Eye Disease.* 1989 ISBN: 0-7923-8908-5
14. T.J. Hamblin (ed.). *Immunotherapy of Disease.* 1990 ISBN: 0-7462-0045-5
15. D.B. Jones and D.H. Wright (eds.). *Lymphoproliferative Diseases.* 1990
    ISBN: 0-85200-965-8
16. C.D. Pusey (ed.). *Immunology of Renal Diseases.* 1991 ISBN: 0-7923-8964-6
17. A.G. Bird (ed.). *Immunology of HIV Infection.* 1991 ISBN: 0-7923-8962-X
18. J.T. Whicher and S.W. Evans (eds.). *Biochemistry of Inflammation.* 1992
    ISBN: 0-7923-8985-9
19. T.T. MacDonald (ed.). *Immunology of Gastrointestinal Diseases.* 1992
    ISBN: 0-7923-8961-1
20. K. Whaley, M. Loos and J.M. Weiler (eds.). *Complement in Health and Disease, 2nd Edn.* 1993
    ISBN: 0-7923-8823-2
21. H.C. Thomas and J. Waters (eds.). *Immunology of Liver Disease.* 1994
    ISBN: 0-7923-8975-1
22. G.S. Panayi (ed.). *Immunology of Connective Tissue Diseases.* 1994
    ISBN: 0-7923-8988-3
23. G. Scadding (ed.). *Immunology of ENT Disorders.* 1994 ISBN: 0-7923-8914-X
24. R. Hohlfeld (ed.). *Immunology of Neuromuscular Disease.* 1994 ISBN: 0-7923-8844-5
25. J.G.P. Sissons, L.K. Borysiewicz and J. Cohen (eds.). *Immunology of Infection.* 1994
    ISBN: 0-7923-8968-9